OAT

COMPLETE PREPARATION FOR THE OPTOMETRY ADMISSION TEST™

2000 Edition

THE SCIENCE OF REVIEW™

AFTAB S. HASSAN, Ph.D.

Contributing Authors

LEON ANDERSON, Jr., D.M.D.
RUTH E. LOWE GORDON, B.S.
JEFFREY D. ZUBKOWSKI. Ph.D.

LIPPINCOTT WILLIAMS & WILKINS
A Wolters Kluwer Company
Philadelphia • Baltimore • New York • London
Buenos Aires • Hong Kong • Sydney • Tokyo

351 West Camden Street
Baltimore, Maryland 21201-2436 USA

227 East Washington Square
Philadelphia, PA 19106

Printed in the United States of America

ISBN: 0-683-30782-7

99 00 01 02 03
2 3 4 5 6 7 8 9 10

CONTENTS

LIST OF FIGURES

PREFACE

Welcome to the 1999 edition of *Complete Preparation for the Optometry Admission Test*. The concepts and skills included here present the latest model of the Optometry Admission Test, according to the American Optometric Association's OAT preparation materials. The extensive practice test items simulate the admission test's format, and terminology of the Optometry Admission Test is used throughout the book.

Complete Preparation for the Optometry Admission Test is organized to facilitate your OAT preparation. The text first introduces practice for reading and math skills renewal, then content review in physics and the natural sciences and, finally, the test-taking experience itself in the form of test-wise strategies and a sample examination. In this way, the guide provides the synthesis of knowledge and skills needed for high performance on the test. Each chapter includes clear and abundant examples, practice questions, and exercises.

- Chapter 1 includes information for undergraduate or preoptometry students preparing for the test. It contains study skills information, time management suggestions, and memorization techniques.

- Chapters 2 and 3 consist of skills practice materials in reading comprehension and quantitative reasoning. Each of the skills development sections includes sample questions to help you judge how much time you will need to finish your preparation.

  The skills development materials in chapters 2 and 3 begin with reading comprehension because it takes longer to develop this skill than to develop quantitative reasoning ability. Some students underestimate the level of reading skills required for a major admission test like the OAT and overestimate the skills they have acquired. A strong section on math is provided in the quantitative reasoning chapter because your math skills need constant brushing up. Practice will bring them back to the level required for the exam. The math review also trains you to work physics problems in chapter 4.

- Chapters 4 and 5 outline the natural sciences and physics required of a knowledge review for the OAT. Chapter 4 is the physics review. Chapter 5 is a condensed, thorough summary of basic concepts in biology, general chemistry, and organic chemistry. Each section in these chapters is followed by OAT prototype test questions. Discussion of answers is also included in each chapter for use in further review and self-assessment to aid you in discerning your individual strengths and weaknesses. Use your science textbooks for a detailed review.

- Chapters 6 and 7 of *Complete Preparation for the Optometry Admission Test* provide test-taking skills practice and a sample exam. Chapter 6 provides information on how the test is scored, as well as actual strategies for use on the test day itself. This includes test-wise suggestions for attaining the best possible scores on the OAT.

  Chapter 7 provides a sample OAT for practice and evaluation. You will know you are ready for the test when you have developed a strong science knowledge base, good reading and math skills, efficient speed, and a time management plan to serve you while taking the actual test.

- Appendix A is presented to help you focus on specific exam topics. It provides a detailed outline keyed to each topic and shows an itemized distribution of content. This information is based on the American Optometric Association's test preparation booklet.

How To Use This Manual

The content outline, study materials, and related skills practice included in *Complete Preparation for the Optometry Admission Test* are presented in a manner that is thorough yet condensed. When you review the natural sciences, you may begin with those OAT concepts that were not covered in your college curriculum. Or, you may choose to start with the ones you failed to master because of time constraints or a personal dislike for the subject. As an example, for the student who does not understand polarity in organic chemistry or the integumentary system in biology, *Complete Preparation for the Optometry Admission Test* provides an opportunity to master these concepts or others that may have been glossed over in the past.

Each OAT concept, such as photosynthesis, neural modulation of the heart, and so forth, can be learned in five essential steps:

1. definition or description,
2. examples,
3. equations, formulas, or drawings
4. comparison and contrast, with key conclusions, and
5. applications including questions and vocabulary/skills checklists for review.

Study skills recommended for OAT preparation are given in chapters 1, 2, and 3. Test-taking strategies for the OAT are included in chapter 6 because both skills and content review material must be mastered fully before the test day arrives. Prepare for the examination by using the skills chapters (1, 2, and 3) before learning OAT science concepts. This will help you review efficiently for the sciences and improve your performance on the actual test.

Organized preparation using this manual will also help you get ready for the rigors of optometry school. **Your best overall strategy is to learn from this guide as thoroughly as you possibly can, then to practice what you have learned until your performance is quite natural.** Remember that the skills and the OAT concepts provided here will be essential prerequisites for high achievement, regardless of any changes that may occur in test format.

Proposed Changes in the OAT

You should know that changes are being considered for many of the nation's standardized tests, including the Optometry Admission Test. Williams & Wilkins' Science of Review products are unique in that they respond relatively quickly to changes in the examinations, including up-to-date information for this guide incorporated right up to press time. Williams & Wilkins will continue to revise *Complete Preparation for the Optometry Admission Test* as needed. We encourage users of this guide to write or call Williams & Wilkins if they detect errors or omissions, or if changes are required. Suggestions from readers are always evaluated by our specialists for future editions.

ABOUT THE AUTHORS

Aftab S. Hassan, Ph.D., Doctorate Water Resources and Hydraulics, Columbia Pacific University (UCLA Program); doctoral scientist in Ocean, Coastal and Environmental Engineering, George Washington University. Dr. Hassan is an educational specialist in the health and life sciences and has strongly supported active learning and problem based teaching through his extensive teaching experience. Dr. Hassan also specializes in hydrodynamics, pollutant transport, and coastal engineering. He was formerly affiliated with George Washington University School of Engineering and Applied Science, and with Georgetown University, Department of Community and Family Medicine. He has been actively involved in MCAT and DAT teaching for students at Georgetown University, Washington, D.C., and Charles R. Drew University of Medicine and Science, Los Angeles, California. In addition, he has given active learning workshops (including physician assistant programs) for approximately thirty-five other schools across the U.S. He has taught, tutored, and advised premedical, medical, and engineering students for over twenty-two years.

Leon Anderson, Jr., D.M.D., Assistant Professor of Restorative Dentistry, University of Mississippi School of Dentistry. Bachelor and Master of Science degrees in Biology from Jackson State University and Doctor of Dental Medicine from the University of Mississippi School of Dentistry. He is presently the attending dentist at the University of Mississippi Medical Center in restorative dentistry and also the director of minority student affairs. Dr. Anderson served in the Jackson Public School System as a teacher of Biology for a number of years. He has years of teaching experience and up-to-date knowledge concerning health care and educational needs of students interested in the Health Professions. He has authored numerous publications and abstracts and serves on the Medical and Dental School Admissions Committee.

Ruth E. Lowe Gordon, B.S., Assistant Director/Education Specialist, Office of Minority Student Affairs, University of Mississippi Medical Center. Bachelor of Science Degree in Mathematics and Science from Alabama State University. She has done graduate study work at the University of Illinois. Ms. Gordon has been a mathematics teacher in three countries (the United States, Ghana, and Scotland). She has worked with premedical and predental training programs and has considerable knowledge and familiarity with preprofessional and professional science education and the medical/dental school environment. She has developed and implemented Medical College Admissions Test (MCAT) and Dental Admission Test (DAT) preparation workshops at numerous undergraduate schools.

Jeffrey D. Zubkowski, Ph.D., Associate Professor of Chemistry, Jackson State University. Bachelor of Science in Chemistry from the University of Pittsburgh, and the Doctor of Philosophy in Chemistry from Indiana University. He is an Associate Professor of Chemistry at Jackson State University, where he teaches freshmen- and senior-level chemistry. Dr. Zubkowski was a post doctoral fellow at the University of Toronto, Ontario, Canada, and has authored and co-authored a number of scientific publications.

INTRODUCTION

The Optometry Admission Test evaluates your level of knowledge in biology, general chemistry, organic chemistry, and physics. It also measures your skills in reading comprehension, quantitative reasoning, and taking tests.

Complete Preparation for the Optometry Admission Test contains specific information on each subject of the Optometry Admission Test. It describes the topics covered by the test in details that focus on optometry school requirements. In addition, to further inform you in advance of the exam, a sample practice test similar in form and content to the actual OAT is given in chapter 7.

What is the Optometry Admission Test? When Is the OAT Administered?

The OAT testing program is conducted by the Council on Optometry Education of the American Optometric Association. Examinations are given twice yearly in February and October at many testing centers in the United States and in foreign countries. It is advisable for students to take the exam during the spring of the year before applying to optometry school.

How Do I Register To Take the Exam?

Registration materials are available for the two annual administrations of the OAT. The registration booklet contains all the information you need to register for the exam. You may obtain this information by contacting your preoptometry advisor or by writing to:

Optometric Admission Testing Program
211 East Chicago Avenue, Suite 1846
Chicago, IL 60611-2678.
Phone: (312) 440-2693

What Is the Structure of the Optometry Admission Test?

Students report at 8:00 a.m. and usually the examination begins at 8:20 a.m. and lasts until 1:40 p.m. The actual (allocated) test time for all four subtests is 235 minutes. The total number of items tested on the OAT is 240. This gives an average time of approximately 58.7 seconds per item (which includes reading the item, solving the problem, and marking the answer sheet). The allotted time for each of the examination subtests is as follows:

Examination Section	Number of Questions	Maximum Time (Minutes)	Average (Seconds/item)
1. Survey of the Natural Sciences	100	90	(54 secs/item)
- Biology	40	25*	(37 secs/item)
- General Chemistry	30	30*	(60 secs/item)
- Organic Chemistry	30	35*	(70 secs/item)
2. Physics	40	50	(75 secs/item)
3. Rest	—	15	—
4. Pretest (not scored)	—	25	—
5. Reading Comprehension	50	50	(60 secs/item)
6. Quantitative Reasoning	50	45	(54 secs/item)

*Recommended times

What Types of Questions Are Covered on the Exam?

The Survey of the Natural Sciences is an achievement test that uses standard multiple-choice questions with one best answer for each science problem. The content consists of subject matter covered by first-year courses in biology, general chemistry, and organic chemistry. The three sciences are tested as subsections of Survey of the Natural Sciences and are listed at the beginning of the test booklet as biology (1–40), general chemistry (41–70), and organic chemistry (71–100). It is important that you pace yourself, since separate subscores will be given for each science section.

The Reading Comprehension test consists of three optometry school reading passages (approximately 1,300 words each), each containing sixteen to seventeen items. The passages are typical of new descriptive information that might be read in the first-year of optometry school. You must read and understand the material to answer the questions, which are based on the details in the passage. Highlighting pens are allowed.

The Quantitative Reasoning test measures the ability to reason with numbers, manipulate numerical relationships, and perform well on quantitative word problems.

The Physics Test is also an achievement test. The focus of the test is problem solving in a two-semester physics course. Standard multiple-choice questions are used on this test. A total of 40 test items is used to evaluate your mastery of physics. There is *no calculus* on the physics test.

How Do I Prepare for the OAT?

To prepare for the Optometry Admission Test, you may select from the several methods described below, including self-preparation, commercial or college preparation courses, or any combination of them, depending on individual circumstances. In any case, you must organize your study. Initially, it is important to identify the subject areas where you lack competency. It is advantageous to continue to identify your weak and strong areas throughout your study period. This can be determined from the following: 1) review old examinations, 2) self-administer sample OAT examinations, and 3) review the topics given here in *Complete Preparation for the Optometry Admission Test*. A detailed preparation plan and good study habits are described in Chapter 1.

After determining your weak areas, begin to organize your efforts. First, begin by studying your weakest subjects. This will help to raise your competency in weaker areas to the level of your stronger ones. Next, study weak and strong subjects together, emphasizing the topics you need to strengthen. Content outlines and the special skills needed for each examination area are given in chapters 2 through 6.

You are more likely to prepare successfully with an organized approach to your study. Self-motivation is an important factor in success so keep a clear goal always in mind and achieve it through concentrated preparation. Preparation alternatives are shown below.

Commercial Preparation. A major disadvantage of commercial preparation courses is expense. Research studies have shown mixed results regarding their effectiveness. Some advantages include the chance to meet other optometry applicants, to obtain condensed course work pertinent to the OAT, to study from material or notes using condensed material as a guide, and better attendance as a result of the expense. You should ask questions about the timeliness of the materials.

Preparatory Programs Sponsored by a College or University. Cost of this method is minimal to intermediate and there are few disadvantages. The major disadvantage is attendance on the part of the student. The advantages include the possible involvement of professors who regularly teach at the university, an environment and teaching staff already familiar to the students, and the teaching staff's awareness of each student's weak and strong areas. The opportunity to participate in group study sessions is also frequently very helpful.

Self-study. Self-study is a method that uses your own organized study plan along with notes, texts, and preparation materials specific to the OAT. The expense of this method is relatively low. It may be the more difficult means to test preparation, but the one that will yield the best results when it is well planned and diligently pursued. A major factor in the advantage of self-study is the development of a disciplined study approach that will also serve you well in optometry school. It is important that you have complete class notes, course outlines, access to textbooks, and the AOA's Optometry Admission Test materials to use as references and guides. Other advantages include: 1) a familiarity with class notes at the onset of study, which enhances your ability to develop a working knowledge of the information, 2) using a guide such as this manual, which provides study protocols and excellent practice for OAT-type problems, and 3) progressing at your own rate and at a time that is most convenient to you.

This manual is designed to stimulate self-study for the OAT. Read and review the basic principles that precede each subtest. The sample test questions will familiarize you with the actual examination because the practice questions are similar to those found in the OAT.

The authors and editors of this book offer no promises or guarantees as to your performance on the OAT. The value you will derive from the use of this book as a study aid is directly related to the amount and quality of time you invest in review. The important point in preparing to take any examination is to have a definite plan in mind before you begin.

How Is the OAT Scored?

Each of the examinations used in the optometry admission testing program yields a raw score that is the sum total of your correct answers. The raw score is converted to a standard score so test takers can compare their performance on one subtest with another (such as comparing Reading Comprehension with Quantitative Reasoning) and across different administrations of the OAT (autumn versus spring). The range of scores for the OAT is 200 to 400 with an average of 300. Scores from an earlier optometry exam (OCAT) are not equivalent to the new OAT scores.

How Are the Scores Reported?

At the written request of test candidates, test scores for the OAT are reported to optometry schools in terms of standard scores rather than raw scores. Scores from the *four* most recent attempts and the total number of times you took the OAT will be reported.

How Are Scores Used?

Through the use of standard scores it is possible to compare the performance of one applicant with the performance of all applicants on any or all of the measures included in the OAT. The conversion of raw scores to standard scores is based on the underlying ability defined by test items.

ACKNOWLEDGMENTS

Complete Preparation for the Optometry Admission Test, formerly known as *The Betz Guide,* is the result of a publishing project directed to helping students understand the level of skills and knowledge required for high performance on the Optometry Admission Test. Leon Anderson, Jr., D.M.D., a professor, DAT preparation teacher, and advisor, agreed to join with Aftab Hassan, Betz Publishing Company's Director of Scientific Research, Ruth Gordon, and Jeffrey Zubkowski in developing the first edition of *Preparing for the DAT*. As the OAT closely parallels the dental admission test, *Complete Preparation for the Optometry Admission Test* is based on the original *Preparing for the DAT* manuscript. The Betz research team carefully reviewed and followed the OAT specifications in creating the original version of this book.

In undertaking this project, we are grateful for the encouragement of the American Optometric Association (AOA), Association of Schools and Colleges of Optometry, Inc. (ASCO) and their Optometry Admission Testing Program booklets and reports. The publications mentioned below provided both insight and essential information. We want to encourage students preparing for the OAT to obtain copies of the Optometry Admission Testing Program's *Application and Preparation Materials,* published by the Optometry Admission Testing Program, Division of Educational Measurements, 211 East Chicago Avenue, Chicago, Illinois 60611.

We truly appreciate the timely review of the first edition by Brian Chou. We also share sincere appreciation for the work of Clyde Brown, Rhonda Thigpen, and Ervin Fox for testing the math problems and evaluating other portions of the manuscript. For typing assistance in preparing the original manuscript, out thanks go to Bruttie Jean Allen.

PART 1

OAT Study Skills

Chapter 1:

Preoptometry Preparation and Study Skills

1.0 INTRODUCTION TO PREOPTOMETRY PREPARATION

The Optometry Admission Test (OAT) accentuates the importance of developing good reading, OAT interpretation, and problem solving skills. These are skills that take a long time to acquire and cannot be crammed into a month or two of preparation. For this reason, what you do in college, high school, and even before will help prepare you for the OAT (and the optometry profession) as much as any review manual or review course. If you feel your reading/study/interpretation skills are weak and your school or college offers a course specifically directed at this, then take it. If you can select your own courses, select those courses that demand interpretive and inferential reading (such as literature, philosophy, and history courses). Also, select science courses that require you to understand and apply principles and interpret data rather than those that demand only memorization.

Read outside your classroom assigned texts, especially newspapers, news magazines, and scientific journals. Although the OAT content has been largely covered in your coursework, remember that the OAT stresses test items linked to optometry preparation and education, perhaps to a greater degree than your classes. When you read, force yourself to draw conclusions, interpret the graphs and charts, predict trends in data, and assay the limitations and errors presented in the data or opinions expressed. When reading an article, check the data and conclusions against other texts. As humans, we understand and learn best in complex webs of information, not in atomized facts.

You can learn to develop specific preoptometry education goals and interests that may last you a lifetime. Furthermore, synthesis of preoptometry education goals and skills will help you achieve a high level of performance on the OAT, in optometry school, and as a practicing professional.

1.1 THE ROLE OF THE OAT IN THE ADMISSION PROCESS

The OAT is a standardized test designed to measure the cognitive skills and scientific knowledge that are important for optometry education. As an objective measure, OAT scores can be reviewed and compared rapidly to more lengthy recommendations and the personal interview. Some schools may require other equivalent tests, such as GRE, in addition to or instead of the OAT, so be sure to check carefully the admissions requirements of the schools to which you apply.

In addition, it is essential that you write to the American Optometric Association to obtain materials for OAT preparation. Pay special attention to the section on Application Regulations and Procedures found in the Optometric Admission Testing Program (application brochure). This chapter teaches you how to develop study skills for high performance on the OAT.

1.2 STUDY SKILLS FOR OAT PREPARATION

It is important to emphasize that the best background for taking the OAT is good preparation in high school and college, especially in reading comprehension, solving algebra word problems, and working with geometry. But even if this is lacking, a well-planned review can improve your performance on the test. It is perhaps best to view OAT preparation time as an opportunity to master those skills and concepts that you failed to master previously. These concepts and skills will provide a solid foundation you will need as an optometry student and a practicing optometrist. A positive attitude toward test preparation is helpful.

Some general and specific study strategies are provided below and can be applied to all portions of the test. Suggestions for managing your preparation time immediately before the test and for the test-day itself appear in Chapter 6.

1.2.1 Make a Schedule

Make a realistic, well-planned schedule that provides appropriate time to study for all natural science subjects. This will help correct for natural tendencies, such as avoiding what you don't like. If you don't like to study a subject, plan to study that subject *first*. Find the reasons that keep you from studying that subject (for example, the material is too difficult, you don't have good books, you don't conceptualize the subject, etc.). You *need* that subject to do well on the OAT, whether you like it or not. Make a schedule for each day with a checklist of "Things *To Do* Today" and "Things *Done* Today." Before going to bed, check off what you actually finished. Make sure that things not reviewed one day are reviewed the next day. This should help you gauge how realistically you have planned your time. See figure 1.1 for sample checklists and keep these daily checklists with you until the OAT is over. These checklists will serve as "tickler memos" during your preparation.

Make a study schedule for each day; the more detailed the better. Use the course content outline found in the Optometry Admission Testing Program application brochure. Block out available time for OAT study and list as precisely as you can what you plan to study in each session. Use your lecture or laboratory class time wherever possible to link with your OAT preparation. If you are taking organic chemistry, for example, review while you study for class. The two activities can be mutually beneficial. (Remember that many questions in the organic chemistry subtest will integrate laboratory experience with the lecture material (e.g., the NMR spectroscopy labs).) Finally, if you regularly have Sunday dinner out, do not schedule around that time for harder subjects such as organic chemistry unless you are really going to forgo the dinner.

THINGS TO DO (Sample)

TODAY

1. Read TIME magazine article on biofeedback instruments.
2. Learn probability concepts.
3. Learn anatomy of the eye and physics section on optics.
4. Review carboxylic acids and their stereochemistry.
5. Learn the differences among virus, virion, bacteriophage, and bacteria.
6. Take GRE test for reading comprehension.

THINGS DONE (Sample)

TODAY

1. Read TIME magazine article in a hurry; didn't understand it.
2. Learned probability concepts.
3. Learned various parts of the eye + developed a correlation between the convergent/divergent lenses.
4. Took and graded GRE test for reading comp.
5. Did some probability problems.
6. Skipped 4+5 on Things To Do Today List due to lack of time, interest, + resources.

Figure 1.1 — Scheduling with daily checklists

Even if the time is theoretically available, do not schedule a twelve-hour OAT preparation day. Six to eight hours of study time is maximum. If you still have "free" time, practice reading comprehension, science and math word problems, and practice on building a good scientific vocabulary. Dictionaries in biology, chemistry, and physics are available from Betz Publishing Company.

Of all the areas you will be tested on, reading comprehension will probably be the slowest to improve. The reason is that the best way to improve your reading abilities is to read more, both in terms of time spent and in terms of varied scientific and technical materials and lab reports. Forgoing television during your OAT preparation time will free your time for reading.

Lastly, do not schedule study time later than 10:00 p.m., even though you may consider yourself a "night person." You learn best when you are fresh, and, of course, the OAT is not given at night. If you are not ready for sleep after 10:00 p.m., read journals such as *Science*, *The New York Times*, *Time*, *Scientific American*, or optometry and medical journals. Do not watch television after 10 o'clock.

1.2.2 Develop a Disciplined Approach

The Natural Sciences Subtest on the OAT is divided into 40 items in Biology, and 30 items each in General Chemistry and Organic Chemistry. Out of these 100 questions, some will be easier and some will be harder and more time consuming. Although separate subscores will be given for each science, the Survey of the Natural Sciences is sequentially mixed in the 100 items and are undifferentiated (items 1–40 are in biology, items 41–70 are in general chemistry, and items 71–100 are in organic chemistry). This means that you must be as disciplined in taking this part of the test as you will need to be when you study for it. For example, many students don't like organic chemistry. If this is true for you, you may be in no hurry to study organic chemistry and on the test day you may find that you are in no hurry to get to that section of the test. As a result, you may spend a longer time in Biology than is appropriate (which does not necessarily guarantee a high biology score). You will realize that you must hurry through General Chemistry (increasing the risk of careless errors) to complete the Survey of the Natural Sciences, thus shortchanging Organic Chemistry. Correlate and intermingle various sciences to avoid duplication of learning common scientific concepts (e.g., gas laws in physics and chemistry are identical). Becoming disciplined and test-wise begins with organized habits.

1.2.3 Use Test Items Efficiently and Effectively

When practicing test items, practice only on a small number of items at a time (one reading passage and follow-up questions or ten test items in any of the other areas). To improve, you need to analyze your errors in order to remember the reasoning you used as you worked the problems.

When analyzing your errors, use the answer key first. Only use the answer analysis section as a last resort and to check yourself after you can explain the keyed response. Once you have decided why the keyed response is correct, check your reasoning against the answer analysis section.

Keep a written record of your errors by making a check mark (√) next to the appropriate topic in the outline found in the Optometry Admission Testing Program application brochure. Errors can be classified in a number of ways. For example, specific content errors (e.g., genetics problems in biology) as well as specific question format errors (e.g., multiple choice) can give you trouble. This "error journal" will help you use your time most efficiently, since you will know where you need to review the most or develop more successful strategies for answering the questions.

As you work problems, note where the test emphasis lies. Once again the outline in the Optometry Admission Testing Program application brochure will help. For example, you may find that genetics is an important topic, so time spent on reviewing Mendelian genetics and application of the Hardy-Weinberg principle will repay the effort; conversely, you do not need to take a course just so you can answer a single obscure question from a topic that only appears once.

1.2.4 Prepare for the Optometry Admission Test Skills Areas

Short daily practice sessions in the skills areas of the test (reading, quantitative, and problem solving) are better than long but infrequent blocks of sustained practice. Plan to spend 30- to 45-minutes daily on skills development, perhaps alternating daily your practice on Reading Comprehension, Quantitative Reasoning, and solving Science Problems. Plan to spend more time on the skills you find to be the most difficult to master.

If you have forgotten basic math skills used in quantitative reasoning, you need to schedule additional time for basic math review. (Scholastic Aptitude Tests may be used for additional practice items. Old tests are available from the Educational Testing Service, Princeton, NJ 08541-6000, in books of five and ten tests.) It is also good practice to learn how to estimate a reasonable answer. If you usually work with a calculator, stop using it while you are preparing for the OAT.

The most basic and essential way to improve reading is simply to read more and understand the underlying assumptions, hypotheses, inferences, and conclusions. In addition to practicing test items, read daily at least one of the following: *Time, The New York Times* (especially the Tuesday edition that regularly has a science and education section), *Discover, USA Today, Science,* and optometry journals such as the *Journal of the American Optometric Association.* After you read an article, summarize it. One way to do this is to explain the author's main points to a friend. You can form a reading group that will discuss articles or you can write a five-minute critical summary.

You can work test items for the Reading Comprehension, Quantitative Reasoning, and Science Problems for the test as though they were "warm-up" exercises, or you can use the practice as a break from your science review.

1.2.5 Review the Natural Sciences

Once you know your skill levels in Reading Comprehension, Quantitative Reasoning, and Problem Solving, then determine how much time you will need to develop these skills further. When you are ready to begin your science review, be sure to include exercises in verbal comprehension, applied mathematics and in developing a basic problem-solving approach.

Review at least *one* topic in each of the four science content areas every day—even if you spend the bulk of your study time on only *one* topic. Do not set a schedule that reserves a week for biology, a week for general chemistry, and a week for organic chemistry. Do not schedule any single day devoted to one subject. Instead, spend at least some time on each subject each day. You need to put this basic information into your long-term memory. The best long-term memory development technique is constant review.

In general, most of us like to work on what we do best; we tend to review what we already know. In preparing for the OAT, you need to develop strategies to correct for these natural tendencies. Keep in mind the following suggestions as you plan your review for the OAT's Survey of the Natural Sciences. Study your *least* favorite subject first. If you schedule a four-hour block of time for your OAT preparation on a given day, divide the time as follows: older content review, new skills review, new content review, and older skills review. This is the most efficient review pattern. First, divide the four hours between content review and skills development. Second, if you have scheduled three months for your OAT preparation, keep in mind that you will be tested on what you review at the beginning of your preparation as well as on what you review immediately before the test; therefore, spend some time each day staying current with the material you reviewed earlier as well as reviewing any new material.

1.2.6 Anticipate OAT-Type Questions: Conceptual Learning

When you study or read, try to formulate OAT-type questions and possible responses. For example, for each test item and the corresponding responses, think about what is false, or the exception, as well as memorize what is true. This is especially important when the text provides a concept and one or two examples. The examples are important for understanding, but not really for rote memorization because the test maker is unlikely to use those precise examples in a test item. Rather, the test maker will check to see if you can understand "new" examples by applying your understanding of the examples you have been given in textbooks or in class notes. The entire OAT review can be grouped into "single concepts." Each concept can be learned using its five analytical components (see Figure 1.2)

D	Define or describe the concept. [What is molarity? Define molarity and its relation to concentration measurements.]
E	Example of the concept. [Prepare a 0.5 M solution for NaCl or HCl or NaOH and determine pH value of solution.]
F	Find a formula, equation, or sketch for the concept. [Is there an equation for molarity? Is there a formula to find molarity? Can you draw "molarity" on a volume diagram? Yes, molarity is defined as moles/liter. It can also be drawn as shown across.]
IN	Investigate the concept in detail. [Compare and contrast molarity, molality, pH, normality, etc. Relate this to usage on the OAT.]
E	Expand your conceptual horizon by application. [Concept of molarity applied to titration problems; also review Acids, Bases, and Salts.]

"Molarity" Drawing

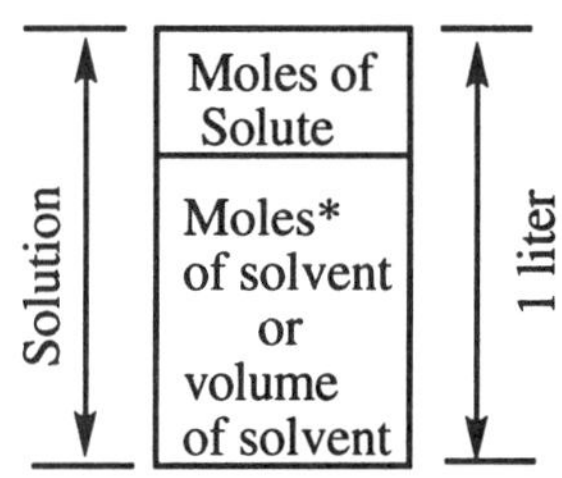

* Density of solvent is required to determine moles.

Figure 1.2 — Components of a OAT Concept: D - E - F - I - N - E

1.2.7 Look for Patterns of Error

Remember that student errors will be spread evenly across all the distracters (incorrect responses or words that catch a test-taker's attention) in an ideal multiple-choice item. This means that each distracter ideally represents typical errors students tend to make. To complicate things further, each of us tend to have patterns of errors that we continue to repeat unless an intervention strategy is introduced.

When you make an error, note whether you react with something like "I always have trouble with Boyle's law" or whatever. This is usually followed with a rationalization, "It's not that I don't know it, it's just that the wording of the test item confuses me." We sometimes confuse "recognition" with "knowing" or "understanding." If you cannot explain a concept clearly to someone who knows it well and who can therefore check your reasoning and accuracy, you really do not know it. Use graphic or visual skills to reinforce and remember each concept when you forget it.

The first step in correcting error patterns is to recognize when they occur. The second step is to develop a mnemonic, a memory device, that you will apply every time you see an item in the category you have identified. For example, it may help you to remember Boyle's law by thinking of your car. As you step on the accelerator, the piston is pushed down; as the volume decreases, the pressure increases. You can even draw a picture in the margin to remind yourself. If you need a mnemonic, you need to apply it every time that topic comes up. Patterns of error tend to be well developed and they do not lend themselves to correction by rote memorization alone.

1.2.8 Develop Your Concentration

The OAT requires a full morning of concentrated problem solving involving knowledge and perception. You need to work on applying yourself without a break for an entire morning. Without practice, concentrating on problem solving can be unexpectedly difficult. The OAT tests your problem-solving abilities and during the test the problem-solving aspects increase while your concentration may decrease.

To increase your concentration, begin with an honest self-assessment. Work with a clock in front of you. Notice the time you begin and the time you would normally take a break. A break can be both *conscious* and *unconscious*. Getting coffee would be an example of a conscious break; reading a page or more without knowing what you have read constitutes an unconscious break.

The next step to improving your concentration is to legitimize your breaks. It is important that you take conscious breaks. Give yourself permission to stop when you cannot concentrate on problems. Remember that without permission, your brain will take a break anyway, only you won't always be aware of what you missed. If you can only concentrate for 15 minutes at a time, then 15 minutes is the base-line from which you will build. (Commercial television, among other influences, has shortened the concentration time span for viewers to brief episodes that fit between advertisements.)

The third step is to build your concentration slowly. If you start with 15 minutes, work for 20 minutes, then 25 minutes, and so on, until you can work without losing concentration for two full hours.

The fourth step is to be self-aware. Which subjects are hardest for you to concentrate on? What time of day do you concentrate best? When is your concentration worst? Does the food you eat affect your concentration? How about background noise or the lack of it? Does stress in school or your job affect your concentration? Does your working place or study area affect your concentration?

Concentration requires both endurance and discipline to correct for variables. It helps to limit the time you plan to work. Avoid open-ended study sessions, the kind where you say, "I'm going to work on this organic chemistry until I've finished it, all night if I must." Open-ended study sessions give permission to daydream. Instead, say to yourself, "I have exactly one and one-half hours to finish this organic chemistry. If it isn't finished by then, too bad." Then stop. Limitless sessions encourage a lack of focus; limiting the time you spend on specific material encourages you to manage your time and concentrate harder.

1.2.9 Find a Study Partner

Explaining difficult material to someone else is a good way to check your understanding of what you have read. Find a study partner who is strong in your weak subjects and weak in your strong subjects. If your study partner is having difficulty, you can act as listener. It is the job of the critical listener to make sure that what the speaker says is accurate, complete, precise, and to the point. Working with someone provides a check that is less punitive than waiting to check your knowledge on the test day. It is important to realize that the weaker student in a given topic *cannot* serve as a critical listener for the stronger student in that topic. The weaker student should use a textbook, class notes, or course outlines to evaluate your understanding.

1.2.10 Develop Your Long-Term Memory

In general, the ability of some American students to memorize information is very poor compared with other societies. This is partly because we rely heavily on the written word to build information cumulatively, little by little. Thus the science courses you took before college were supposed to build a foundation for those you took in college. Now both are supposed to provide a foundation for optometry school.

Very little attention is given to developing memory in school. Some students acquire useful strategies accidentally or by trial and error, but in general there is no formal instruction or guidance to help you. Reading several texts for comparison, for example, can help boost your understanding and your memory.

In a cumulative information model of how our memory works, there is an assumed distinction made between long-term memory and short-term memory. An example of short-term memory might be when you make an appointment to see the dentist. Once you have kept the appointment, you immediately "erase" the date and time. When you sit down and simply memorize materials without conceptualizing them for a test the next day, they tend to be stored in your short-term memory. Immediately after the test the memory of these new materials is erased just as the optometry appointment is erased. In fact, almost everyone has experienced this in some particular course or seminar in school. The point to remember here: rote memorization alone is a short-term memory technique.

Long-term memory, on the other hand, is based on understanding what it is you have read or learned. Thus you tend to retain the information you really understood, such as the biology you took in high school. The understanding is what formed the foundation for subsequent learning. But note: those areas in high school biology that you didn't really understand you probably handled by using rote memorization. This helped you pass the tests, which is fine, but it did not create a strong foundation for subsequent learning. A better approach to learning biology would be to use the OAT concept model presented in section 1.2.6. When you understand what you are learning the information stays with you longer. The best way to check your understanding is to explain the topic to someone who knows enough about the subject to act as a critical listener.

It is also true that we remember best what we enjoy (this is based on what we *want* to remember, not what we *need* to remember) and we tend to like what we understand. When someone says, "I never liked mathematics," he or she is really saying, "I never fully understood it." Their lack of understanding may be caused by a poor teacher or bad classroom experience. Math, science, and Shakespeare are all topics too large and important to dismiss with a statement like: "I never liked math..., etc."

Understanding a topic contributes to liking it, and liking it contributes to how long you will retain it. If you think you don't like a subject, pretend that you do. That is, look for reasons to find it interesting and remember that you need it for the OAT. Make connections with it and other subjects that you do like. Every time you say to yourself, "I don't like this," you are making learning more difficult.

Understanding information also works in favor of your long-term memory because it allows you to build a complex web of information. The hardest memory task is memorizing a list of discrete and unconnected statements or items. The more connections we make then, the easier it is to memorize. Teach yourself to look for connections or pathways to enhance your ability to learn.

Long-term memory is also enhanced by increasing the different ways in which you can absorb and express the information you are learning. You have probably experienced the truth about this already. When you particularly like a course in school, you tend to discuss it; in talking about it, you reinforce what you learned, clarify your conceptual understanding, and increase the precision of your use of details. Although you may have done this unconsciously in the past, use it now to enhance learning. If you read difficult information in a textbook, can you express that information in a simpler way in a letter to your grandmother? Can you explain it to a friend over lunch?

Immediate review is also important for long-term memory. Research shows that unless you review what you have read or heard before you go to sleep at night, you will forget more than 90 percent of it twenty-four hours later. High school is structured to take advantage of this, because most classes are held each day. But when you go to college, classes are held less frequently. To improve your retention, you need to review your class notes every night before bed, or tell a friend about your class over lunch. If you are preparing for the OAT, the same principle applies. Unless you review what you did that day, you will not remember it. You will still know those topics that you understood and learned to like (beginning with high school), but the study preparation time for the OAT will be wasted unless you build immediate review time into your schedule. As shown in figure 1.1 above, you may want to combine your chart of "Things Done Today" with a review of "Things Learned Today."

Finally, constant use contributes to long-term memory. Your chemistry teacher knows a great deal about chemistry and has a remarkable amount of information that he or she can talk about easily without referring to notes or books. This is partly because your chemistry teacher works with chemistry every day both in lecture and the lab. If your teacher stopped using chemistry for a while, much information would fade. While preparing for the OAT, work with various subject areas every day and apply them in solving complex problems.

1.2.11 Distinguish Short-Term From Long-Term Memory Tasks

Ideally, most of your learning would be long-term. As an example, learning the circulatory system is a long-term memory task. It requires you to understand what happens at each step as the blood enters and leaves various chambers in the heart. As you talk about it, explaining it to your study partner, you will be storing it in your long-term memory. Drawing a flow diagram (another mode of expression) as you explain it will also help. Go to a grocery store and purchase animal organs, such as heart and kidneys. Hold each organ under a water faucet in your kitchen or bathroom and fill it up with water. Feel and observe the shape, size, and texture of the organ and various parts of the organ by cutting it and observing water flow through each organ, thus making a model for blood or fluid circulation. This will help improve or strengthen your visual skills, which is an aid to long-term memory.

When you visit a drugstore and look at the labels of prescription and nonprescription drugs, try to remember chemical names, symbols, and units of measurement for chemical compounds. This will give you real-life exposure to chemicals and a basic preparation in stoichiometry. For example, what are the ingredients in aspirin? Can you draw the molecules of the ingredients? Different approaches to the same topic help you retain the details as well as understand the related concepts. Explaining biological concepts or regurgitating your lessons or review material along with drawings and *actual* observation improves your long-term memory. *Repetition* and *conceptual drawing* are keys to long-term learning. Organic chemistry might sound really hard, but buying plastic model molecules and observing changes in structure by changing atoms or groups is a very useful tool. This way, you can actually *observe* and *remember* what kinds of mistakes you make in organic chemistry. Three-dimensional perception can be improved tremendously with these organic molecular structures. Organic chemistry then can become a part of your long-term memory.

Short-term memory is also useful. Short-term memory items are forgotten as soon as finish using them. Do not waste time memorizing short-term memory information three months before the test. Seldom-used equations or a chart comparing smooth, skeletal, and cardiac muscles might constitute short-term memory tasks. When working with items that require short-term memory information, solve the problem with the information in front of you. During the last few days of your study time just before taking the OAT, commit to memory what you have identified as short-term memory tasks. And on the test day itself, take a few minutes just after the exam begins to write out some of those short-term items so you have them for your use without having to concentrate on holding them in your memory.

Although you are now ready to go on to chapter 2, refer again to this study skills section from time to time to reinforce your good study habits and to find which of these study skills is most useful.

1.3 REFERENCES

1. Whimbey, Arthur, and Jack Lochhead, *Problem Solving & Comprehension*, 5th edition. Lawrence Erlbaum Associates, Publishers, 1991.
2. American Optometry Association, *Optometry Admission Testing Program* (application brochure) 1992.
3. Miller, L.L., *Increasing Reading Efficiency,* 5th edition. Holt Rinehart & Winston, Inc., 1984.
4. Harris, Albert J., and Edward R. Sipay, *How to Increase Reading Ability,* 8th edition. Longman, 1985.

Chapter 2

Reading Comprehension Skills

2.0 INTRODUCTION TO READING COMPREHENSION SKILLS

The reading comprehension section of the OAT measures (but is not limited to) your ability to read, organize, analyze, and remember new information in the basic sciences and optometry research. It is designed to test your reading ability (comprehension, evaluation, and analysis) through multiple-choice questions. Reading comprehension passages are selected from books and journals describing scientific information. These materials are typical of materials encountered in the first year of optometry school. No prior knowledge of the science topic is required for the reading comprehension test. This section of the OAT consists of three passages (approximately 1,300 words each). Each passage is followed by sixteen or seventeen items that test the comprehension skills and analytical skills required to understand concepts and ideas developed in the passage.

2.1 PREPARATION FOR READING COMPREHENSION IN THE OAT

Special reading skills may be learned and developed to prepare for the Reading Comprehension examination of the Optometry Admission Test. You will need an average of one to two hours per day to develop such skills and it is useful to know what they consist of before preparing to master them. This manual describes the major reading comprehension topics related to the OAT and then further refines and expands upon them, as shown below in section 2.1.1.

According to the AOA, the OAT Reading Comprehension exam tests four major skills areas. These are given as the ability "to read, organize, analyze and remember...." As shown in the outline that follows, these major skills have been expanded into practice topics that are explained in greater detail in the text of this chapter. In addition to the major OAT skills, the authors of this manual have added subsections enumerating the expansion of these major skills areas. With practice, these expanded topics will permit you to master the primary skills more completely.

2.1.1 Reading Comprehension Skills

I. Comprehension of "New" Information (2.2)
- **A.** Introduction (2.2.1)
- **B.** Reading (2.2.2)
  - scanning and correlating
  - understanding new words
  - developing speed and rhythm
- **C.** Organizing (2.2.3)
  - underlining and marking techniques
  - developing quick charts (mind mapping)
  - remembering important concepts
- **D.** Analyzing (2.2.4)
  - reading test items with choices
  - eliminating wrong answers
  - choosing the *best* answer
- **E.** Remembering (2.2.5)
  - vocabulary familiarity
  - visual maps and charts
  - extraction of information

II. Comprehension of "Current" Information (2.3)
- **A.** Introduction (2.3.1)
- **B.** Developing reasoning and problem-solving skills (see Chapter 4)
  - **1.** Analytical
  - **2.** Synthetic
  - **3.** Associative/analogical
  - **4.** Comparative
  - **5.** Intuitive
  - **6.** Visual

7. Logical
8. Quantitative
9. Proportional

C. Some uses of logic in testing (2.4)

D. Comprehension of scientific information (2.5)
1. Extracting the central idea
2. Cause-effect statements
3. Developing intra-relationships including chronological mapping
4. Developing comparison/contrast abilities
5. Understanding assumptions
    a. Direct or stated
    b. Indirect or unstated
6. Conclusions
    a. Direct or obvious
    b. Indirect or implied
7. Errors in reading and how to avoid them (2.5.1)

2.2 COMPREHENSION OF "NEW" INFORMATION

New information includes optometry research reports, magazine articles, and even newspapers such as *The New York Times.* These sources of new information are easy to obtain if you visit your school library. Sometimes, new information is provided in your textbook or during lectures by the professor. The OAT requires you to be able to read, organize, and analyze "new" information as you encounter it. "New" means unseen, unrehearsed, and representing information at first glance. "New" does *not* mean unknown, unfamiliar, or information never heard before. You may or may not have prior knowledge of the topic presented.

2.2.1 Introduction

Following is a suggested list of sources to read on a regular basis. These sources will provide you with "new" information passages.

1. *The New York Times* (daily newspaper)
2. *Scientific American* (monthly magazine)
3. *Discover* (monthly magazine)
4. *American Scientist by Sigma Xi* (bimonthly magazine)
5. *The New England Journal of Medicine* (weekly journal)
6. *Encyclopaedia Britannica* (latest edition)
7. *Journal of the American Optometric Association*
8. *USA Today*

2.2.2 Reading

Reading ability, a difficult concept to define, depends on the difficulty of the passage, your concentration level at the time you read it, your interest in the subject matter of the passage, your speed in reading and understanding the text, and, finally, your retention of various parts of the passage to make connections. The difficulty of the passage results from unfamiliar vocabulary (author's word choice) and minute details of content. Construct a vocabulary notebook and record on a daily basis the new words you encounter. Vocabulary expansion on a short-term basis is possible with constant review.

Use analytical reasoning while you read. This will make you more critically inclined when reading various types of complex and detailed information. When reading a passage requiring conceptual understanding, break the sentences into short, understandable phrases. Analytical reasoning consists of breaking a complex passage into short, understandable pieces. Analytical reasoning is covered later in this chapter in section 2.3.2, "Developing Reasoning Skills."

OAT reading passages should be encountered as typical comprehension exercises using reading ability skills, which include scanning, correlating, understanding vocabulary, and developing speed and rhythm. Before elaborating on these skills, attempt the following sample OAT passage. This passage is similar in format and style to OAT passages used in previous examinations.

PRACTICE EXERCISE IN COMPREHENSION OF OPTOMETRY MATERIAL

Use the following reading techniques during this exercise:

1. Skim the passage first—approximately 30 seconds. Find out the main topic covered.
2. Read the questions to get clues (do not read the responses or choices).
3. Take about three to five minutes to read the passage and develop connections among various parts (use light underlining or highlighting).
4. Answer the questions, consulting the passage as necessary.

Typical Sample Passage
Reading Comprehension Test

Connective Tissue:
General Characteristics and Functions

Connective tissue allows movement and provides support. In this tissue there is an abundance of intercellular material called matrix, which is variable in type and amount and is one of the main sources of difference between the types of connective tissue. It consists of various fibers embedded in a ground substance.

Loose Connective Tissue

The fibers of loose connective tissue are not tightly woven. The tissue, filling spaces between and penetrating into the organs, is of three types: areolar, adipose, and reticular.

Areolar Tissue. The most widely distributed connective tissue is pliable and crossed by many delicate threads; yet, the tissue resists tearing and is somewhat elastic. Areolar tissue contains fibroblasts, histiocytes (macrophages), leukocytes, and mast cells.

Fibroblasts are small, flattened, somewhat irregular cells with large nuclei and reduced cytoplasm. The term fibroblast refers to the ability of a cell to form fibrils. Fibroblasts are active in repair of injury. It is generally believed that suprarenal steroids inhibit and growth hormones stimulate fibroblastic activity. **Histiocytes** are phagocytic cells similar to leukocytes in blood; however, they perform phagocytic activity outside the vascular system. The histiocyte is irregular in shape and contains cytoplasmic granules. The cell is often stationary (or "fixed"). **Mast cells,** located adjacent to small blood vessels, are round or polygonal in shape and possess a cytoplasm filled with metachromatic granules. Mast cells function in the manufacture of heparin (an anticoagulant) and histamine (an inflammatory substance responsible for changes in allergic tissue). Depression in mast cell activity results from the administration of cortisol to patients. Areolar tissue is the basic supporting substance around organs, muscles, blood vessels, and nerves forming the delicate membranes around the brain and spinal cord and comprising the superficial fascia, or sheet of connective tissue, found deep in the skin.

Adipose Tissue. Adipose tissue is specialized areolar tissue with fat-containing cells. The fat or lipid cell, like other cells, has a nucleus, endoplasmic reticulum, cell membrane, mitochondria, and one or more fat droplets. Adipose tissue acts as a firm yet resilient packing around and between organs, bundles of muscle fibers, nerves, and supporting blood vessels. Since fat is a poor conductor of heat, adipose tissue protects the body from excessive heat loss or excessive rises in temperature.

Reticular Tissue. Reticular fibers consist of finely branching fibrils taking a silver stain as observed under the microscope. The primary cell of the reticular fiber is the reticular cell. Reticular fibers form the framework of the liver, lymphoid organs, and bone marrow.

Dense Connective Tissue

Dense connective tissue is composed of closely arranged tough collagenous and elastic fiber. It can be classified according to the arrangement of the fibers and the proportion of elastin and collagen present. Examples of dense connective tissue having a regular arrangement of fibers are tendons, aponeuroses, and ligaments. Examples of dense connective tissue having an irregular arrangement of fibers are fasciae, capsules, and muscle sheaths.

Specialized Connective Tissue

Cartilage. Cartilage has a firm matrix consisting of protein and mucopolysaccharides. Cells of cartilage, called **chondrocytes**, are large and rounded with spherical nuclei. Collagenous and elastic fibers are embedded in the matrix, increasing the elastic and resistive properties of this tissue. The three types of cartilage are hyaline, fibrous, and elastic.

In utero, **hyaline cartilage**, the precursor of much of the skeletal system, is translucent with a clear matrix caused by abundant collagenous fibers (not visible as such) and cells scattered throughout the matrix. Hyaline cartilage is gradually replaced by bone in many parts of the body through the process of ossification; however, some remains as a covering on the articular surfaces. The hyaline costal cartilages attach the anterior ends of the upper seven pairs of ribs to the sternum. The trachea and bronchi are kept open by incomplete rings of surrounding hyaline cartilage. This type of cartilage is also found in the nose.

Fibrous cartilage contains dense masses of unbranching, collagenous fibers lying in the matrix. Cells of fibrous cartilage are present in rows between bundles of the matrix. Fibrocartilage is dense and resistant to stretching; it is less flexible and less resilient than hyaline cartilage. Fibrous cartilage, interposed between the vertebrae in the spinal column, is also present in the symphysis pubis, permitting a minimal range of movement.

Elastic cartilage, which is more resilient than either the hyaline or the fibrous type because of a predominance of elastic fibers impregnated in its ground substance, is found in the auricle of the external ear, the auditory tube, the epiglottis, and portions of the larynx.

Bone is a firm tissue formed by impregnation of the intercellular material with inorganic salts. It is living tissue supplied by blood vessels and nerves and is constantly being remodeled. The two common types are **compact**, forming the dense outer layer, and **cancellous**, forming the inner lighter tissue of the shaft of a long bone.

The **dentin** of teeth is closely related to bone. The crown of the tooth is covered by enamel, the hardest substance in the body. Enamel is secreted onto the dentin by the epithelial cells of the enamel organ before the teeth are extruded through the gums. Dentin resembles bone but is harder and denser.

Blood and Hematopoietic Tissue. Marrow is the blood-forming (hematopoietic) tissue located in the shafts of bones. The red blood cells (erythrocytes) and most white blood cells (leukocytes) originate in the capillary sinusoids of bone marrow. Some leukocytes are formed in the lymphoid organs. Blood is a fluid tissue circulating through the body, carrying nutrients to cells, and removing waste products.

Lymphoid tissue is found in the lymph nodes, thymus, spleen, tonsils, and adenoids. The germinal centers of lymph tissue produce plasma cells and lymphocytes. Lymphoid tissues function in antibody production.

Connective tissues perform many functions, including support and nourishment for other tissues, packing material in the spaces between organs, and defense for the body by digestion and absorption of foreign material.

Reticuloendothelial system. Connective tissue cells, carrying on the process of phagocytosis, are frequently referred to as the reticuloendothelial system. The cells ingest solid particles similar to the manner in which an amoeba takes in nourishment. Three types of phagocytic cells belong to this classification: reticuloendothelial cells lining the liver (Kupffer's cells), spleen, and bone marrow; macrophages, termed tissue histiocytes or "resting-wandering" cells; and microglia, located in the central nervous system. The reticuloendothelial system is a strong line of defense against infection.

Synovial Membranes. Synovial membranes line the cavities of the freely moving joints and form tendon sheaths and bursae.

1. Which of the following is not a type of areolar connective tissue?
A. mast cells
B. histiocytes
C. plasma cells
D. leukocytes
E. fibroblasts

2. The connective tissue forming the framework for the liver is classified as
A. specialized connective tissue.
B. loose connective tissue.
C. synovial membranes.
D. fibrous cartilage.
E. areolar tissue.

3. Mast cells function in the production of
A. heparin.
B. histamine.
C. cortisol.
D. **A** and **B** only.
E. all of the above.

4. Which of the following is not a function of specialized connective tissue?
A. Carrying nutrients to cells.
B. Producing plasma cells and lymphocytes.
C. Phagocytosis.
D. Protecting the body from an excessive increase or decrease in temperature.
E. Producing blood cells.

5. Which of the following terms does not apply to any connective tissue?
A. squamous
B. areolar
C. reticular
D. bone
E. lymphoid

6. Which of the following is not a characteristic of the reticuloendothelial system?
   A. Kupffer's cells
   B. microglia cells
   C. macrophages
   D. serve as framework for bone marrow and liver
   E. defense against infection

7. Which of the following type(s) of tissue is largely characterized by the nature of material that lies between the cells?
   A. epithelium
   B. connective tissue
   C. smooth muscle tissue
   D. nervous tissue
   E. pseudostratified tissue

8. The most widely distributed connective tissue is
   A. reticular connective tissue
   B. dense connective tissue
   C. adipose connective tissue
   D. areolar connective tissue
   E. specialized connective tissue

9. The type of connective tissue that acts as a precursor to much of the skeletal system is
   A. hematopoietic tissue.
   B. hyaline cartilage.
   C. fibrous cartilage.
   D. elastic cartilage.
   E. synovial membrane.

10. Cartilage cells are called
    A. osteocytes.
    B. histiocytes.
    C. erythrocytes.
    D. chondrocytes.
    E. mast cells.

1. Control passage as it branches from the intro paragraph — Keep looking for differences in structure (S) and function (F).
2. Develop a mental layout of passage as it expands in content.

Approx. 500 words

Connective Tissue: General Characteristics and Functions

Connective tissue allows movement and provides support. In this tissue there is an abundance of intercellular material called matrix, which is variable in type and amount and is one of the main sources of difference between the types of connective tissue. It consists of various fibers embedded in a ground substance.

Loose Connective Tissue

The fibers of loose connective tissue are not tightly woven. The tissue, filling spaces between and penetrating into the organs, is of three types: areolar, adipose, and reticular.

Areolar Tissue. The most widely distributed connective tissue is pliable and crossed by many delicate threads; yet, the tissue resists tearing and is somewhat elastic. Areolar tissue contains fibroblasts, histiocytes (macrophages), leukocytes, and mast cells.

Fibroblasts are small, flattened, somewhat irregular cells with large nuclei and reduced cytoplasm. The term fibroblast refers to the ability of a cell to form fibrils. Fibroblasts are active in repair of injury. It is generally believed that suprarenal steroids inhibit and growth hormones stimulate fibroblastic activity. **Histiocytes** are phagocytic cells similar to leukocytes in blood; however, they perform phagocytic activity outside the vascular system. The histiocyte is irregular in shape and contains cytoplasmic granules. The cell is often stationary (or "fixed"). **Mast cells**, located adjacent to small blood vessels, are round or polygonal in shape and possess a cytoplasm filled with metachromatic granules. Mast cells function in the manufacture of heparin (an anticoagulant) and histamine (an inflammatory substance responsible for changes in allergic tissue). Depression in mast cell activity results from the administration of cortisol to patients. Areolar tissue is the basic supporting substance around organs, muscles, blood vessels, and nerves forming the delicate membranes around the brain and spinal cord and comprising the superficial fascia, or sheet of connective tissue, found deep in the skin.

Adipose Tissue. Adipose tissue is specialized areolar tissue with fat-containing cells. The fat or lipid cell, like other cells, has a nucleus, endoplasmic reticulum, cell membrane, mitochondria, and one or more fat droplets. Adipose tissue acts as a firm yet resilient packing around and between organs, bundles of muscle fibers, nerves, and supporting blood vessels. Since fat is a poor conductor of heat, adipose tissue protects the body from excessive heat loss or excessive rises in temperature.

Reticular Tissue. Reticular fibers consist of finely branching fibrils taking a silver stain as observed under the microscope. The primary cell of the reticular fiber is the reticular cell. Reticular fibers form the framework of the liver, lymphoid organs, and bone marrow.

Dense Connective Tissue

Dense connective tissue is composed of closely arranged tough collagenous and elastic fiber. It can be classified according to the arrangement of the fibers and the proportion of elastin and collagen present. Examples of dense connective tissue having a regular arrangement of fibers are tendons, aponeuroses, and ligaments. Examples of dense connective tissue having an irregular arrangement of fibers are fasciae, capsules, and muscle sheaths.

Specialized Connective Tissue

Cartilage. Cartilage has a firm matrix consisting of protein and mucopolysaccharides. Cells of cartilage, called **chondrocytes**, are large and rounded with spherical nuclei. Collagenous and elastic fibers are embedded in the matrix, increasing the elastic and resistive properties of this tissue. The three types of cartilage are hyaline, fibrous, and elastic.

In utero, **hyaline cartilage**, the precursor of much of the skeletal system, is translucent with a clear matrix caused by abundant collagenous fibers (not visible as such) and cells scattered throughout the matrix. Hyaline cartilage is gradually replaced by bone in many parts of the body through the process of ossification; however, some remains as a covering on the articular surfaces. The hyaline costal cartilages attach the anterior ends of the upper seven pairs of ribs to the sternum. The trachea and bronchi are kept open by incomplete rings of surrounding hyaline cartilage. This type of cartilage is also found in the nose.

Fibrous cartilage contains dense masses of unbranching, collagenous fibers lying in the matrix. Cells of fibrous cartilage are present in rows between bundles of the matrix. Fibrocartilage is dense and resistant to stretching; it is less flexible and less resilient than hyaline cartilage. Fibrous cartilage, interposed between the vertebrae in the spinal column, is also present in the symphysis pubis, permitting a minimal range of movement.

Elastic cartilage, which is more resilient than either the hyaline or the fibrous type because of a predominance of elastic fibers impregnated in its ground substance, is found in the auricle of the external ear, the auditory tube, the epiglottis, and portions of the larynx.

Bone is a firm tissue formed by impregnation of the intercellular material with inorganic salts. It is

remember elasticity and springs from Physics (are density and elasticity related?)

dense outer layer (next page)

living tissue supplied by blood vessels and nerves and is constantly being remodeled. The two common types are **compact**, forming the dense outer layer, and **cancellous**, forming the inner lighter tissue of the shaft of a long bone.

The **dentin** of teeth is closely related to bone. The crown of the tooth is covered by enamel, the hardest substance in the body. Enamel is secreted onto the dentin by the epithelial cells of the enamel organ before the teeth are extruded through the gums. Dentin resembles bone but is harder and denser.

Blood and Hematopoietic Tissue. Marrow is the blood-forming (hematopoietic) tissue located in the shafts of bones. The red blood cells (erythrocytes) and most white blood cells (leukocytes) originate in the capillary sinusoids of bone marrow. Some leukocytes are formed in the lymphoid organs. Blood is a fluid tissue circulating through the body, carrying nutrients to cells, and removing waste products.

Lymphoid tissue is found in the lymph nodes, thymus, spleen, tonsils, and adenoids. The germinal centers of lymph tissue produce plasma cells and lymphocytes. Lymphoid tissue function in antibody production.

Connective tissues perform many functions, including support and nourishment for other tissues, packing material in the spaces between organs, and defense for the body by digestion and absorption of foreign material.

Reticuloendothelial system. Connective tissue cells, carrying on the process of phagocytosis, are frequently referred to as the reticuloendothelial system. The cells ingest solid particles similar to the manner in which an amoeba takes in nourishment. Three types of phagocytic cells belong to this classification: reticuloendothelial cells lining the liver (Kupffer's cells), spleen, and bone marrow; macrophages, termed tissue histiocytes or "resting-wandering" cells; and microglia, located in the central nervous system. The reticuloendothelial system is a strong line of defense against infection.

Synovial Membranes. Synovial membranes line the cavities of the freely moving joints and form tendon sheaths and bursae.

What is most difficult in this passage? ⇒ classification of tissues, bones, cartilage, and other anatomical features, e.g., types of cells.

Figure 2.1 — Marked-up Passage

Answers to Connective Tissue Passage Questions
(All answers are found within the passage.)

1. **(C)** Paragraph two under loose connective tissue. Topic: areolar tissue.

2. **(B)** Paragraph six under loose connective tissue. Topic: reticular tissue.

3. **(D)** Paragraph three under loose connective tissue. Topic: areolar tissue.

4. **(D)** The functions of specialized connective tissues are found under that heading. As explained under the topic adipose tissue, response **D** is a function of this type of connective tissue.

5. **(A)** This is covered adequately in the passage.

6. **(D)** Found under the topic Reticuloendothelial System.

7. **(B)** Paragraph one under connective tissue.

8. **(D)** Found under the topic areolar tissue.

9. **(B)** Found under the topic specialized connective tissue. Topic: cartilage.

10. **(D)** Found under the topic specialized connective tissue. Topic: cartilage.

PRACTICE EXERCISE IN PASSAGE MARKING AND MAPPING

If you have fewer than five correct answers to the questions above, use this section to reinforce your skills in passage analysis. Try to answer the following questions about the passage; then proceed to the marking and mapping suggestions presented below.

a. How long (in words) is the passage?
b. How much time did you spend reading the passage?
c. What is the main idea conveyed in the passage?
d. Did you make scratch notes (highlight, underline, etc.) as you extracted information from the passage?
e. Do you remember 20 vocabulary words (difficult ones) or terms? (Do not look at the passage again!)
f. Are you ready to write a short summary of the passage?
g. Which parts of the passage were the hardest?
h. Did you find any irrelevant information in the passage?

Marking: After you finish answering all the above questions, look at the marked-up passage (Figure 2.1). The marks include underlining, circles, and other relevant marks that illustrate active reading. As you read the passage, you should have marked it actively to highlight important points. Questions **a** through **h** above may be answered at this stage. Use the following hints to check your answers. To answer question **a** above, count the average number of words per line and multiply by the number of lines in the passage. The connective tissue passage is approximately one and one-half typed pages and about five hundred words long. The answer to question **b** will vary according to your insights into the subject matter of the passage, your underlining, notes taken, and other factors. For this kind of information, reading should take about five minutes (no more). On the actual OAT you are given 50 minutes for three passages and 50 items. An average student would read the passages and work the 50 items in the times shown below:

15 min.	Passage 1 ≈ 5 min.	16 items ≈ 10 min.	30 min.
	Passage 2 ≈ 5 min.	17 items ≈ 10 min.	
	Passage 3 ≈ 5 min.	17 items ≈ 10 min.	

Figure 2.2 — Suggested Time Distribution for Reading Comprehension in the OAT

This time distribution assumes that all passages and items are of equal difficulty and length. Note that passage reading time is usually half the item reading/answering time. The total of 15 minutes for passages plus 30 minutes for working the items equals 45 minutes. This leaves five minutes to review difficult items or to readdress any part of a passage that may have confused you. It helps to save time by noting important terms as you encounter them in the passage.

Mapping: To answer question **c**, refer to the Mind Map given below. The Mind Map shows that the passage relates structure, function, and examples of various types of connective tissue. A mind map helps you make the right connections to various parts of a passage if you have forgotten any term or definition used there. The purpose of question **d** is to make sure you highlighted or underlined the passage for very fine details. Use long arrows or leaders to connect various ideas or thoughts in the passage. For example, look at the arrows connecting the use of words such as "fibroblasts" and "histiocytes." The mind map helps you to manage the details of the passage right from the start and it traces major ideas as you scan or read them. It is a useful tool for developing a layout for the entire passage.

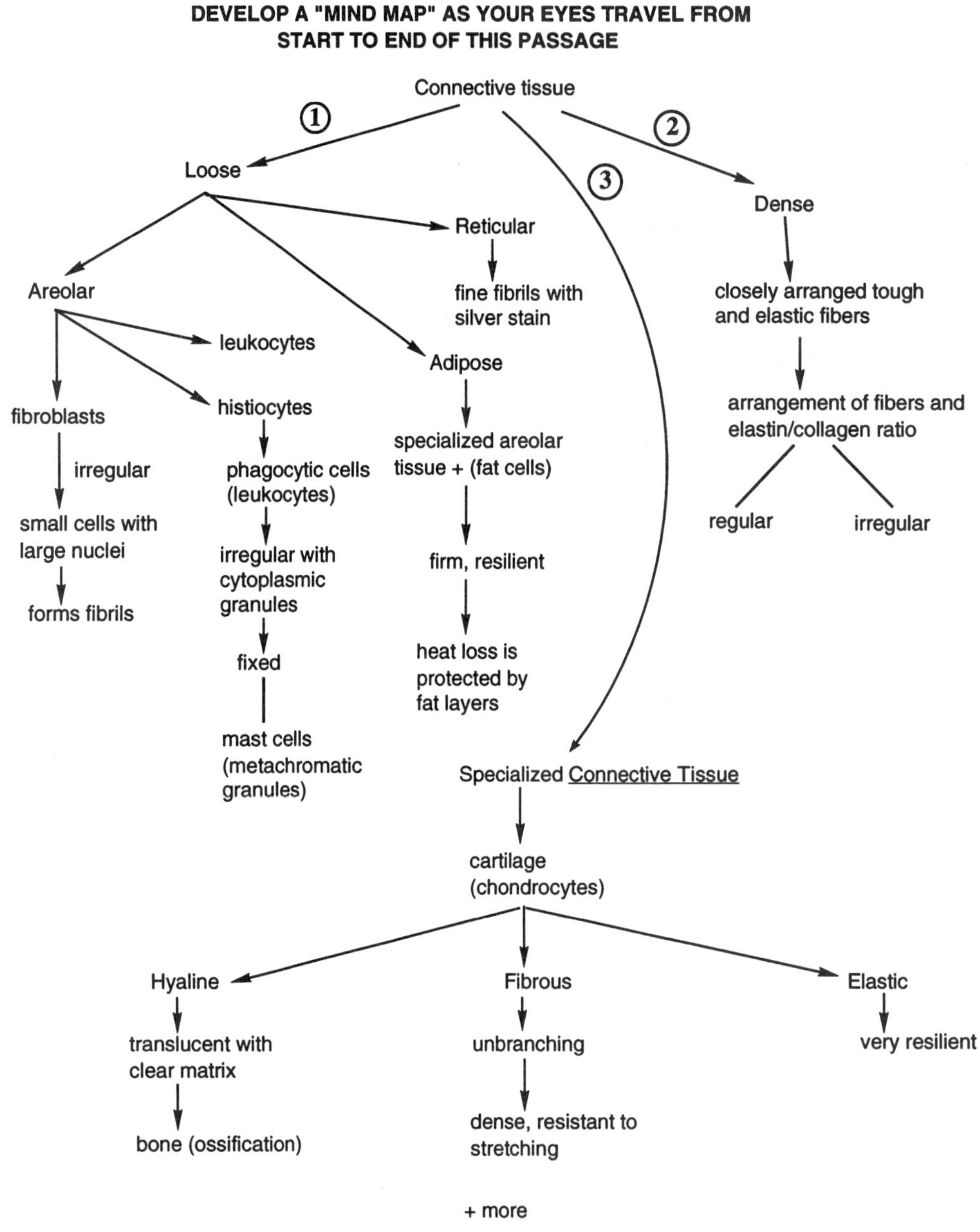

Figure 2.3 — Mind Map

A mind map, like the one illustrated here, traces and records your ideas as your eyes travel through a reading passage. Mind maps are very useful for extracting basic detail and rearranging it for later use. Mind maps should produce a schematic chart of your observations as you read a passage. Construct mind maps for every article you read. After a while, you will be able to draw such maps quickly and accurately. The mind map shown here was made from the earlier connective tissue reading passage. Mind maps also lead and connect you to the right segment or paragraph when you answer the questions at the end of active reading.

To answer question **e**, use the mind map in figure 2.3 to find the twenty vocabulary words, which could include the following: loose tissue, dense tissue, areolar, adipose, reticular, fibroblasts, fibrils, histiocytes, cytoplasmic granules, mast-cells, metachromatic granules, hyaline, ossification, cartilage, chondrocytes, fibrous cartilage, elastic cartilage, elastin/collagen ratio, phagocytic cells, leukocytes, resilient, and so on. Record in a notebook all the new words added to your vocabulary. Referring again to the mind map to answer question **f**, write a brief summary (one or two paragraphs) based on the marked up connective tissue passage (fig. 2.1). This summary more or less repeats important ideas in the passage and writing it will improve your short-term memory.

In response to questions **g** and **h**, by marking the passage you have located hidden information there. Look at the use of the word "where?" in the marked-up passage that asks, "Where is that kind of connective tissue found in the body?" The key word is "where?" because the introduction does not stress it. Irrelevant information is usually limited in such passages (textbook or encyclopedia information). Information you do not use to answer questions is unused information, but do not consider it irrelevant.

Your reading ability should now improve—you have learned to scan information, mark a passage, correlate information using a mind map, and increase your working vocabulary. You have also taken steps to develop your speed, which is based on developing a rhythm while you work that allows you to integrate all the above skills. Such rhythm comes from practice and a heightened interest in improving your reading ability. You should now answer questions more confidently.

2.2.3 Organizing

The elements of a good organization system include drawing constructive mind maps using the right amount of detail and preparing a vocabulary notebook. Use underlining, circles, brackets, parentheses, and other marks that help you locate information quickly. The mind maps are quick charts to trace your thoughts.

AIDS TO RECALLING FACTS AND DETAIL

To remember important concepts, follow these information-locating aids:

1. Read with interest. This will help you recall facts. Associate facts and details with your needs regarding the outcome of the OAT. These may include achieving a good OAT score or being accepted into optometry school. This level of interest will keep facts at the surface of your memory for instant recall and use.
2. Observe and concentrate to develop good recall. A person remembers best those things that he or she finds interesting, that require careful examination, and that invoke serious thought.
3. Read with the intention to recall facts. As you read, decide which facts are important; not all printed facts are worth recalling. It is impractical to try to recall everything you read.
4. Develop optimal speed. This is tied to your rate of reading. Your rate of reading should never be so high as to interfere with understanding. Comprehension should never be sacrificed in favor of speed. Excessive speed will only compound problems for a student who has difficulty comprehending ideas and recalling facts. Your reading rate will increase over time as techniques improve. Taking a speed reading course will hurt and not help you to improve reading comprehension.

2.2.4 Analyzing

This section relates to developing special skills in reading test questions and the corresponding choices or responses. It shows you how to eliminate bad answers and how to choose the *best* answer, not just a good one.

The conventional multiple-choice question is composed of a stem and a set of five answer choices. Multiple-choice items appear to be made in much the same way on tests from high school-level SATs right through the National Optometry Boards. The test maker puts a correct answer in one of the slots. Then the trickiest, hardest wrong answer is added. This most difficult wrong answer tends to be very close to the right answer—which is why we call it the "almost-right" answer. The test maker knows that the closer the almost-right answer is to the correct answer, the more difficulty you will have distinguishing one from the other. For example, if the question stem says, "All of the following are functions of the liver EXCEPT," the exception might be a function of the spleen, one that the test maker knows that students tend to ascribe to the liver. In many cases, thinking of difficult, almost-right answers is hard work, so the test maker tends to fill in the remaining letters with relatively easy-to-eliminate wrong answers.

Because there tend to be at least two seemingly right answers, the test taker who leaps for a single answer can easily be misled. For example, under the pressure of the real OAT, you might be tempted to choose the first answer choice that seems correct, but it may turn out to be the almost-right answer, or what the test makers call "the most likely distracter." You need to read *all* the answer choices. If you do not see at least two possibly correct responses (that is, if you don't see what the test maker thought was difficult) you are probably in trouble.

"What if I know the answer? Shouldn't I just mark the answer sheet and keep going?"

The OAT eliminates contestants by posing a large variety of questions around a limited basic content. Taking the OAT is therefore more like running a marathon than a sprint. When running a sprint, the contestant simply runs as fast as possible from starting gun to finish line. In running a marathon, on the other hand, the contestant develops an overall plan well in advance with appropriate strategies for each part of the race. The runner then practices those strategies so that performance in the actual race is deliberate yet automatic. In preparing for and in taking the OAT, you will do best if you have an overall plan and well-practiced specific strategies for reading comprehension. When you have decided on a strategy for answering multiple-choice questions, for example, it is less time-consuming and less risky to use that strategy consistently rather than sometimes using it and sometimes not. Remember that "consistently" means "every time" or "without exception." It is also a word that appears in other questions. The meaning of "consistently" must be distinguished from "trend."

When working with multiple-choice questions, we recommend that you use the following strategies consistently until they become habit:

- Eliminate clearly wrong answers by putting a slash mark (/) through the identifying number.
- Once you have identified at least two "right" answers, SLOW DOWN to make the best possible choice.

A word of warning: in many ways much of a student's classroom training runs counter to the deliberate, careful strategies suggested here for best performance on multiple-choice items. From junior high school on, many students have competed not only for the right answer, but for getting it faster. This focus on speed encourages students to rely on rote memory and intuitive leaps rather than rewarding those who carefully work their way to the correct answer. To benefit from what is recommended here, you will need to practice deliberate strategies consistently until they are automatic. But if the answer choices require so much thought, how can you find enough time in the reading subtest deliberately to select the right answer? We recommend that you learn to use the question analysis strategy below.

QUESTION ANALYSIS STRATEGY

For most readers, even good ones, recall is insufficient to pick the best answer on the OAT reading subtest. In using the question analysis strategy, however, you read the question first so you know what to look for; then you search the passage for the passage sentence (usually only one) that gives the answer. Note that this step always follows after you have carefully highlighted the passage and drawn your mind map of the passage.

You will know when you have found the right passage sentence because of the number of important words (primarily *significant* nouns) that it has in common with the question. For example, if a question asks, "In what historical period was U.S. population growth the lowest," you can scan the passage given for "population growth" and "lowest." The passage sentence that provides the answer in this case reads: "This was the lowest rate of population growth recorded until the 'Great Depression' when the net growth rate fell to 7 per 1,000 population during the 1930–1935 period." Once you have found the passage sentence, which you can learn to do quickly with practice, choosing the right answer depends on precise understanding—which, once again, may require you to SLOW DOWN.

At first, you may find the question analysis strategy awkward and time-consuming. After all, it is unlikely you have read this way before. However, practice will perfect this skill, which in turn will both increase your accuracy and ensure that you have enough time to complete this section of the test.

Question analysis is a bit like going to a grocery store with a shopping list. You can zip through the aisles checking items off on the list instead of wandering around and backtracking as you try to recall where you have seen the items you need.

With the question analysis strategy, follow these six steps:

1. Read the question first, working with one question at a time.
2. Underline the significant words in the question, primarily the nouns and active verbs.
3. Scan the passage looking for the passage sentence that contains the same words that you have underlined. Note that these words may appear in the passage sentence in a different order than the way they appear in the question, but you know you have found the right passage sentence by the number of words it shares with the questions.
4. Put the number of the question in the margin of your test booklet.
5. You can learn to do steps 1–4 quickly, but now SLOW DOWN because you are looking for what the test maker thought was difficult, that is, you need to look for the right answer and the "almost right" answer.
6. Answer the question carefully, working back and forth between passage and question. Pay special attention to the remaining words in the sentence, especially to the precise meaning of conjunctions, qualifiers such as adverbs and adjectives, and restrictive phrases.

Since part of your strategy is to read the questions first, analyze each question for the following:

- Can you pick out the significant nouns and verbs?
- Can you begin to anticipate where the difficulty in choosing the right answer might lie?

Look to the marked passage (Fig. 2.1) for examples of what to look for in the passage. In addition, leave ample space for your own notes when you read passages.

Don't worry yet about speed: you need to get the correct answer consistently before you attempt to get it quickly!

2.2.5 Remembering

Memorization is linked to diagramming and reasoning skills. Developing your reasoning skills will help to improve your short-term memory. Read section 2.3.2 for direction in developing vocabulary, drawing visual maps and charts, and learning how to extract information. The mind mapping skill you practiced earlier should then be integrated with your reasoning abilities to help you to become a highly skilled critical reader.

2.3 COMPREHENSION OF "CURRENT" INFORMATION

2.3.1 Introduction

Current information includes but is not limited to lecture notes, laboratory notes, information from friends and news media, your textbooks, and study guides. To master any sort of information, the first step is to comprehend it and discover various forms of reasoning embedded within the information. Good comprehension aims at developing reasoning skills, developing inter-relationships between various forms and types of information, understanding given and implied assumptions, and, finally, deriving direct and indirect (or implied) conclusions. The material below includes sections on reasoning skills, logic, and comprehension skills.

2.3.2 Developing Reasoning Skills

The following series of exercises will help you systematically to organize the knowledge and skills areas you need to review for the OAT subtests, including Reading Comprehension, Problem Solving, Quantitative Reasoning, and the Survey of the Natural Sciences. The diagramming and reasoning approaches described below will help you to review, but from different and possibly more challenging directions.

DIAGRAMMING SKILLS

Venn or association diagrams help you to improve your concentration and to focus on concepts. They help you think about the difference between *some* and *all*, and about *what is not* as well as *what is.* In a way, a Venn diagram is a visual representation of an outline.

Example: The statement "All roses are red" can be diagrammed as follows:

– things that are red
– roses (all red)
– things that are red but are not roses

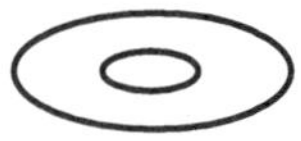

In a Venn or association diagram, a circle entirely contained within another circle means that all the members of the inner group belong in the outer group as well. Circles, ovals, or squares may be used to construct Venn diagrams. In the diagram representing "All roses are red," the inner circle denotes *roses* (and all of them are red) and the outer circle denotes *things that are red.* (Note: Look only at the relationship given in the statement; for the purpose of this diagram it does not matter that in real life not all roses are red.)

Example: The statement "*Some* roses are red" can be diagrammed as follows:

– roses
– red things

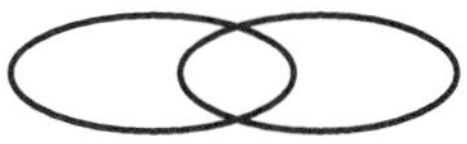

If you look at the lines of the ovals, you can see the relationship between red things and roses, only some of which are red. But if you look at the spaces rather than the lines, you see the relationships between three categories:

– roses that are not red (the space on the left)
– *some* roses that are red (the space in the middle)
– red things that are not roses (the space on the right)

Example: The statement "*No* roses are red" can also be diagrammed as follows:

– roses (none of which are red)
– red things (which include no roses)

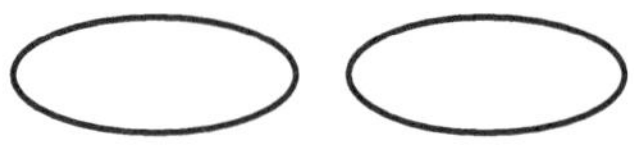

Exercise 1: Make a Venn diagram to illustrate the relationship between the following:

– mothers
– daughters
– grandmothers
– aunts

(This is not an easy relationship to diagram. As a hint, start with mothers and daughters only, and remember that any circle that is contained within another circle means that *all* its members belong to both groups. When you have that relationship represented by Venn diagrams, add a circle for grandmother. Then add aunts.)

When you have completed your drawing, turn to the solution in section 2.4.1 and compare your drawing with the one shown.

What has this to do with OAT preparation? Consider the following narrative reprinted from *The Betz Guide: A Complete Preparation for the MCAT*, latest edition.

REVIEW PASSAGE ON CARBOHYDRATES

"Carbohydrates have the general formula $C_n (H_2O)_m$ where n and m are whole numbers. Monosaccharides are the basic units of carbohydrates. They are classified by the number of carbons they contain, i.e., hexoses (C_6), pentoses (C_5), etc. Hexoses and pentoses exist in predominantly ring forms called pyranoses (six membered rings) or furanoses (five membered rings) in equilibrium with the open-chain forms. Ring forms are hemiacetals; open-chain forms are polyhydroxyl aldehydes. In the ring forms, a- or b-anomers are possible. The pyranoses exist in the stable chair conformation with most, if not all, of the hydroxyls in equatorial positions. When two monosaccharides differ by the configuration of one hydroxyl group, they are called epimers. If n is the number of asymmetric carbons, then 2^n is the number of optical isomers (based on open chain).

"Hexoses usually have n = 4 and pentoses usually have n = 3. Sugars are given a relative configuration on the basis of the orientation of the next to last carbon's hydroxyl group as compared to D-glyceraldehyde. Most naturally occurring sugars have the D configuration. A ketose is a carbohydrate with a ketone group; an aldose has an aldehyde group.

"Monosaccharides bond together to form disaccharides. The new bond is called a glycosidic bond and is between the hemiacetal carbon and an hydroxyl group of the other sugar; water is released when the bond is formed. Hydrolysis (breaking) of the bond requires water. The glycosidic bond is an acetal grouping. Sucrose (common sugar) is made of glucose and fructose. Lactose (milk sugar) is made of galactose and glucose. Maltose (α-1,4 bond made of two glucose units and is an hydrolysis product of starch or glycogen. Cellobiose (β-1,4 bond) is also made of two glucoses, and it is the breakdown product of the cellulose.

"Polysaccharides are many monosaccharides joined by glycosidic bonds; they may be branched also. Starch (plant energy storage), glycogen (animal short-term energy storage), and cellulose (plant structural component) are all made from glucose. Cellulose has β-1,4 bonds not found in the other two. Starch and glycogen both have α-1,4 bonds but differ in the frequency and position of branch points (alpha-1,6 bond).

"Insulin is a polymer of fructose."

Exercise 2: Using the passage above, draw an association diagram using the following words : carbohydrates, monosaccharides, disaccharides, starch, glucose, polysaccharides, fructose, sucrose, lactose, maltose, cellobiose, glycogen, and cellulose.

When you finish turn to section 2.4.1 and check to see if your association diagram reflects the same relationships as the one shown.

Below are three more exercises. The more you work these problems the more proficient you will become. In working them, first decide what information belongs in the diagram to help you remember the concept, then be as careful and precise as possible. Check especially what each *space* represents.

(a) Draw a Venn diagram illustrating the characteristics of eukaryotic cells and prokaryotic cells.
(b) Draw Venn diagrams that illustrate the relationship between isomers, stereoisomers, and enantiomers.
(c) Draw Venn diagrams to illustrate the relationship between diastereomers and meso compounds.

Remember, problem areas present opportunities for learning. Use your textbook or other resource to clarify any word or term that is difficult for you.

REASONING SKILLS

A conscious awareness of reasoning skills can improve your understanding of the material you study and result in improved test performance. As you read the section that follows, think about what you are reading. Continue to refer to it during your review, consciously applying the different forms of reasoning described. Also review reasoning and problem-solving skills from Chapter 4 of this book.

1. **Analytical Reasoning**

Analysis involves breaking something down into its component parts. This is as true of chemical analysis as it is of textual analysis. Taking notes in class is one way to use analytical reasoning in your academic life. A good note taker is able to select out the main points (the primary information) and the supporting details, and, at the same time, indicate by means of an outline the relationship between the two. Underlining is also a tool for analyzing text. The good student selectively underlines key words. At the same time, he or she makes notes in the margin or uses numbers to indicate the relationship of one piece of information to another and especially how both relate to the whole. Analysis identifies significant terms (often nouns) or pieces of information, but the work is incomplete unless the relationship of the part to the whole also is recognized—and this is where you use reasoning.

If analysis involves identifying key nouns as indicators of primary and secondary information, reasoning often requires a focus on words that the careless or hurried reader can overlook. These are qualifying words such as *always, some, for example, most likely, probably, however, consequently, as a result of, or* (as distinguished from *and*), etc. These words are the traffic lights and road signs for reading. As you work practice test items, circle these qualifying words and think about what they are telling you—how to proceed, what to look for, which of your stored information is relevant, which is irrelevant, etc.

To strengthen your analytical skills, we recommend two additional books: for reading power, Whimbey and Lochhead's *Problem Solving and Comprehension* and, for underlining and outlining, Pauk's *How to Study in College.* If you feel that your reasoning skills are weak, we recommend that you work the practice items in any available manuals that prepare students to take the LSAT (Law School Admission Test) and/or the GRE (Graduate Record Exam). The above titles, (except LSAT titles) may be ordered from Betz Publishing Company.

2. **Synthetic Reasoning**

Learning is incomplete unless analysis is followed by synthesis. Can you summarize the main points read in a textbook? Can you write in complete sentences the notes you wrote in class? Can you explain to a classmate what was covered in class? Can you clearly explain a concept (e.g., entropy) to someone in your family who may not understand it? All these things require you to synthesize what you've learned. Synthesis is thus the test or proof of your learning. In addition, you are expected to synthesize facts from various subjects to construct new possibilities, e.g., in the way that human physiology may be seen in light of what you have learned in physics, chemistry, biology, math, reading, visualization, and common sense. In memorizing concepts, try to link the key words together. Thus, the words synapse, axon, neuron, dendrite, effector organ, and neurotransmitter belong *together* and should be associated in memory to provide an interrelated web of information. For practice, make a list of words to memorize with pancreatic duct. Then check the accuracy of your list in reference books.

3. **Associative/Analogical Reasoning (especially useful during science review)**

Associative reasoning is also a tool recommended for improving memory by remembering similar or analogical situations. For example, it is easier to remember a difficult list if you associate the items on the list with something you know very well, such as the rooms in your house. Another example is to associate the action of driving a car with Boyle's law. In Boyle's law, pressure is inversely proportional to volume. When you push on the accelerator, you are decreasing the volume and increasing the pressure in the piston. Conversely, when you let up on the accelerator, the volume in the piston increases and the pressure decreases.

Analogical reasoning uses associations in a particular way. To better understand a concept, an unknown is compared to something known. You can use associative reasoning to transfer concepts from one subject to another, as in learning biology principles within a chemistry framework. For example, does the movement of blood inside veins and arteries relate to the concept of chemical structure of hemoglobin in organic chemistry? Explain. Can you make an analogy between biological cells and chemical cells? Explain.

Understanding by analogy is often a creative tool used by scientists and developed through years of practice. It is not by accident that the discovery of the structure of DNA was presented as a visual analogy (in a dream) of two snakes coiled around each other.

4. **Comparative Reasoning**

Associative reasoning leads naturally to comparison/contrast. We tend to compare things that are similar in some ways and dissimilar in others. That is, no one bothers to compare an orange and a truck. But textbooks do present comparisons and contrasts between smooth muscles and skeletal muscles, or between afferent and efferent nerves. When reading how two things are different, remember that they are being contrasted because they also have similarities. To memorize comparison/contrast information, you also need to organize it in a way that will enable you to separate in your mind the things being compared. It is easy to confuse the functions of the liver with those of the spleen, for example, as every test maker knows.

Comparison/contrast test items are often very difficult to answer correctly, partly because students tend to read textbooks passively without doing the active work that would enable them to anticipate comparison/contrast questions. You can avoid this by constructing a comparison/contrast chart or table whenever a textbook compares and contrasts, e.g., look at the table of similarities and differences between liquids, solids, and gases; or eukaryotic and prokaryotic cells.

For the following comparison/contrast exercises, think up aspects that are or are not shared and make a yes/no list for each. Then check your list against information in *The Betz Guide: A Complete Preparation for the MCAT* or other reference or textbooks.

(a) Electrolytic, galvanic, and concentration cells
(b) Heterozygous and homozygous genes

(c) Period and group for the atomic table
(d) Entropy and enthalpy

5. **Intuitive Reasoning**

Creative use of the imagination to solve problems is a subject rarely mentioned in the classroom because we know neither how to teach it nor how to test it. Basically, creative imagination makes an intuitive leap (usually unasked for and instantaneous) that was not logically apparent. Thus, a doctor might have a preliminary diagnosis that is systematically and carefully checked with further questions, examination, tests, etc. The scientist who discovered the way stars age did so by making an intuitive connection between aging stars and humans.

If you would like to develop your creativity further, you might work some of the exercises in Edwards' *Drawing On the Right Side of the Brain.* Meanwhile, Vitale's *Unicorns are Real: A Right-Brained Approach to Learning* also includes information about individual learning styles.

6. **Visual Reasoning (especially useful during science review)**

There is experimental evidence that very young infants can reason visually—well before they have acquired language. Although the ability to reason visually is the key to solving many science problems, some students find they have neglected their visual reasoning skills.

Picture a first-floor apartment and a sixth-floor apartment in the same building. Which apartment is likely to have better water pressure in the shower? Why? Which apartment is likely to have the better bathtub drainage? Why? How could you improve water pressure or drainage?

Now try some more exercises:

- Visualize the Krebs Cycle. Can you explain in one sentence what causes the cycle to work?
- Draw the molecules of epimers and anomers to help you conceptualize them in your mind.
- Visualize Doppler effect as a fire engine approaches a building.

As you work other science problems, notice how many require visual reasoning skills. Visual reasoning skills are directly tied to your perceptual abilities. Perceptual ability can be developed both directly and indirectly. Direct observation of mechanisms or processes makes you reinforce pictures in your memory. Perceptual ability is a useful aid in understanding abstract terms, such as orthoptics, monocular blindness, electromagnetic induction, coefficient of static friction, surface tension, drag force on a moving trailer, effusion, passive transport, chemical bond length, etc. Drawing small scale, freehand sketches or views of large scale objects (e.g., bioreactors, houses, trains, and trailers) makes you develop visual insight and also learn to simplify details. Indirect observation is more or less imagining mechanisms, molecules, or systems, e.g., drawing a sketch to illustrate words or concepts such as antigen-antibody interactions; pressure; molecular arrangement of chemicals in a cup of coffee; path of a bolus of food through the digestive system; bee's extraction of nectar from a flower; etc. Direct and indirect observation leads to improved perception. *Develop scientific concepts using sketches, diagrams, and easy-to-remember illustrations.*

7. **Logical Reasoning**

Because it is concerned with proof, logical reasoning is a way of thinking that is associated with the development of science and scientific methods. Logical reasoning provides a systematic means of testing or proving a hypothesis or conclusion. Conclusions come in three degrees of certainty: hypothesis, conclusion suggested, and conclusion confirmed. Conclusions can be valid or invalid.

There are many books available that provide the formal rules of logic and exercises to practice them. We recommend that you consult them to improve your logical reasoning ability. A recommended text is S. Morris Engel's *With Good Reason: An Introduction to Informal Fallacies.*

8. **Quantitative Reasoning (especially useful for math review)**

An improvement in quantitative reasoning depends primarily on the ability to estimate a reasonable answer before calculating it. Unfortunately, much skill in this area has been lost as a result of using calculators. (Calculators are not allowed while taking the OAT, so begin now to practice estimating reasonable answers.)

Quantitative reasoning is involved when you quickly and precisely carry out mathematical operations in your head. For example, multiply 41×41. Quantitative reasoning is also used to translate words to numbers and numbers to words. For example, looking only at a graph or chart in a newspaper, can you tell what the accompanying story is about? Conversely, can you read the article and picture the graph or chart?

9. **Proportional Reasoning (especially useful for science review)**

Proportional reasoning may be used to solve problems in biology and chemistry, such as flow of blood in arteries or veins of varying diameters, acid-base concentrations, etc. Proportional reasoning is also used to measure changes in one variable relative to another, as in problems applying Boyle's law. Both flow and concentration problems often require you to use proportional reasoning. In the OAT quantitative reasoning subtest, questions about population tables or charts can also require proportional reasoning.

Proportional reasoning is often aided by visualization or the ability to picture the elements of a problem (see Visual Reasoning, item 6 above). Schematic drawings in the margin sometimes are helpful.

2.4 SOME USES OF LOGIC IN TESTING

In our culture generally, and on national standardized tests in particular, form and syntax in written text are governed by the language and rules of logic. Thus, we use logical reasoning both to understand what we read and to determine the way we organize our thoughts when we write. Logical reasoning should also govern our understanding of test questions, of what is being asked and how to choose an answer.

In logic, there are premises, at least three by convention. "Premise" is a logician's term. Although each academic discipline is governed by the use of logic, each has developed its own specialized language. In the law, for example, the word for premise is "evidence"; in medicine, "symptoms"; in biology, "data." No matter what the discipline, logic supplies the rules; that is, although the "labels" might change from discipline to discipline, the "rules" of academic thinking stay the same. Thus, if you recognize a pattern in the data, the evidence, or the symptoms, you might draw a conclusion. In logic, recognizing a pattern to draw a conclusion is called "making an inference." Just as each discipline has its own word for premise, so each has its own word for conclusion. In law, this would be "verdict"; in medicine, "diagnosis"; in biology "results" or "conclusions"; and in an essay, it would be "thesis."

Conclusions come in three degrees of certainty. First, a hypothesis is a conclusion drawn that has not yet been tested. Second, a conclusion suggested is one that has been tested somewhat, but not enough to make it a conclusion confirmed. The third and most certain is a conclusion confirmed.

Premises (Valid or Invalid)			Conclusions (Direct or Indirect)
premise #1	→		hypothesis
premise #2	→	inference →	conclusion suggested
			-----------------
premise #3	→		conclusion confirmed
evidence	→		verdict
data	→		results/conclusion
facts	→		conclusion/decision
symptoms	→		diagnosis
supporting sentences	→		thesis

Figure 2.4 — Model of a Logical Argument

The broken line between "conclusion suggested" and "conclusion confirmed" represents a standard we often set for ourselves. This helps determine when a conclusion moves from one that is suggested to one that is confirmed. For example, the Food and Drug Administration sets the standard that governs when a medicine is declared effective and can be put on the market. That is, if a certain percentage of patients taking the drug are made to feel better, and the side effects are acceptable, and when a certain amount of time has passed to make sure that there are no undesirable long-term side-effects, etc., the medicine is declared effective, or, in the language of the model, the conclusion suggested becomes a conclusion confirmed.

In a text, you can tell whether a sentence is a conclusion suggested or a conclusion confirmed by the syntax. That is, if the sentence is a conclusion suggested, it will contain the conditional verbs: may, seem, can (as in "it *can* be inferred"), etc.; or adverbs such as *probably, primarily, most likely, most nearly,* etc. In logic, these conditional verbs and/or adverbs signify to you, the reader, that you are to read the sentence according to the rules of inductive logic, that is, the conclusion is to be judged according to probability. This is different from a deductively phrased statement that you are to judge according to logical validity. Logical validity states that if the premises are true, then the conclusion must also be true.

Perhaps an example will help: you ask me to dinner at your house and I say "I may come." This is a very different statement from if I say "I will come." The first statement is to be read as "I may, or I may not" and you must judge whether to expect me or not on the basis of probability. On the other hand, if I say "I will come," I mean "All other things being equal, I will be there."

Many students are uncomfortable with inductively phrased questions and their conclusions, which are based only on probability. For everyone, in real life as in the OAT, probability causes trouble in at least two related ways. First, in an inductively phrased multiple-choice question, there can be more than one possible right answer, but one will be more probable than the other. Second, probability is a sliding scale. Consider a brown paper bag that contains 10 blue marbles, 3 green marbles, and 4 yellow marbles. If I reach in my hand and pick one at random, what is its most probable color? Blue, of course. But now I add 5 orange marbles and 8 white marbles. Again, I reach in my hand and pull one out at random. What is the most probable color of this second marble? The answer is still blue simply because there are more blue marbles than any other color, but the probability is less. As I add different colored marbles, "blue" will remain the correct answer as long as there are more blue marbles than any other color, but the answer "blue" will feel less and less certain, until only the deliberate application of the rules of probability will help you to answer. As the probability lessens, you will no longer feel as certain as to which answer is right.

Clever students have an additional difficulty. They tend to look for the obscure but possible answer rather than choosing the probable answer that seems too easy. This can be corrected if you understand the nature of probability and if you understand that the syntax of the question stem tells you that you must make your answer selection based on probability only. Do not base your answer on either possibility or certainty. Remember: the directions on the OAT tell you to pick the "one best answer."

SOLUTIONS TO THE DIAGRAMMING EXERCISES

Exercise 1: In the left-hand drawing, the outer circle is "daughters" because all mothers are daughters, but daughters are not necessarily all mothers. The space between the two circles thus becomes "daughters who are not mothers."

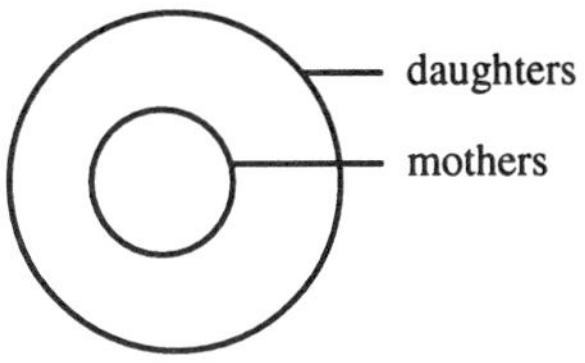

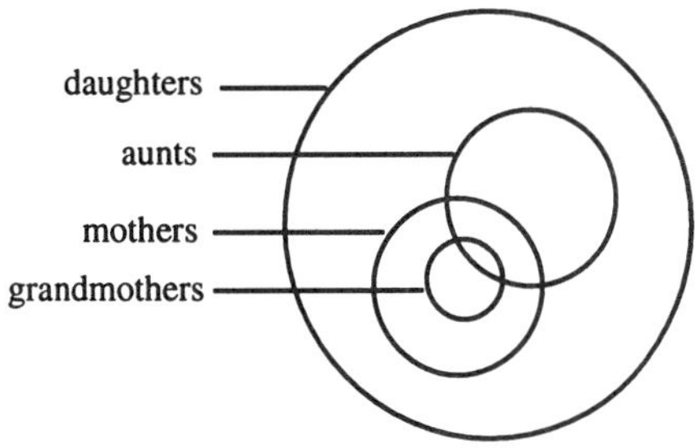

Exercise 2:

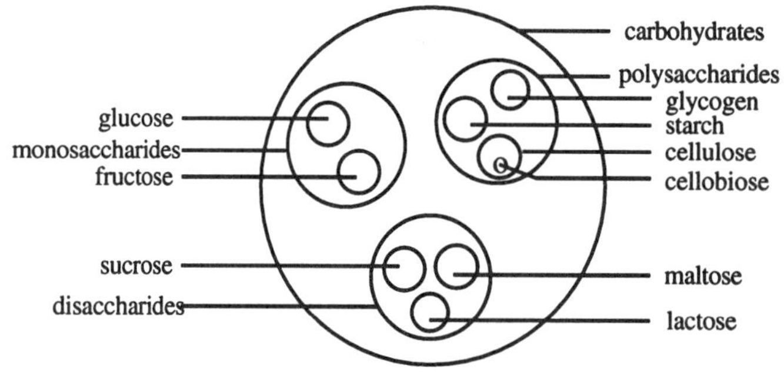

2.5 COMPREHENSION OF SCIENTIFIC INFORMATION

Reading comprehension skills can be defined by the following questions:

1. How is the central idea extracted from a passage?
2. Which statements in the passage are related as cause and effect? Mark them with the symbol C/E for use in answering test items.
3. Is there a set of time-related events in the passage? Draw a time-line to develop a chronological map to understand the variations with time.
4. Are there compare/contrast items or issues? Look through the practice passage on connective tissues and review the skills that were taught there.
5. Are there any direct or stated assumptions?
6. Are there any indirect or unstated assumptions?
7. Are there any direct or obvious conclusions?
8. Are there any indirect or implied conclusions?

This section is written to help you understand your reading error patterns and how to overcome them. It should help you answer the above questions relating to reading comprehension skills.

Some students find that they frequently score less than 80 percent correct even though they are working for accuracy rather than for speed. If this is true for you, take time to work on your basic reading skills. A speed reading course will not help. Rather, we recommend *Analytical Reading and Reasoning* by Arthur Whimbey. In addition, especially if your verbal SAT scores were low, you might want to review basic reading vocabulary beyond what is presented in Dr. Whimbey's book. Finally, *Vocabulary for the College-Bound Student* is a good basic reading vocabulary book. To improve your critical reading ability we recommend *Active Reading in the Arts and Sciences* by Shirley Quinn and Susan Irvings (the book can be directly ordered from Betz Publishing Company).

One key component in learning to read better is to try reading new and difficult materials. Work out a program for active reading by selecting new material from school texts. In addition, we recommend that you read at least one of the weekly national scientific magazines such as *Scientific American.* These magazines and *Encyclopaedia Britannica*, for example, are especially good reading resources for OAT preparation for the following reasons:

- they are approximately the same difficulty as OAT passages;
- they are similar to the information given in your textbook; and
- they are written for a generally well-educated but not necessarily scientifically educated audience. This means that each article helps you to review the basic scientific knowledge that is tested in the OAT. Reading a scientific magazine each week has the added bonus of keeping you abreast of current issues in science.

2.5.1 Errors in Reading and How to Avoid Them

1. **Continued Analytical Reading Problems**

Students are not accustomed to the precise, problem-solving approach of reading analytically. If you have trouble reading the questions precisely enough to reason out the correct answer, you need to obtain a copy of *Problem Solving and Comprehension* by Arthur Whimbey and Jack Lochhead. Almost any college student can benefit from doing the exercises they prescribe.

2. **Careless Reading of the Question**

Do you read the question analytically? Do you circle important qualifiers such as "some"? In compare/contrast questions, do you pay attention to which set the question refers to? Do you recognize when a question has more than one proposition? If your errors result from reading the question, SLOW DOWN until you are getting all or nearly all of the answers correct; then slowly build for speed.

3. **Careless or Hasty Reading of the Passage**

Are you finding the correct sentence in the passage but still failing to get the correct answer? Finding the correct passage sentence is only the first step. Learn to do this quickly. After that SLOW DOWN to make sure that you thoroughly understand what is said, carefully working back and forth between the passage sentence until you are certain of the meaning. The passage should be read as evidence and you, as the reader, are the detective looking for very precise clues.

4. **Variations in Degree of Concentration**

Do you find some passages more interesting and some less interesting than others? This is natural. Nonetheless, finding the passage *too* interesting can cause you to waste precious time, while finding the passage uninteresting can cause you to lose concentration. Instead, approach each passage and its attendant set of questions as though it were an enclosed puzzle.

For the OAT, as a first step to improve your concentration, eliminate unconscious breaks by taking a deliberate break as soon as you need it. Work with a clock in front of you. Make your break deliberate by standing, stretching, or moving around for 2 to 5 minutes. Then, when you get back to studying, try to concentrate for just a little longer before your next break. Just as you need to build your speed slowly, you should also increase your concentration little by little. To prepare for the OAT in its entirety, you need to work on building your concentration.

When you analyze practice tests (or class tests), do you notice that your correct answers and wrong answers tend to come in groups? That is, you will be doing well and then suddenly get three or more answers wrong in a cluster? This pattern indicates that you slip in and out of focus. To correct for this, you need to develop your concentration. In this situation, do not blame question difficulty if you get the wrong answers.

5. **Slow Start, Slow Finish**

Do you perform better on the second reading passage than on the first? It is a good idea to bring a practice reading passage (newspaper or journal article) with you on the test day itself. Working on a practice reading set in the last minutes of your break will enable you to get a running start for the reading test.

Does your performance slack off as you progress toward the end of the test? If so, you need to build for stamina. After all, 50 minutes is a long time for sustained concentration when you are not reading for entertainment or pleasure. As with speed, build for stamina slowly.

6. **Early Panic, Late Anxiety**

Do you look at the first question and sense your mind go blank? If so, don't answer it. Move on until you find a question you can answer with confidence. Then come back to the first one. You may find your anxiety rising as the time passes and you become increasingly aware that you are never going to finish unless you speed up. Try to get your pacing under control *before* you take the OAT. Speeding up under pressure tends to increase the number of careless errors. You do not get extra points for answering every question on the reading test. Scores depend on how many you answer ***correctly***. In the real OAT, save the last minute on each subtest to fill in a preselected guess answer (choose **2**, for example, or any number). Unlike the SATs, there is no penalty for wrong answers.

7. **Question Type Preference**
Do you find you do better on one type of question than another? If so, increase your practice on the type that gives you more difficulty. Each of us tends to work hardest on what we do best, so you must practice to reverse that habit. The best learning strategy for improvement dictates that you work to overcome your weaknesses.

8. **Problems with Multiple-Choice Questions**

Multiple-choice questions take more analyzing time than conventional questions (open-ended or true/false). When working multiple-choice questions, you should eliminate three answer choices after careful scrutiny. You should slow down to consider the remaining two out of the five possibilities. When choosing the right answer proves difficult, put slash marks through clearly wrong answers or you will waste time by rereading them. It is a good idea to practice multiple-choice reading questions until you are consistent in both accuracy and speed because multiple-choice questions tend to dominate the reading portion of recent OAT examinations.

9. **Trouble with Negative Stems**

The presence of negative words in a question or answer makes the item more difficult. We are not used to reading for what is not, for what is false, or for the exception. The test maker knows this. You will find more negative-stemmed questions in the biology subtest than in chemistry. Biology does not offer as many options (for definition questions). A test maker creates a problem by posing a negative-stemmed question.

When you see a negative-stemmed item, circle the negative word and SLOW DOWN. You need a separate strategy for these items. Consider each answer and decide whether it is true or false, writing a "T" or "F" next to each. If you aren't sure, mark "?T" or "?F". Force yourself to choose. When you do this, the answer should be apparent—but pay attention when you choose your answer: true answers are easier to approve than false answers.

Especially time consuming are the questions that start, "All of the following are true **EXCEPT**...." As the exam date approaches, if you find you are still working too slowly in the reading section, consider answering all **EXCEPT** questions last. Remember, answering the single hardest or most time-consuming OAT question is not rewarded with extra points. It is a better strategy to spend the same amount of time answering two or three easy questions correctly.

10. **Problems with Keyed-choice (I, II, III) Questions—Usually Not Tested on the OAT**

Although unfamiliar at first, with practice most students see dramatic improvement in this kind of question. Most of the lingering trouble students have is distinguishing between choice II and choice III, two choices that may both appear correct. If you notice that you tend to pick one when it should be the other, try putting the question statement into the passage next to what you have identified as the passage statement. Would it fit logically? Or does the one contradict the other in some way? If it fits in logically, ignore the content; the answer is III. On the other hand, if you put the question statement into the passage and logically it does not fit, the answer is II.

11. **Reasoning Problems**

Many students continue to have problems with inductively phrased questions. If this is true for you, reread section 2.3.2 (Developing Reasoning Skills) above. Compare inductively phrased questions with deductively phrased questions. Do you see why they are written inductively? Do you see how inductive phrasing allows for more than one possible answer? Do you remind yourself that inductive phrasing is a clue to remind you that you should choose the *best* or most likely answer?

If most of your reading has been in textbooks, you may be unfamiliar with inductive reasoning in text. Regular reading of research reports and *Scientific American* will help to familiarize you with this type of reasoning.

If you need more practice with questions that primarily test your reasoning, you can find extra practice materials either in an LSAT or GRE guide (GRE test books are available from Betz Publishing Company.) Whenever an actual test is used it obviously provides the most accurate material from which to study. An excellent first book in learning how to improve reasoning ability is *With Good Reason: An Introduction to Informal Fallacies* by S. Morris Engel.

12. **Language Problems**

Synonyms may cause problems. If you encounter words or phases that appear to be synonymous and you know synonyms cause you trouble, SLOW DOWN and DOUBLE CHECK. Do the words *really* mean the same thing?

To be synonymous, words must be on the same level of classification. As an example, "dog" and "German shepherd" are not synonyms because "German shepherd" is only one kind of dog. A discussion of synonyms is actually a discussion about the relationship between the two terms under consideration. There are three ways to illustrate this relationship: by outlines, Venn diagrams, and analogical reasoning.

• An outline would look like this:

I. Canine
  A. Dog
    1. German shepherd
    2. poodle
  B. Wolf
    1. red
    2. grey

• A Venn diagram illustrating the same relationship would look as follows:

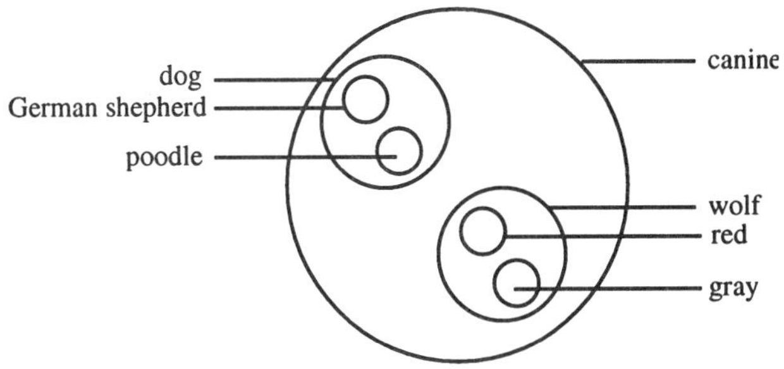

Learn how to draw Venn diagrams if they are unfamiliar to you. Venn diagrams can clarify the concept "not." Practice exercises using Venn diagrams can be found in both the LSAT and GRE practice guides.

13. **Double Propositions**

Questions with more than one proposition, or answers with more than one variable, can also cause trouble. Once again, SLOW DOWN. Remember the correct answer must satisfy all the conditions given.

14. **Proportional Reasoning**

Students often have trouble with questions that include the words "increase" and "decrease," especially when they require proportional reasoning. This is true in the OAT Survey of the Natural Sciences and Quantitative Reasoning examinations as well. Make a little chart in the margin and use arrows to help you visualize what is being asked and facilitate choosing the right answer.

15. **Speed, Accuracy, and Concentration**

The most common OAT error pattern is misunderstanding the outcomes of speed, accuracy, and concentration. Managing time during the exam is a complex matter. Figuring out how many minutes per question on average you have for each section of the test does not help, simply because the test maker does not expect you to spend the same amount of time on each question. Rather, the test maker carefully balances relatively quick-to-answer questions with those that take longer. As a sophisticated test taker, you need to develop a question/timing sense.

Moreover, keep in mind that speed is always a trade-off for accuracy. This is as true on the OAT as it is on the highway. Too many students confuse the two; that is, they believe their primary problem on tests is speed, whereas they really have an accuracy problem that must be dealt with first. If you work on speed first, you will only get the wrong answer faster. Once your accuracy is high, then (and *only* then) build for speed SLOWLY.

Negative-stem test questions (i.e., questions that contain **false** or **not** or **except**) usually take longer to answer because you must be careful in checking your answer against what is being asked. Negative-stem questions cause added difficulties simply because students neither slow down nor change strategy when answering them. When you see a negative-stem question, SLOW DOWN first, then ask yourself whether each answer choice is TRUE or FALSE and put a "T" or "F" next to the letter. If you are not sure, guess with a "?T" or an "?F"; when you are finished, check your answer choice against the question stem one more time.

In the reading passages, both interest and disinterest in the content can slow you down. Take each passage and its questions as an enclosed logic game that challenges your wits against the wits of the test maker. If he can slow you down unnecessarily, he wins; if he can speed you up inappropriately, he also wins. Remember that the OAT

is a long exercise in concentration that requires much stamina. Stamina can only be developed over time, and OAT stamina is both physical and mental. For example, students often find during the Survey of the Natural Sciences subtest that when the mind begins to tire it takes a break of its own accord. This can happen several ways: either the student begins to think about something else (the rest of the weekend, for example) or he or she begins to read a single question over and over again.
Do not let your unconscious mind determine when you take your breaks. Rather, go into the examination knowing that after every thirty questions or so you are going to sit back and stretch and roll your head around to ease the strain in your neck and shoulders. If you do this, you will be taking the test rather than letting the test take you!

Finally, remember to analyze your errors! As you continue to work reading passages, add your errors to the error journal you started in Chapter 1 (section 1.2.3) and analyze the data for repeated error patterns. An important part of improving your performance is developing your skills as a self-conscious test taker.

When you study, you should spend about two-thirds of your time working to correct your errors, that is, working from your error journal, and only one-third of your time reviewing what you already know or do well. Unless you do this deliberately, you will tend to work longest on what you already know and can do well. After all, success feels better than concentrating on errors. Correcting error patterns is not easy because we all tend to revert carelessly to old habits. Breaking error patterns requires long-term dedicated and conscious effort, but it can be done! To gain more practice and familiarity with OAT items, try the model OAT test in Chapter 7.

2.6 REFERENCES

1. Giroux, James A., and Glenn R. Williston, *Comprehension Skills, Isolating Details to Recalling Specific Facts*, Advanced Level. Jamestown Publishers, Providence, Rhode Island, 1974.
2. *Diagnostic Microbiology,* 7th Edition. Finegold & Baron 1986; Mosby Yearbook Publishers.
3. Flesch, R.F., *The Art of Clear Thinking.* Harper & Row, 1973.
4. Quinn, Shirley, and Susan Irvings, *Active Reading in the Arts and Sciences,* Allyn and Bacon, Boston, 1991.

Chapter 3:

Quantitative Reasoning Skills

3.0 INTRODUCTION TO QUANTITATIVE REASONING SKILLS

The Quantitative Reasoning examination is forty-five minutes long and contains fifty items. To prepare successfully for the quantitative reasoning exam, you need to develop your ability to reason with numbers, manipulate numerical relationships, and apply information appropriately in situations involving quantitative material.

This chapter, which follows the AOA outline, presents mathematical concepts and exercises in various topics. Speed and accuracy are necessary for proficiency on this section. No mathematical tables, rulers, measuring devices, calculating devices, calculators, slide rules, etc., are allowed inside the testing center. Therefore, it is recommended that you prepare for the OAT without such aids. The Quantitative Reasoning examination has items that are divided into two groups: mathematical problems and applied mathematics. Mathematical problems test your knowledge of arithmetic, algebra, geometry, and trigonometry. The applied mathematics consist of practical word problems.

3.1 QUANTITATIVE APPROXIMATION SKILLS

The abilities to approximate, estimate, and round off numbers in mathematical calculations are useful skills for the OAT. Regarding approximation and estimation, work with these skills carefully because alternative answer choices may be very close. During practice compare your estimated answer to the actual answer. Experience and practice will make you a better estimator. Review section 3.7.2 to understand precision and accuracy in measurements.

Learn to express a decimal in fewer digits, an approximation called rounding. In some cases doing mental arithmetic by changing an arithmetic problem to an equivalent problem can be done easily (without pencil or paper). This type of approximation is called number rounding.

(a) Rounding down skill:
Round off 3.1416 to two decimal places. (Answer: 3.14)
If the first digit to be dropped is less than five, then the last retained digit is unchanged (rounding down).

(b) Rounding up skill:
Round 0.4536 to three decimal places. (Answer: 0.454)
If the first digit to be dropped is greater than five, then the last retained digit is increased by one.

(c) Number rounding skill:
Numbers may be rounded to the nearest ten, hundred, thousand, etc.

246 → Rounded to nearest ten is 250.
→ Rounded to nearest 100 is 200.

(d) Sum estimation skill:
(i) Estimate sums by rounding to the nearest ten.
$789 + 42 = 831
790 + 40 = 830
(ii) Estimate sums by rounding to the nearest 100.
428 + 583 = 1,011
400 + 600 = 1,000
(iii) Numbers can be added by conversion to simpler numbers.

$$\begin{aligned} 789 + 42 &= (700 + 89) + (40 + 2) \\ &= (700 + 40) + (89 + 2) \\ &= (740 + 80) + 9 + 2 \\ &= 820 + 11 = 831 \end{aligned}$$

(e) Multiplication by rounding numbers:
Simplification is made easier by taking each number and rewriting it as a sum or difference of equivalent numbers, i.e., 58 = 50 + 8 and 66 = 60 + 6, therefore using the form (a + b) (a + b) = a^2 + 2ab + b^2, the result is as follows:

(i) $58 \times 66 = (50 + 8)(60 + 6)$
$= 3{,}000 + 300 + 480 + 48$
$= 3{,}000 + 300 + 400 + 80 + 40 + 8$
$= 3{,}700 + 128$
= 3,828 (exact answer)

Approximate answer:
$58 \times 66 = 60 \times 65$
$= 3{,}900$

(ii) Find the approximate quotients:

$\frac{89}{58} \cong \frac{90}{60} \cong 1.50$

$\frac{89}{58} = 1.53$ (exact answer)

3.2 FRACTION INTERPRETATIONS AND FACTOR DETERMINATION SKILLS

A fractional number is a ratio of two numbers expressed as a/b in which *a* can be any positive or negative number and *b* can be any positive or negative number except 0. The fraction is made up of two parts, the numerator and the denominator. In $\frac{3}{7}$ the numerator is 3, which indicates how many of the 7 equal parts are considered. In $\frac{5}{6}$, 6 is the denominator that indicates the number of equal parts. Factors are associated with fractional operations and interpretations.

3.2.1 Concepts Related to Interpretation of Fractions

(a) When the numerator is less than the denominator, the fraction is called a *proper fraction,* otherwise the fraction is called an *improper fraction.*

Proper fractions: $\frac{1}{2}, \frac{3}{4}, \frac{7}{9}, \frac{11}{13}$

Improper fractions: $\frac{5}{3}, \frac{6}{6}, \frac{10}{5}, \frac{8}{5}$

(b) A *mixed number* has a whole number part and a fraction part.

$3\frac{1}{4}$ 3 = whole number part +

$\frac{1}{4}$ = fractional part

(c) Equivalent fractions reduction skill:
Equivalent fractions are fractions with the same value but different numerators and denominators.

Examples: $\left(\frac{2}{6} \text{ and } \frac{1}{3}\right), \left(\frac{3}{4} \text{ and } \frac{9}{12}\right), \left(\frac{1}{2} \text{ and } \frac{3}{6}\right)$

(d) Fraction multiplication skill:
Multiplying a numerator and denominator by the same whole number can produce equal fractions:

$\frac{1}{2} = \frac{3}{6}$ because $\frac{3}{3} \times \frac{1}{2} = \frac{3}{6}$

$\frac{3}{4} = \frac{9}{12}$ because $\frac{3}{3} \times \frac{3}{4} = \frac{9}{12}$

(e) Reciprocal fractions:
Reciprocal fractions are two fractions whose numerators and denominators are reversed. Their product is always equal to 1.

$\frac{1}{5}$ and $\frac{5}{1}$ are reciprocals, $\frac{1}{5} \times \frac{5}{1} = 1$

$\frac{3}{4}$ and $\frac{4}{3}$ are reciprocals because $\frac{3}{4} \times \frac{4}{3} = 1$

3.2.2 Concepts Related to Determining Factors

The factors of a whole number are those whole numbers that divide *evenly* into the given number. A whole number is even if it can be divided evenly by 2, otherwise it is odd.

Example: Write the factors of 8
8: 1, 2, 4, 8
Example: Write the factors of 28
28: 1, 2, 4, 7, 14, 28

(a) Divisibility skills:
When is 2 a factor? 2 is a factor of a number if the last digit in the number is even.
When is 3 a factor? 3 is a factor of a number if the sum of the digits in the number is divisible by 3.
When is 4 a factor? 4 is a factor of a number if the last 2 digits in the number are divisible by 4.
When is 5 a factor? 5 is a factor of a number if the last digit in the number is 0 or 5.
When is 6 a factor? 6 is a factor of a number if the last digit is even and the sum of the digits is divisible by 3.

(b) Common factors and how to find them:
Common factors are identical factors that are common and contained in two or more numbers.
Example: Write all the factors of 8 and 28
8: 1, 2, 4, 8
c c c
28: 1, 2, 4, 7, 14, 28
Common factors: 1, 2, and 4

(c) GCF finding skill:
The greatest common factor (GCF) is the greatest or largest of the common factors found in two or more numbers.
Example: Write the GCF of 24 and 32
Factors of 24: 1, 2, 3, 4, 6, 8, 12, 24
Factors of 32: 1, 2, 4, 8, 16, 32
Common factors: 1, 2, 4, 8
GCF: 8
A fraction is said to be in simplest form when the GCF of the numerator and denominator is 1.

(d) GCF simplification skill:
Dividing the numerator and denominator of a fraction by the GCF does not change the value of a fraction. It simply reduces the fraction to a simpler form.
Example: $\frac{6}{8} = \frac{6}{8} \div \frac{2}{2} = \frac{3}{4}$
GCF of 6 and 8 is 2
6 = 1, 2, 3, 6
8 = 1, 2, 4, 8
GCF = 2

Example: Reduce $6\frac{8}{12}$ to lowest term

$$6 + \frac{8}{12} \div \frac{4}{4} = 6 + \frac{2}{3} = 6\frac{2}{3}$$

(e) Common multiple finding skill:
The multiple is the product of a given number and a whole number. To find the multiples of a number, multiply it by each integer number, e.g., 1, 2, 3, 4, etc.
Example:
Multiples of 3 are 3, 6, 9, 12, 15...
Multiples of 4 are 4, 8, 12, 16, 20...
If one number is divisible by another, it is a multiple of that number. When the multiples of two or more numbers have a value in common, this value is called a *common multiple* of the numbers.
3: 6, 9, 12, 15
5: 10, 15
15 is a common multiple of 3 and 5

(f) Least common multiple finding skill:
The smallest common multiple of two or more numbers is called the Least Common Multiple (LCM).

2 = 2, 4, 6, 8, 10, 12
3 = 3, 6, 9, 12
4 = 4, 8, 12

LCM = 12

The Least Common Denominator of two or more fractions is the LCM of the denominators of the fractions.

Example: Find the LCD of $\frac{1}{4}$ and $\frac{1}{5}$

$\frac{1}{4}$ = 4, 8, 12, 16, 20, 24

$\frac{1}{5}$ = 5, 10, 15, 20, 25

LCD = 20

3.3 OPERATIONAL MATH WITH FRACTIONS

3.3.1 Addition of Fractions

(a) Like denominator adding skill:
To add fractions that have common denominators, add their numerators and keep the same common denominator.

Example: Determine the sum of $\frac{1}{4}+\frac{5}{4}+\frac{3}{4}$ by adding the numerators: 1 + 5 + 3 = 9 keeping the same common denominator, 4.

$$\frac{1}{4}+\frac{5}{4}+\frac{3}{4}=\frac{9}{4}=2\frac{1}{4}$$

(b) Unlike denominator adding skill:
To add fractions with unlike denominators, determine the least common denominator. Express each fraction in equivalent form with the LCD. Then perform the addition.

Example: Determine $\frac{1}{2}+\frac{3}{4}+\frac{2}{8}$

LCD = 8

The sum with the fractions in equivalent form is

$$\frac{4}{8}+\frac{6}{8}+\frac{2}{8}=\frac{12}{8} \text{ or } \frac{3}{2} \text{ or } 1\frac{1}{2}$$

(c) Mixed number adding skill:
To add mixed numbers calculate the sum of the integers separately from the sum of the fractions. Then add the sums.

Example: Add the mixed numbers $7\frac{1}{6}$ and $2\frac{3}{4}$

First, add the integers: 7 + 2 = 9

then add the fractions, $\frac{1}{6}+\frac{3}{4}=$?

$$\text{The LCM} = 12\text{:}\quad \frac{1}{6}+\frac{3}{4}=\frac{2}{12}+\frac{9}{12}=\frac{11}{12}$$

$$7\frac{1}{6}+2\frac{3}{4}=9\,\frac{2+9}{12}=9\frac{11}{12}$$

3.3.2 Subtraction of Fractions

As with addition, before two fractions can be subtracted they must have a common denominator.

Example: $\frac{3}{4}-\frac{2}{3}$

The LCD is 12. The subtraction with the fraction in equivalent form gives: $\frac{3}{4}\times\frac{3}{3}-\frac{2}{3}\times\frac{4}{4}=\frac{9}{12}-\frac{8}{12}=\frac{1}{12}$

3.3.3 Multiplication of Fractions

(a) How to multiply skill:
To multiply two or more fractions multiply their numerators to obtain the numerator of the product. Multiply the denominators to obtain the denominators of the product.

Example: Multiply $\frac{3}{7} \times \frac{2}{5}$

The desired product is $\frac{3 \times 2}{7 \times 5} = \frac{6}{35}$

(b) Common factor canceling skill:
Calculations are greatly simplified and the product put in simplest terms by cancellation of common factors.

Example: $\frac{2}{5} \times \frac{10}{3} \times \frac{6}{7}$

Express all the numerators and denominators in factored form, cancel the common factors, and carry out the multiplication of the remaining factors. Cancellation lets you work with smaller rather than larger numbers in the numerator and denominator, which decreases the chances of error.

$$\frac{2}{5} \times \frac{2 \times 5}{3} \times \frac{2 \times 3}{7} = \frac{8}{7}$$
$$= 1\frac{1}{7}$$

(c) Mixed number multiplication skill:

Every integer, $\frac{a}{b}$ where $b \neq 0$, can be written as a fraction. An integer divided by 1 is equal to the integer.

Example: $\frac{3}{5} \times 6 \Rightarrow \frac{3}{5} \times \frac{6}{1} = \frac{3 \times 6}{5} = \frac{18}{5} = 3\frac{3}{5}$

To multiply mixed numbers, convert them first into fractions and then apply the rule for multiplication of fractions.

Example: Multiply $1\frac{3}{4}$ by $3\frac{1}{7}$

Convert $1\frac{3}{4}$ and $3\frac{1}{7}$ into common or improper fractions (an improper fraction is one in which the numerator is larger than the denominator, otherwise it is a proper fraction) and multiply:

$1\frac{3}{4} = \frac{4}{4} + \frac{3}{4} = \frac{7}{4}$

$3\frac{1}{7} = \frac{21}{7} + \frac{1}{7} = \frac{22}{7}$

$\frac{7}{4} \times \frac{22}{7} = \frac{7}{2 \times 2} \times \frac{2 \times 11}{7} = \frac{11}{2} = 5\frac{1}{2}$

3.3.4 Division of Fractions

(a) How to divide skill:
To divide one fraction by another, invert the second fraction after the division sign, which is the process of interchanging the numerator and denominator of the second fraction and multiply the fractions. This gives the reciprocal of a fraction.

The reciprocal of $\frac{a}{b}$ is $\frac{b}{a}$, where, $a \neq 0$, and $b \neq 0$. e.g., The reciprocal of $\frac{3}{2}$ is $\frac{2}{3}$

(b) Reciprocal finding skill:
To find the reciprocal of a whole number, first write the whole number as a fraction with a denominator of 1; then find the reciprocal of that fraction:

The reciprocal of 5 is $\frac{1}{5}$, because $5 = \frac{5}{1}$

The reciprocal of a number is 1 divided by the number. It follows from the definition that the product of a number and its reciprocal is 1.

Example: the reciprocal of $\frac{a}{b}$ is $\frac{b}{a}$, therefore $\frac{a}{b} \times \frac{b}{a} = \frac{ab}{ab} = 1$

Division by Zero
It is important to emphasize that division by zero is impossible, therefore a fraction cannot have zero as a denominator.

Example: Divide $\frac{3}{5}$ by 7

The division operation can be obtained by $\frac{3}{7} \div \frac{7}{1}$, rewriting 7 as $\frac{7}{1}$.

Applying the rule for division of fractions, the result is:
$\frac{3}{5} \div \frac{7}{1} = \frac{3}{5} \times \frac{1}{7} = \frac{3}{35}$.

(c) Mixed numbers dividing skill:
To divide mixed numbers, convert them first to fractions and apply the rule for division.

(d) Miscellaneous examples:
Example: What is the value of $\frac{1}{6} - \frac{3}{8} - \frac{2}{3} + \frac{3}{4}$

A. $\frac{1}{24}$
B. $-\frac{3}{24}$
C. $\frac{21}{24}$
D. $-\frac{1}{24}$

The correct answer is **B.**

Solution: Find the LCD of 6, 8, 3, 4
6 = 6, 12, 18, 24 (multiples)
8 = 8, 16, 24 (multiples)
3 = 3, 6, 9, 12, 15, 18, 21, 24 (multiples)
4 = 4, 8, 12, 16, 20, 24 (multiples)
LCD = 24

$$\begin{aligned} \frac{1}{6} - \frac{3}{8} - \frac{2}{3} + \frac{3}{4} &= \frac{4(1) - 3(3) - 8(2) + 6(3)}{24} \\ &= \frac{4 - 9 - 16 + 18}{24} \\ &= \frac{-5 - 16 + 18}{24} \\ &= \frac{-21 + 18}{24} \\ &= -\frac{3}{24} \end{aligned}$$

Example: Multiply $5\frac{3}{7} \times 3\frac{1}{2}$

A. $\frac{2}{7}$
B. $\frac{19}{7}$
C. 19
D. $\frac{7}{2}$
E. 9

The correct answer is **C.**

Solution: Change both mixed numbers to improper fractions.

$$5\frac{3}{7} = \left(\frac{35+3}{7}\right);\ 3\frac{1}{2} = \frac{6}{2} + \frac{1}{2} = \frac{7}{2}$$

Multiply using rule for multiplying fractions: $\frac{38}{7} \times \frac{7}{2} = \frac{2 \bullet 19}{7} \times \frac{7}{2} = 19$

3.4 PERCENTS, DECIMALS, AND FRACTIONS

Remember the following conversion model for percents, decimals, and fractions:

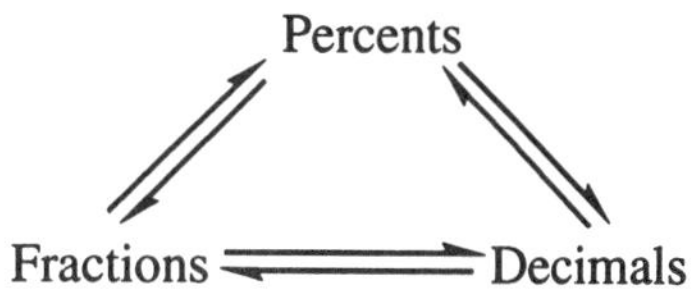

Figure 3.1 — Conversion Model for Percents, Decimals, and Fractions

Percent means "part of 100," one one-hundredth. If you consider that a quantity is subdivided into 100 equal parts, a certain percent of the quantity is the number of these hundredth parts involved. The word *rate* is sometimes used for percent.

Thus, a percent is really a fraction: 25% is 25 parts of 100, or $\frac{25}{100}$, or $\frac{1}{4}$.

Percentage results from taking a specified percent of a quantity. The process of using percent in calculations is called percentage operations. *Base* is the number of which a given percent is calculated. When percent is involved, it is the quantity that is divided into 100 parts.

3.4.1 Conversion Skills for Percents, Decimals, and Fractions

Percent is a special type of fraction with 100 as a denominator. The symbol for percent is %. Thus, 20 percent (20%) means 20 hundredths or $\frac{20}{100}$, 60 percent (60%) 60 hundredths or $\frac{60}{100}$. A percent may always be reduced to a fraction and then this fraction may in turn be expressed in decimal form. Thus, 25 percent represents the same fractional measure as $\frac{25}{100}$ or $\frac{1}{4}$ or the same decimal measure as 0.25. A fractional measure can always be expressed as a percent by writing an equivalent fraction with 100 as its denominator.

Thus, $0.24 = \frac{24}{100} = 24\%$ and $1.15 = \frac{115}{100} = 115\%$

Skills for converting a decimal fraction to a percent and vice versa are as follows:

(a) Decimal to percent conversion:
To convert a decimal fraction to equivalent percent, multiply the decimal fraction by 100. This means that the decimal point has to be moved two places to the right. For example, express 2.15 as a percent. Multiply by 100, which means moving the decimal point two places to the right.

$2.15 \times 100 = 215\%$.

(b) Fraction to decimal conversion:
To convert a fraction to a decimal fraction, divide the numerator by the denominator using long division, e.g., express $\frac{1}{4}$ as a decimal by dividing 4 into 1. Four does not divide into 1, hence add a zero and put a decimal point in the quotient, $\frac{1.0}{4} \approx 0.2$. Add another zero to get $\frac{1.00}{4} = 0.25$ to two decimal places. Memorize a few common conversions for the OAT: $\frac{1}{4} = 0.25$; $\frac{1}{2} = 0.50$; $\frac{3}{4} = 0.75$; $\frac{1}{8} = 0.125$; $\frac{3}{16} = 0.1875$; $\frac{3}{8} = 0.375$.

(c) Fraction to percent conversion:
To convert a fraction to percent, convert the fraction so that its denominator is 100. The numerator of the new fraction is the percent. The fraction also may be converted into its decimal equivalent using long division.

Example: Express $\frac{6}{25}$ as a percent by multiplying the fraction by $\frac{4}{4}$. $\frac{6}{25} \times \frac{4}{4} = \frac{24}{100} = 24\%$.

Example: Express $\frac{3}{7}$ as a percent by converting $\frac{3}{7}$ to its decimal equivalent, $\frac{3}{7} = 3 \div 7 = 0.42857.... \cong 42.86\%$.

3.4.2 Word Problems Using Percent Rate, Percentage Change

All percentage problems can be reduced to three types.
1. Calculating the percent of a given quantity, = percentage.
2. Determine the rate or percent rate, = rate.
3. Calculating the base or the quantity, = base.

Most percent problems involve three quantities:
The rate, **R**, which is followed by a percent (%) sign.
The base, **B**, which follows the word "of" or a preposition.
The amount of percentage, **P**, which usually follows the word "is" or a verb.
Thus a basic equation or formula can be used to solve most types of percentage problems.

$\frac{R}{100} = \frac{P}{B}$, where

R = Rate or %
B = Base
P = Percentage

Example: What is 5.7% of 160?

Using the formula $\frac{R}{100} = \frac{P}{B}$, noting R = 5.7%, P = unknown, and B = 160

$$\frac{5.7}{100} = \frac{P}{160}$$
$$100\,P = 160\,(5.7)$$
$$P = \frac{10 \times 16\,(5.7)}{10 \times 10} = \frac{91.2(10)}{10 \times 10} = 9.12$$

Answer: P = 9.12

Example: 72 is what percent (%) of 120?

Using the formula $\frac{R}{100} = \frac{P}{B}$

R = unknown
P = 72
B = 120

$$\frac{R}{100} = \frac{72}{120}$$
$$120\,R = 72\,(100)$$
$$R = \frac{72\,(10)\,(10)}{12\,(10)} = \frac{720}{12} = 60$$

Answer: R = 60%

Example: A copper compound contains 80% copper by weight. How much copper is there in a 1.95 g sample of the compound?
1. 15.60
2. 156
3. 1.56
4. 15.0
5. 150

The correct answer is **3.**

Solution: Using the formula $\frac{R}{100} = \frac{P}{B}$,

R = 80%
P = Unknown
B = 195

$$\frac{80}{100} = \frac{P}{1.95}$$
$$100\,P = 80\,(1.95)$$
$$P = \frac{(10)\,(8)\,(1.95)}{(10)\,(10)}$$
$$P = \frac{15.60}{10} = 1.56$$

Therefore, the given sample contains 1.56g of copper.

Special Percent Skills

(a) Percent change, percent increase, and percent decrease are special types of percent problems in which the difficulty is in making sure to use the right numbers to calculate the percent. The full formula is:

$$\frac{(\text{New Amount}) - (\text{Original Amount})}{(\text{Original Amount})} \times 100 = \text{Percent change}$$

(b) Where the new amount is less than the original amount, the number on top will be a negative number and the result will be a *percent decrease.* When a percent decrease is asked for, the negative sign is omitted.

(c) Where the new amount is greater than the original amount, the percent change is positive and is called a *percent increase.* The percent of increase or decrease is found by putting the amount of increase or decrease over the original amount and changing this fraction by multiplying with 100.

Example: Mrs. Morris receives a salary increase from $25,000 to $27,000. Find the percent increase.
Using the formula,

$$\frac{(\text{New Amount}) - (\text{Original Amount})}{(\text{Original Amount})} \times 100$$

$$\frac{\$27000 - \$25000}{\$25000} \times 100 = \frac{2000}{\$25000} \times 100$$
$$= \frac{20}{250} \times 100$$
$$= \frac{200}{25} = 8\%$$

The percent increase is 8%.

(d) A percentage is just an alternative way of representing a fraction or ratio as explained earlier. The statement "x is P percent (P%) of y" means that:

$$x = \frac{P}{100} \cdot y \quad \text{or, equivalently,} \quad P = \frac{x}{y} \cdot 100$$

Important: A percentage is a fraction with a denominator of 100, e.g., a nickel is 5% of a dollar.

Percentages are typically used to express the fractional part that one quantity is of another; for example, if there are 16 women in a class of 25 students, then alternatively one can say that P = (16/25)(100) = 64% of the students in the class are women. Percentages are also used to express a change in a quantity in terms of its percent increase or decrease. By definition, if x_2 is the result when x_1 is increased by P%, then:

$$x_2 = x_1 + \frac{P}{100} \cdot x_1 = x_1 \cdot \left(1 + \frac{P}{100}\right);$$

if x_2 is the result when x_1 is decreased by P%, then:

$$x_2 = x_1 - \frac{P}{100} \cdot x_1 = x_1 \cdot \left(1 - \frac{P}{100}\right).$$

It is important to note that in both of these definitions the change in the variable is expressed as a percentage of its original value (x_1), not its final value (x_2).

Example: What is the percent increase or decrease in a quantity x when its value is: a) doubled, b) halved, c) reduced by a third, d) reduced to a third of its original value, and e) reduced to a fifth of its original value?

(a) $x_2 = 2x_1 \; ; \; 2x_1 = x_1\left(1 + \frac{P}{100}\right)$ P = 100% increase

(b) $x_2 = \frac{1}{2}x_1 \; ; \; \frac{1}{2}x_1 = x_1\left(1 - \frac{P}{100}\right)$ P = 50% decrease

(c) $x_2 = \frac{2}{3}x_1 \; ; \; \frac{2}{3}x_1 = x_1\left(1 - \frac{P}{100}\right)$ P = $33\frac{1}{3}$% decrease

(d) $x_2 = \frac{1}{3}x_1 \; ; \; \frac{1}{3}x_1 = x_1\left(1 - \frac{P}{100}\right)$ P = $66\frac{2}{3}$% decrease

(e) $x_2 = \frac{1}{5}x_1 \; ; \; \frac{1}{5}x_1 = x_1\left(1 - \frac{P}{100}\right)$ P = 80% decrease

3.5 OPERATIONS WITH SCIENTIFIC NOTATIONS (EXPONENTIALS)

Scientific Notation
A number is said to be in scientific notation if it is expressed as the product of a number between 1 and 10 and some integral power of 10. For example, 1,000 is written in scientific notation as 1×10^3 or more simply, 10^3; 0.0001 is written as 10^{-4}; $1247 = 1.247 \times 10^3$; $0.000786 = 7.86 \times 10^{-4}$.

3.5.1 Conversion to and From Scientific Notation (General Skill)

Since the decimal point of any number can be shifted at will to the left or to the right by multiplying by an appropriate power of 10, any number can be expressed in scientific notation. In general, if **n** is any number, we write $n = a \times 10^z$, where **a** is a number between 1 and 10 and **z** is an integer, positive or negative.

Example: Write 10,000,000 in scientific notation. The decimal point in 10,000,000 is after the last zero. The first significant digit is 1. Move the decimal point to the left seven places (1.000 000 0) multiplying by 10^7 gives the number in scientific notation as: $10{,}000{,}000 = 1 \times 10^7$, usually written 10^7

Example: Write 0.005329 in scientific notation. The decimal point is moved to the right three places. The resulting number is $0.005329 = 5.329 \times 10^{-3}$.

3.6 PROBABILITY AND STATISTICS CONCEPTS

Probability values range from one to zero. A value of 1 stands for absolute certainty, and zero indicates there is no chance at all that the event will occur. There are very few things in life about which we can be absolutely certain. Most things in life, however, have probability values of their occurrence somewhere between 1 and zero.

If you take a new coin that has not been mutilated and toss it, we can state that the probability of obtaining a head is one out of two. This can be written as $P = \frac{1}{2}$, or 0.5.

It is also true that the probability of obtaining a tail is $\frac{1}{2}$, or 0.5.

In this situation, only one of these two outcomes can occur. Notice that the sum of the two probabilities is equal to 1. We designate the probability of an event occurring by use of the symbol **p** and the probability of it not occurring by the **q**. The sum of **p** + **q** is always equal to 1.

Example: Take a die with six sides and toss it into the air. What is the probability of any single side coming up? The probability of any single side coming up is $\frac{1}{6}$ or 0.167. That is when we toss a die, the chance of throwing a six spot is one in six. There are five chances in six chances of some other number appearing on the upturned face.

In this case, $\mathbf{p} = \frac{1}{6}$ and $\mathbf{q} = \frac{5}{6}$, therefore $\mathbf{p} + \mathbf{q} = \frac{1}{6} + \frac{5}{6} = \frac{6}{6} = 1$

Example: There are 6 yellow marbles and 2 blue marbles in a bag. If Sara draws a marble out of the bag without looking, what are the chances that it will be blue?

A. $\frac{2}{8}$

B. $\frac{6}{8}$

C. $\frac{2}{6}$

D. $\frac{6}{2}$

E. $\frac{8}{2}$

The correct answer is **A.**

Solution: Let **p** = number of favorable outcomes, which is 2
q = number of unfavorable outcomes, which is 6
p + **q** = total outcomes, which is 2 + 6 = 8

$$\frac{\mathbf{p}}{\mathbf{p}+\mathbf{q}} = \frac{2}{8}$$

3.6.1 Statistical Data Analysis Skills

Data from two experiments are presented and analyzed. Statistical analysis at an elementary level is being illustrated.

Experiment A: A psychology experiment designed to test the difficulty of a particular maze for rats is done by having ten rats run the maze. The results for their solution times to the nearest 0.1 seconds are:

8.3, 7.1, 8.8, 11.1, 7.0, 13.7, 9.5, 10.3, 10.8, 9.9

Experiment B: Two groups of 35-year-old subjects, one of men and one of women, have their blood cholesterol levels (mg/100 ml) measured. The data obtained (rounded to the nearest 1 mg/100 ml) are:

Group I (men): 195, 198, 199, 196, 195, 196, 191, 194, 195, 196
Group II (women): 196, 193, 194, 201, 202, 205, 204, 202, 199, 204

Having this data, the problem now becomes one of how to organize and analyze them so that they can be interpreted/presented to someone else clearly and meaningfully. The information above reflects two types of data that are commonly encountered in raw form (as taken during an experiment and not manipulated into graphs, means, ranges, etc.). In Experiment A, the data are of a **continuous** nature because all decimal values of time are possible (e.g., 8.003, 9.1083, etc.) even though they are not recorded. **Count** data is important for integer values such as age of a person, or number of times teeth are brushed each day. In experiment B, cholesterol level is a continuous variable but it is being rounded to compare cholesterol count of two groups.

Problem 1: Are the data in Experiment A count data or continuous data?

Simple Data Analysis

Often it is a good idea, when presented a set of data, to make some simple observations. The easiest way to do this is to organize the data in ascending or descending order (or groups). Experiment A's data will be organized into an ascending order:

7.0, 7.1, 8.3, 8.8, 9.5, 9.9, 10.3, 10.8, 11.1, 13.7

Next, get a feeling for the data in Experiment A by using the simple steps below:

Experiment A:

(1) smallest value = 7.0
(2) largest value = 13.7
(3) range is 7.0 to 13.7: 13.7 – 7.0 = 6.7
(4) average might be about 10: $\frac{13.7 + 7.0}{2} \cong 10$

These simple observations, which can be made rapidly, gives you an idea about the limits of the data, the average value of the data, the variability of the data, and the distribution of the data over its possible values.

Problem 2: Do the same type of simple analysis on the data for Groups I and II in Experiment B as was done for Experiment A.

3.6.1.1 STRUCTURING THE DATA

If it has not already been done, the next steps in the analysis will probably be to construct graphs and/or tables from the data; our concern now is mostly with tables. When interpreting **tables**, like interpreting graphs, it is essential to read the headings at the tops and sides of the tables to determine what is being presented. Then, survey the whole table to get a feel for the data and any noticeable general trends there. Next, look for more specific points or regions of data that may be of interest. Whether or not in conjunction with a table, another simple way to structure a set of data is to determine what **percentages** (or proportions) of it meet specified classifications. This is best illustrated by **examples**:

Experiment A:

(i) For some reason, you are interested in the percentage of rats with times less than 9.0 seconds:

$$\text{\% with times less than 9.0 seconds} = \frac{4}{10} \times 100 = 40\%$$

(ii) You are told that 40% of the rats ran the maze in times greater than 10.0 seconds. How many rats, T, ran the maze in times greater than 10.0 seconds?

$$T = \frac{40}{100} \times 10 = 4$$

Problem 3: What are the respective percentages of subjects in Groups I and II of Experiment B who had blood cholesterol levels of 196 or lower?

3.6.1.2 STATISTICAL ANALYSIS

Once a set of data is structured in a desired format and preliminary analysis has been done, more formal statistical calculations can be made to describe it. Statistically, the two key features of a set of data are its central tendency and its variation.

3.6.1.3 CENTRAL TENDENCY

The central tendency of a set of data is the value it seems to approach. It is also called the "expected value." It is the one value that is taken to be representative of the whole set of data. The common measures of central tendency are the mode, the median, and the average (or mean). Only the computation of averages is required for the OAT. The mode and the median are not required; however, their definitions will be given if they are needed on the OAT. For this reason, you should be familiar with them beforehand.

The **average** takes into account directly the value of each piece of data. It is calculated by adding together each piece of data and then dividing the sum by the total number of pieces of data:

$$\text{The average} = x = \frac{x_1 + x_2 + ... + x_n}{n},$$

where $x_1, x_2, \ldots, x_n$ = the individual pieces of data and n = the total number of pieces of data. For example:

$$\text{Experiment A: The average} = \frac{7.0 + 7.1 + 8.3 + 8.8 + 9.5 + 9.9 + 10.3 + 10.8 + 11.1 + 13.7}{10}$$

$= (9.65) \approx 9.7$

(remember that the eyeballed average was about 10)

The **median** is the value in a set of data that is positionally halfway between the lowest and highest values in the set. It is determined by listing all the values in the set of data in ascending order and then identifying the one that is positionally in the middle. In general, when there is an even number of values in a set of data, the median is calculated by taking the average of the middle two numbers. Examples of medians are:

Experiment A: The values in ascending order are:

7.0, 7.1, 8.3, 8.8, 9.5, 9.9, 10.3, 10.8, 11.1, 13.7

Since there is an even number of values (10), the two middle values are 9.5 and 9.9.

$$\text{The median} = \frac{9.5 + 9.9}{2} = 9.7$$

The **mode** is the most frequent value that appears in a set of data. It exists only if one value occurs more often than any of the other values. Examples are:

Experiment A: None exists—each value occurs only once.

The question naturally arises as to which measure of central tendency is the best; the answer is that it depends on the distribution of the data. Consider three sets of data, which are presented graphically in histograms, where N = the frequency of a particular value of the variable x:

$$\text{mean} = 2.9 = \frac{7(2)+1(4)+1(5)+1(6)}{7+1+1+1} \approx 3$$

median = 2
mode = 2

data = 2,2,2,2,2,2,2,4,5,6

I

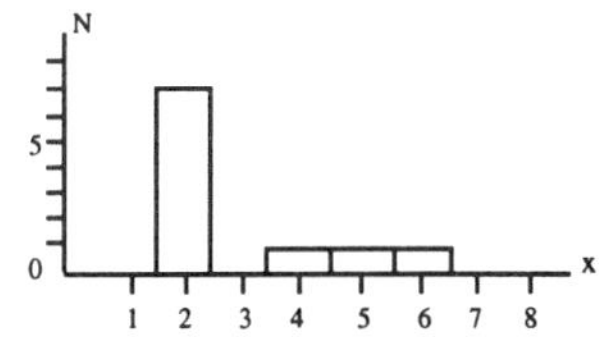

$$\text{mean} = 3 = \frac{2(1)+2(2)+2(3)+2(4)+2(5)}{2+2+2+2+2}$$

median = 3
one mode does not exist
data = 1,1,2,2,3,3,4,4,5,5

II

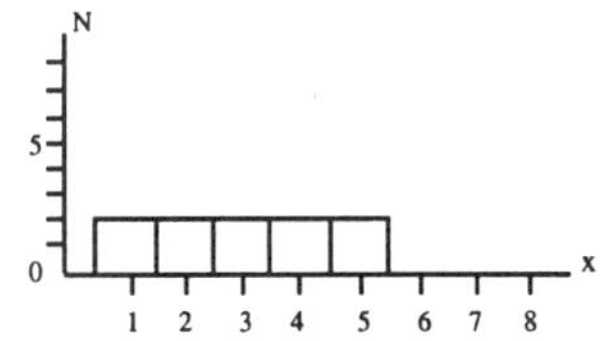

$$\text{mean} = 3.3 \cong 3 = \frac{2(1)+2(2)+3(4)+3(5)}{2+2+3+3}$$

median = 4
two modes = 4,5 (bi-modal)
data = 1,1,2,2,4,4,4,5,5,5

III

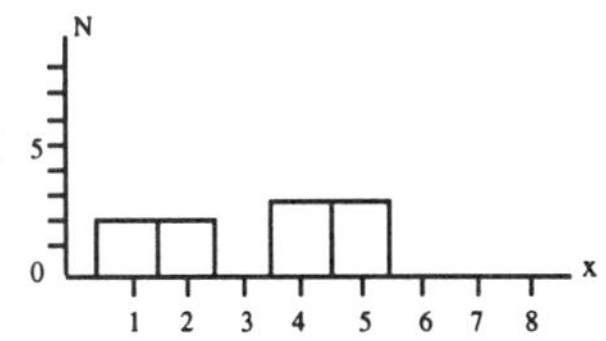

Figure 3.2 — Histograms Illustrating Mean, Median, and Mode

For the data in histogram I, both the mode and the median are good measures of central tendency; the average (mean) is probably not. Whenever the frequency of one value predominates in a set of data, the mode is usually a good measure of central tendency. Unique modes do not exist for the data in histograms II and III. For the data in histogram II, both the average and the median are good measures of central tendency. When the values of a set of data are distributed fairly evenly over the range of the data (as in this case), the average is sometimes considered better because it takes into account directly the value of each piece of data. The median is probably a better measure of central tendency than the average for the data in histogram III. Typically, the median is preferable to the average in cases where the values in a set of data are clustered toward one end of the range, but not in a way where the mode would become a good measure of central tendency as in histogram I.

Problem 4: Calculate the mode, the median, and the average for each group in Experiment B: Identify, if possible, which of the three measures of central tendency is probably best for each group.

Variation or Dispersion Around Average

The measures of central tendency discussed above each give one value to describe a whole set of data. This one value is inadequate to "completely" describe the data because it gives no sense of the variation (or the dispersion) of the data about this value. In other words, we need a knowledge of the variation in a set of data to complement our knowledge of its central tendency. The common measures of variation are the range, the variance, and the standard deviation. Only the computation of the range is required for the OAT. The variance and the standard deviation are not required; however, their definitions will be given if they are needed on the OAT. For this reason, you should be familiar with them beforehand.

The **range** is simply the difference between the highest and lowest values in a set of data. For example:

Experiment A: Range = 13.7 – 7.0 = 6.7

Experiment B: Range = 90 – 50 = 40

Because the range takes into account only the highest and lowest values in a set of data, it is a rough measure of variation. In some cases, it is really not a reasonable measure of variation. When either or both of the extreme values in a set of data are far out of line with the rest of the data, the range is a questionable measure of variation. For example, consider the data presented in the histograms below (N = the frequency of a particular value of the variable x):

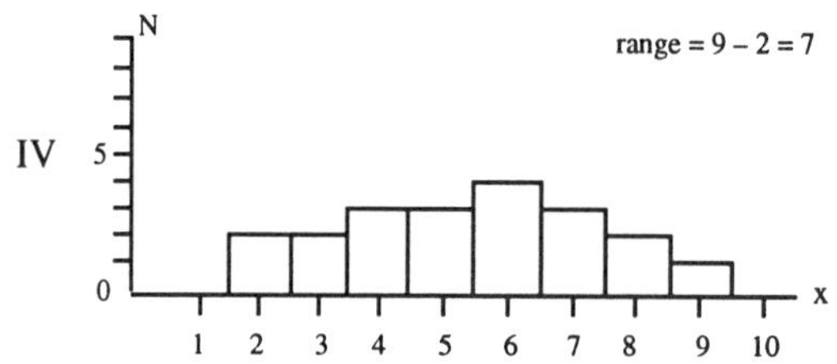

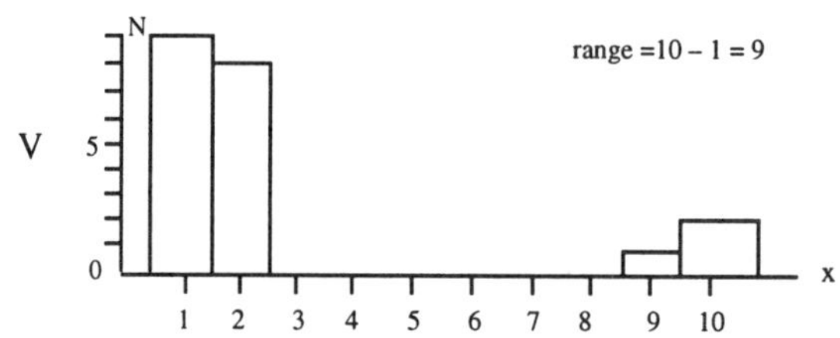

Figure 3.3 — Histograms Illustrating Range and Variation in Data

The range of the data in histogram IV gives a good idea of that data's variability. On the other hand, the range of the data in histogram V does not really give a good idea of that data's variability.

The **variance** (V) and the **standard deviations** (S.D.) are intimately related:

$$S.D. = \sqrt{V}$$

The OAT requires that you understand the concepts, but you will not have to make calculations. The following should be reviewed and understood but need not be memorized.

The variance, like the mean, takes into account each value in a set of data. It is calculated by taking the average value of the squares of the deviation for each data point from the mean:

$$\text{variance} = \frac{(x_1 - x)^2 + (x_2 - x)^2 + \ldots + (x_n - x)^2}{n},$$

where $x_1, x_2, \ldots, x_n$ = values of individual pieces of data, x = the mean, and n = the total number of pieces of data. The standard deviation is simply calculated by taking the square root of the variance so calculated:

$$\text{standard deviation} = \left(\frac{(x_1 - x)^2 + (x_2 - x)^2 + \ldots + (x_n - x)^2}{n}\right)^{1/2}.$$

Examples of calculation of the standard deviation and the variance are:

$$\text{Experiment A: } V = \frac{(7.0\text{–}9.7)^2 + (7.1\text{–}9.7)^2 + \ldots + (11.1\text{–}9.7)^2 + (13.7\text{–}9.7)^2}{10}$$

$$= (3.643) \cong 3.6$$

$$\text{S.D.} = \sqrt{V} = \sqrt{3.6} = 1.9.$$

A rough way to estimate the standard deviation of a set of data is to take its range and divide by 4:

$$\text{S.D.} \cong \frac{\text{Range}}{4}.$$

$$\text{Experiment A: S.D.} \cong \frac{13.7\text{–}7.0}{4} = (1.675) \cong 1.7$$

Comparing these estimates of the standard deviation to the exact calculations above, we can observe that when the range is a good indicator of the variation in a set of data, this S.D. approximation using it is also good.

Problem 5: Calculate the range, the variance, and the standard deviation for each group in Experiment B.

3.6.2 Solutions to Data Analysis Problems

(1) The data in Experiment A are continuous data.

(2) Group I: Put the data in ascending order: 191, 194, 195, 195, 195, 196, 196, 198, 199; then:
- (1) smallest value = 191
- (2) largest value = 199
- (3) range is 199 – 191 = 8
- (4) most values are around 195 or 196, so the average is probably about 195 or 196
- (5) there are few values at the ends of the range (191 and 199), but many at the middle (195 to 196)

(2) Group II: Put the data in ascending order: 193, 194, 196, 199, 201, 202, 202, 204, 204, 205; then:
- (1) smallest value = 193
- (2) largest vale = 205
- (3) range is 205 – 193 = 12
- (4) average might be about 199: $\frac{193 + 205}{2} = 199$
- (5) the values cluster toward the higher end of the range

(3) Group I: Percentage with blood cholesterol levels of 196 or lower = $\frac{8}{10} \times 100 = 80\%$

Group II: Percentage with blood cholesterol levels of 196 or lower = $\frac{3}{10} \times 100 = 30\%$

(4) Group I: A unique mode does not exist, as 195 and 196 both appear three times.

$$\text{The median} = \frac{195 + 196}{2} = 196 = (195.5)$$

$$\text{The average} = \frac{191 + 194 + 3(195) + 3(196) + 198 + 199}{10}$$

$$= 196 = (195.5)$$

Both the average and the median are good measures of the central tendency of Group I's data.

Group II: A unique mode does not exist, as 202 and 204 both appear twice.

The median $= \frac{201 + 202}{2} = 202 = (201.5)$

The average $= \frac{193 + 194 + 196 + 199 + 201 + 2(202) + 2(204) + 205}{10}$

$= 200$

It is a toss-up as to which measure of central tendency, the median or the average, is probably better. Qualitatively, the average tends to reflect the spread of data at the lower end of the range more than the median does, while the median tends to reflect the cluster of data at the high end of the range more than the average does.

(5) Group I: The range = 199 – 191 = 8

$$V = \frac{(191 - 196)^2 + (194 - 196)^2 + \ldots + (198-196)^2 + (199 - 196)^2}{10}$$

$= (4.5) \equiv 5$

S.D. $= \sqrt{V} = \sqrt{5} = (2.236) \equiv 2$

Group II: The range = 205 – 193 = 12

$$V = \frac{(193 - 200)^2 + (194 - 200)^2 + \ldots + 2(204 - 200)^2 + (205 - 200)^2}{10}$$

$= (16.8) \equiv 17$

S.D. $= \sqrt{V} = \sqrt{17} = (4.123) \equiv 4$

(6) See solutions to problems 1 through 5.

3.7 PLANE GEOMETRY CONCEPTS

Geometry deals with measurements of sides, angles, areas, and perimeters and volumes. It can be divided into two branches: plane and solid. Plane and solid geometry are inseparable from two-dimensional and three-dimensional perceptual abilities. You should spend considerable time reviewing principles in plane and solid geometry before going deep into chapter 4. For example, learn the difference between plane angles and dihedral angles by looking at real-life examples. Angles in two dimensions (between two lines or rays) are plane angles. Angles in three dimensions (between two or three surfaces) are dihedral or solid angles. Look at various corners in your room. Each corner forms dihedral or solid angles. Learn to connect dihedral angles to isometric and perspective views of a solid object, such as wings of an airplane.

The most common geometric concepts used in the OAT will be explained in this section.

Angles:

An **angle** is formed by two lines meeting at a point.
Right Angle—an angle that measures 90°
Complementary Angles —two angles, the sum of whose measures is 90°
Supplementary Angles—two angles, the sum of whose measures is 180°
Acute Angle—an angle whose measurement is less than 90°
Obtuse Angle—an angle whose measurement is greater than 90°
Straight Angle—an angle whose measurement is equal to 180°
Perimeter—the distance around a plane figure.

3.7.1 Rules and Formulas

1. The sum of the measure of the angles in a triangle is 180°.

2. Perimeter is the distance around a figure. To find the perimeter, add the length of the sides:
   Perimeter = p; and $p = a + b + c$

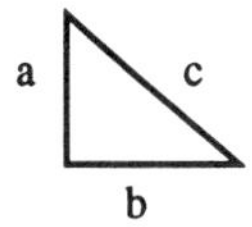

3. Square Perimeter :
   $p = s + s + s + s$
   $p = 4s$

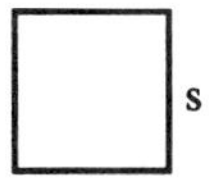

4. Rectangle Perimeter:
   $p = 2 \times \text{length} + 2 \times \text{width}$
   $p = 2L + 2W$

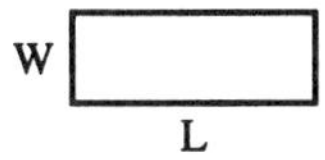

5. Circumference (c) of a circle is the distance around the circle. The diameter is twice the radius times π(pi) or π times the diameter.
   $c = 2 \times \pi \times \text{radius}$
   $c = 2\pi r$
   $c = \pi \times \text{diameter}$
   $c = \pi d$
   $\pi \approx 3.14, \frac{22}{7}$

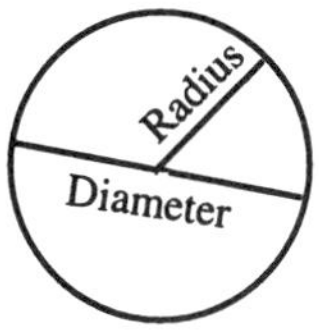

6. Composite geometric figures are made of two or more simple geometric figures:

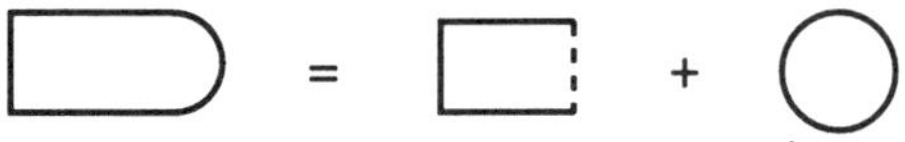

   Composite figure = 3 sides of a rectangle + $\frac{1}{2}$ the circumference of a circle

   Perimeter of the composite figure = $(2 \times \text{length}) + \text{width} + \frac{1}{2} \times \pi \times \text{diameter}$

3.7.2 Similar Triangle Concepts

Similar figures are figures that have the same shape but not necessarily the same size. Similar figures have corresponding sides and angles. The relationship between the sizes of each of the corresponding sides or angles can be written as a ratio, and each ratio will be the same.

The two triangles below, ABC and DEF, are similar. The ratios of corresponding sides are equal.

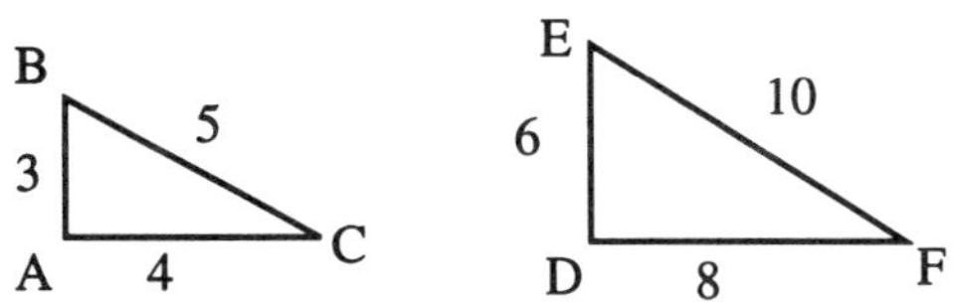

$$\frac{AB}{DE} = \frac{3}{6} = \frac{1}{2}; \frac{BC}{EF} = \frac{5}{10} = \frac{1}{2}; \text{and } \frac{AC}{DF} = \frac{4}{8} = \frac{1}{2}$$

The ratio of the corresponding sides = $\frac{1}{2}$

Since the ratios of corresponding sides are equal, three proportions can be formed:

$$\frac{AB}{DE} = \frac{BC}{EF};\ \frac{AC}{DF} = \frac{BC}{EF} \text{ and } \frac{AB}{DE} = \frac{AC}{DF}$$

Example: Triangles ABC and DEF are similar. Find the perimeter of Δ ABC.

A. 11
B. 12
C. 14
D. 13
E. 10

The correct answer is **B.**

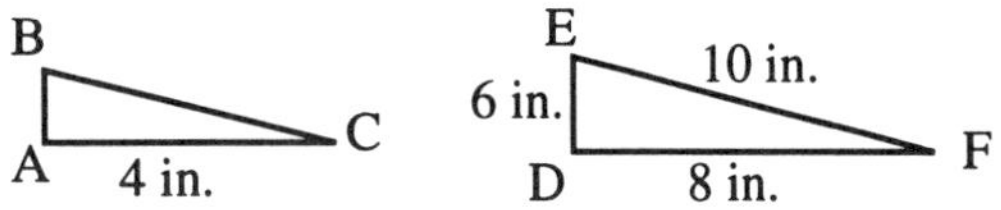

Find the length of BC by using proportion

$$\frac{AC}{DF} = \frac{BC}{EF}$$

$$\frac{4 \text{ in.}}{8 \text{ in.}} = \frac{BC}{EF}$$

$$8\ BC = 40 \text{ in.}$$

$$BC = 5 \text{ in.}$$

$$\frac{BC}{EF} = \frac{AB}{DE}$$

$$\frac{5 \text{ in.}}{10 \text{ in.}} = \frac{AC}{6 \text{ in.}}$$

$$10AB = 30 \text{ in.}$$

$$AB = 3 \text{ in.}$$

The perimeter of Δ ABC $= 4 + 3 + 5$
$= 12$

3.7.3 Cartesian or Analytic Geometry

All graphical representations of data and functions are based on some sort of coordinate system. Even bar graphs (histograms) and pie graphs have an implicit coordinate system in their construction. By far the most commonly used graphs are based on the rectangular (Cartesian) coordinate system that consists of two perpendicular axes, each representing a variable:

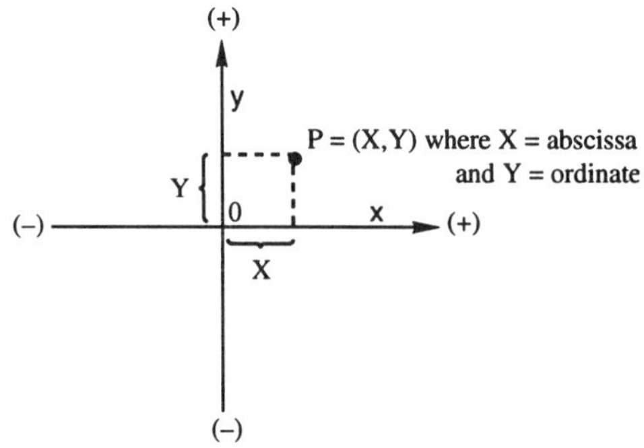

Figure 3.4 — Cartesian Coordinate System

The intersection of the two axes in the Cartesian plane is called the origin (O). The origin splits each axis into two segments that respectively represent positive and negative values of that axis' variable. Usually the ordinate represents the dependent variable (y) and the abscissa represents the independent variable (x). The standard positive and negative segments of each axis are labeled on the graph above; this is also shown by the arrows that indicate the directions of positive change for each axis' variable. Each point in the Cartesian plane is represented by a pair of coordinates (called an ordered pair), each of which represents a distance from the origin along one of the axes [e.g., the point P = (x,y) on the graph above and the origin O = (0,0)].

Slope or Rate of Change:

Probably the most important parameter in interpreting the relationship between the two variables in a graph is the slope. The slope of the line segment between two points is defined as the ratio of the change in the ordinate to the change in the abscissa:

$$\text{slope} = \frac{\text{change in ordinate}}{\text{change in abscissa}} = \frac{\Delta y}{\Delta x} = \frac{\text{Rise}}{\text{Run}} = \frac{\text{change in dependent variable}}{\text{change in independent variable}}$$

A slope exists for every point on a graph whether it is a straight line or a curved line. For each point on a graph, the slope is the rate of change (positive or negative) in the ordinate with respect to the change in the abscissa. It may be constant as for straight lines or portions of curves that are straight, or it may be constantly changing as for curved lines. In practice, the slope is calculated as follows:

For straight lines:

$$\text{slope} = m = \frac{y_2 - y_1}{x_2 - x_1} = \frac{\Delta y}{\Delta x} = \text{constant}$$

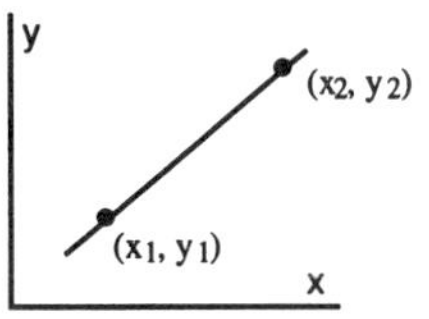

For curved lines:

measure $\Delta x, \Delta y$ for any two points on tangent

$\text{slope} = m = \frac{\Delta y}{\Delta x} \neq \text{constant}$ (changes along the curve)

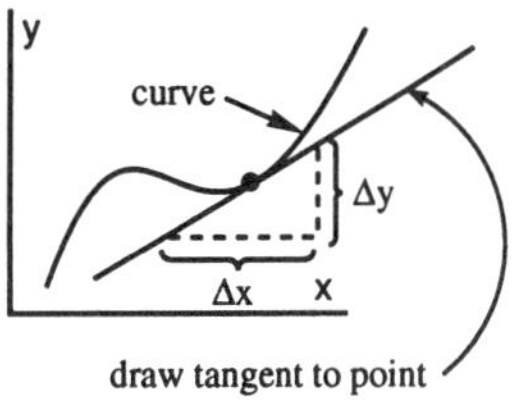

Figure 3.5 — Definition Sketch for Slope

Example 1.
Calculate the slope of the line graphed below:

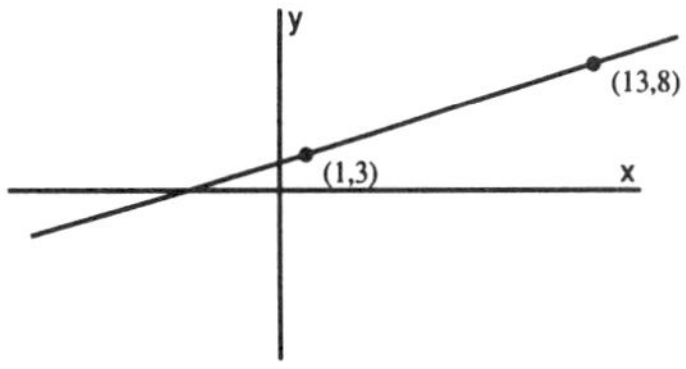

$$m = \frac{y_2 - y_1}{x_2 - x_1} = \frac{8-3}{13-1} = \frac{5}{12}$$

3.8 ALGEBRAIC EQUATIONS AND PROPORTIONALITY PROBLEMS

The solution of a simple equation in one variable usually amounts to the isolation of an "**unknown quantity**" or variable on one side of the equation. Any operation, except multiplication or division by zero, can be used to achieve this "isolation" as long as it is done to both sides of the equation. More generally, the basic rule for solving equations is that whatever is done to one side must be done to the other side so that the equality of the sides is not affected. It is like a weighing scale with two balanced sides or pans. Before considering some examples of solving equations, first it is important to recall that, when manipulating an expression (whether or not it is part of an equation), the order of operations is as follows:

Order of Operations

(1) parentheses
(2) powers or exponents
(3) multiplication and division (whichever comes first from the left side of the expression)
(4) addition and subtraction (whichever comes first from the left side of the expression)

Example 1: Solve for a: $4a + 5 = 13$

$$4a + 5 - 5 = 13 - 5$$
$$4a = 8$$
$$\frac{4a}{4} = \frac{8}{4}$$
$$a = 2$$

Example 2: Solve for m: $\frac{10}{m} - 8 = \frac{5}{3}$

$$\frac{10}{m}(3m) - 8(3m) = \frac{5}{3}(3m)$$
$$30 - 24m = 5m$$
$$30 = 29m$$
$$m = \frac{30}{29}$$

Example 3: Solve for c: $3c^2 = 75d^4$

$$c^2 = 25d^4$$
$$(c^2) = \sqrt{25d^4}$$
$$c = \pm 5d^2$$

Example 4: Solve for q:

$$3[(q + 2)^2 - 4q] = 2q^2 + 13$$
$$3[(q + 2)(q + 2) - 4q] = 2q^2 + 13$$
$$3[q^2 + 4q + 4 - 4q] = 2q^2 + 13$$
$$3q^2 + 12 = 2q^2 + 13$$
$$q^2 = 1$$
$$q = \pm 1$$

Problem 1: Solve for a: $s(a - p) + q = ta + r^2$

Problem 2: Solve for d: $\frac{1}{d-2} + \frac{2}{d+3} = \frac{4}{d-2}$

Problem 3: Solve for x: $3(4x - 2[1 - (x + 5) + 3]) = 13x + 19$

3.8.1 Proportionality

(a) Some problems will be solvable by recognizing that the quantities in question are directly or inversely proportional to each other. Two variables, x and y, are **directly proportional** if their ratio has a constant value, a:

$\frac{y}{x} = a$ or $y = ax$.

(Linear variation)

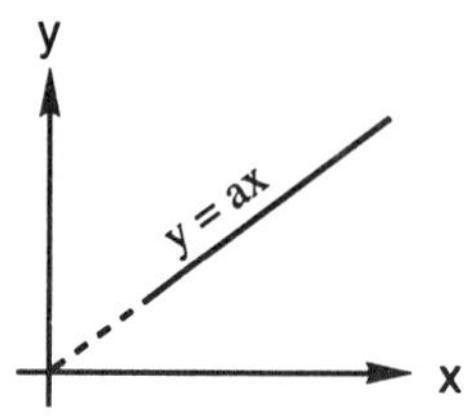

Figure 3.6 — Linear Variation

Consequently, for any distinct values of x, x_1, and x_2, there are corresponding values of y, y_1, and y_2, such that:

$$\frac{y_1}{x_1} = \frac{y_2}{x_2}. \quad \text{(x, y directly proportional)}$$

If we know three of the terms in this proportion, then we can always determine the fourth term.

Example 5: If two moles of compound A react with 5 moles of compound B to form 3 moles of compound C, then how many moles of A are required to react completely with 7 moles of B?

In a chemical reaction, the quantities of reactants/products are directly proportional. (Why?)

Let $x_1 = 2$ moles of A and $y_1 = 5$ moles of B.
Then, x_2 = number of moles of A and $y_2 = 7$ moles of B such that:
$\frac{5}{2} = \frac{7}{x_2}$; $x_2 = 2.8$ moles of A.

Problem 4: In Example 5, how many moles of C are formed?

(b) Two variables, x and y, are **inversely proportional** if their product has a constant value, b:

$$xy = b \quad \text{or} \quad y = \frac{b}{x}.$$

(Nonlinear or hyperbolic variation)

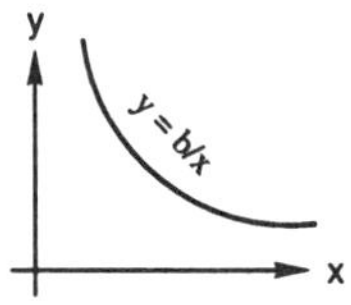

Figure 3.7 — Nonlinear Variation

Consequently, for any distinct values of x, x_1, and x_2, there are corresponding values of y, y_1, and y_2, such that:

$$x_1y_1 = x_2y_2 \quad \text{or} \quad \frac{y_1}{x_2} = \frac{y_2}{x_1} \qquad \text{(x,y inversely proportional)}$$

If we know three of the terms in this equation, $x_1y_1 = x_2y_2$, then we can always determine the fourth term.

Example 6: A car traveling at x mph takes 5 hours to go from city A to city B. Traveling at x – 15 mph, the car makes the return trip in six and two-thirds hours. What was the speed of the car on the return trip?

Since displacement = (speed)(time), d = vt, speed and time are inversely proportional for a constant displacement. Let v_1 = x mph and t_1 = 5 hours; v_2 = x – 15 mph and $t_2 = 6\frac{2}{3}$ hours $= \frac{20}{3}$ hours. Then:

$$5x = (x - 15)\frac{20}{3}$$

$$15x = 20x - 300$$

$$5x = 300$$

$$x = 60 \;;\; v_2 = x - 15 = 45 \text{ mph.}$$

Problem 5: Before an engine tune-up, a car with a gas consumption rate of r gallons/mile can go 400 miles on a full tank of gas. After a tune-up, the same car has a gas consumption rate of r – .01 gallons/mile and can go 500 miles on a full tank of gas. What was the gas consumption rate of the car before it had an engine tune-up?

Problem 6: The ideal-gas law for 1 mole of any gas is pV = RT. Thus, two different macroscopic states of a mole of a particular gas are respectively described by

$$p_1V_1 = RT_1 \quad \text{and} \quad p_2V_2 = RT_2.$$

Write an equation that shows the relationship between these two states. According to this equation, the pressure p is inversely proportional to what quantity?

An important application of proportionality is to use it to find proportional changes in variables that occur when other related variables change. This is called "sensitivity analysis" and is an important part of the OAT on all subjects being tested. It teaches how to think proportionally.

Problem 7: In 1984, a particular item A cost $2,500. In 1986, the price of A rose 20% due to scarcity while in early 1987 there was 10% increase in the price of A over its 1986 price. At the end of 1987, A was put on sale with a 30% decrease in price. What was the sale price of A?

3.8.2 Solutions to Algebra Problems

(1) $a = \dfrac{r^2 + sp - q}{s - t}$;

$$s(a - p) + q = ta + r^2$$

$$sa - sp + q = ta + r^2$$

$$a(s - t) = r^2 + sp - q$$

$$a = \frac{r^2 + sp - q}{s - t}$$

(2) $d = -13$;

$$\frac{1}{d-2} + \frac{2}{d+3} = \frac{4}{d-2}$$ [Multiply through by $(d-2)(d+3)$]

$$d + 3 + 2(d-2) = 4(d+3)$$
$$3d - 1 = 4d + 12$$
$$d = -13$$

(3) $x = \frac{13}{5}$;

$$3(4x - 2[1 - (x+5) + 3]) = 13x + 19$$
$$3[4x - 2(4 - x - 5)] = 13x + 19$$
$$3(4x + 2x + 2) = 13x + 19$$
$$18x + 6 = 13x + 1$$
$$x = \frac{13}{5}$$

(4) $C = \frac{21}{5}$ moles

Let $x_1 = 5$ moles of B and $y_1 = 3$ moles of C;
then $x_2 = 7$ moles of B and y_2 = number of moles of C.
Since B and C are directly proportional:
$\frac{y_2}{7} = \frac{3}{5}$; $y_2 = \frac{21}{5}$ moles of C

(5) $r = .05$ gallons/mile

From the problem, $xy = a$, where:

x = gas consumption rate (gallons/mile),

y = number of miles that the car can go on a full tank of gas,

a = number of gallons in full tank of gas (constant).

Thus, x and y are inversely proportional with $x_1 = r$, $y_1 = 400$, $x_2 = r - .01$, and $y_2 = 500$;

$$r(400) = (r - .01)500$$
$$400r = 500r - 5$$
$$r = .05 \text{ gallons/mile}$$

(6) $\frac{p_1V_1}{T_1} = \frac{p_2V_2}{T_2}$; $\frac{V}{T}$

$p_1V_1 = RT_1$ and $p_2V_2 = RT_2$ can be rewritten as: $\frac{p_1V_1}{T_1} = R$ and $\frac{p_2V_2}{T_2} = R$.

Therefore, the two states are related by:

$$\frac{p_1V_1}{T_1} = \frac{p_2V_2}{T_2}.$$

From the definition of inversely proportional variables, if p is one of the variables, then the other variable is V/T.

(7) Sale price (1987) = \$2,310

1984: cost of A = \$2,500

1986: cost of A $= \$2,500 + \frac{20}{100} \times \$2,500$
$= \$3,000$

1987: cost of A $= \$3,000 + \frac{10}{100} \times \$3,000$
$= \$3,300$

Sale price (1987) $= \$3,300 - \frac{30}{100} \times \$3,300$
$= \$2,310$

3.9 TRIGONOMETRY

3.9.1 Basic Definitions and Facts

Trigonometry is concerned with the relationships between the angles and sides of triangles. Recall that for similar triangles, i.e., triangles that have the same angles but which are not necessarily the same size, the ratios of the corresponding sides are equal:

$X/x = Y/y = Z/z$

$\theta_1, \theta_2, \theta_3$ = angles

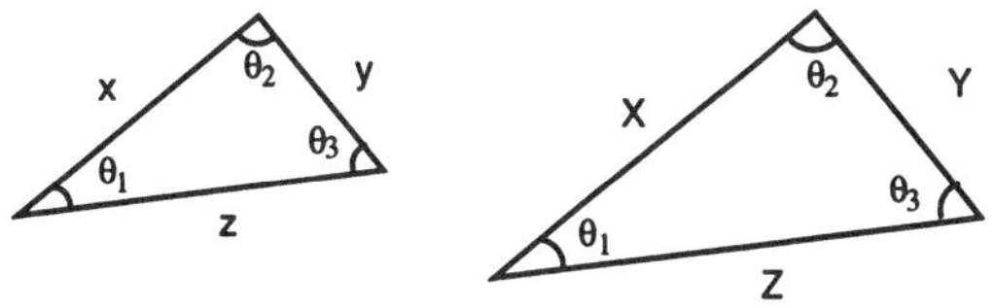

Figure 3.8 — Trigonometric Elements of Similar Triangles

Focusing on right triangles, it can be directly deduced from this that the ratio of any two of the sides of a right triangle is the same for all similar right triangles. In other words, the possible ratios depend only on the angles of the right triangle. Thus, defining the sides and angles of a right triangle as:

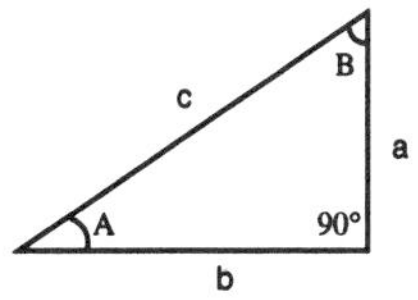

a,b = legs of the right triangle
c = hypotenuse of the right triangle
A,B = angles

Figure 3.9 — Definition Sketch for Trigonometric Functions

The basic trigonometric functions are:

the sine of an angle $= \dfrac{\text{opposite side}}{\text{hypotenuse}}$, i.e., $\sin A = \dfrac{a}{c}$ and $\sin B = \dfrac{b}{c}$

the cosine of an angle $= \dfrac{\text{adjacent side}}{\text{hypotenuse}}$, i.e., $\cos A = \dfrac{b}{c}$ and $\cos B = \dfrac{a}{c}$

the tangent of an angle $= \dfrac{\text{opposite side}}{\text{adjacent side}}$, i.e., $\tan A = \dfrac{a}{b}$ and $\tan B = \dfrac{b}{a}$

Note that these definitions are interrelated; for example, observe that sin A = cos B, sin B = cos A, and

$$\frac{\sin A}{\cos A} = \tan A.$$

$$\cot A = \frac{1}{\tan A}$$

$$\operatorname{cosec} A = \frac{1}{\sin A}$$

$$\sec A = \frac{1}{\cos A}$$

Problem 1: Find sin A, cos A, and tan A.

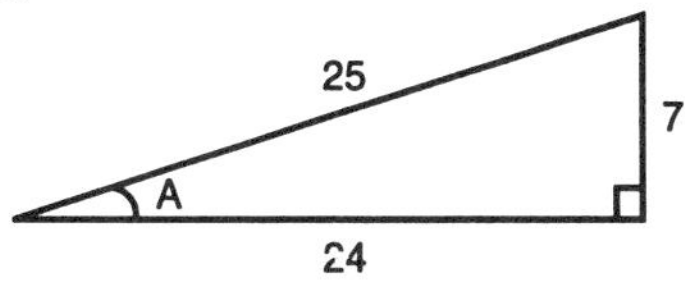

Problem 2: Find sin B, cos B, and tan B.

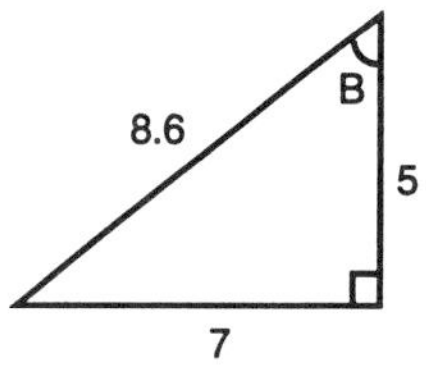

These right triangle definitions of the basic trigonometric functions are restricted to angles between 0° and 90°. However, the definitions of the trigonometric functions can be extended to include all angles. Without showing how this can be done (see textbook treatment of trigonometry), the trigonometric functions for angles between 0° and 360° are graphically represented by:

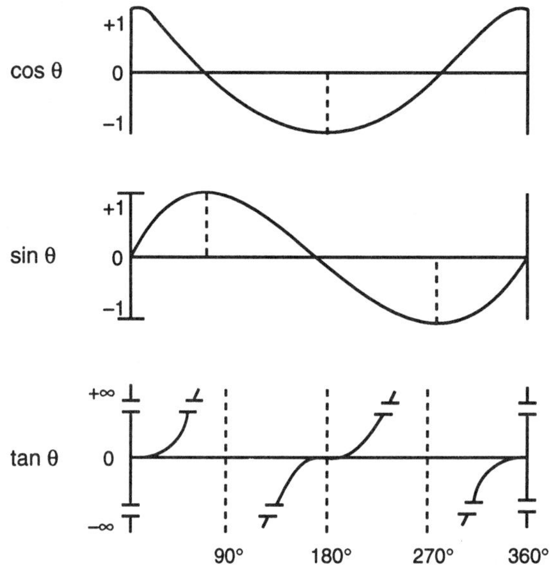

Figure 3.10 — Graphical Representation of Trigonometric Functions

Problem 3: Using the graphs above, find sin θ, cos θ, and tan θ for θ = 0°, 90°, 180°, and 270°.

The trigonometric functions are typically represented graphically for angles between 0° and 360° because they have repeating values, i.e., because they are periodic:

$$\sin(x + 360°n) = \sin x \qquad x = \text{angle}$$
$$\cos(x + 360°n) = \cos x \qquad n = \text{integer}$$
$$\tan(x + 180°n) = \tan x$$

Based on the brief discussion above, two things should be observed and remembered:

(1) Trigonometric functions should logically turn up when considering quantities that are periodic in nature, e.g., waves.

(2) Trigonometry should be useful when it is advantageous to represent a quantity as the hypotenuse or a leg of a right triangle.

The characteristics of a few basic right triangles are shown below. They should be memorized for the OAT along with the values of the trigonometric functions for the angles in them.

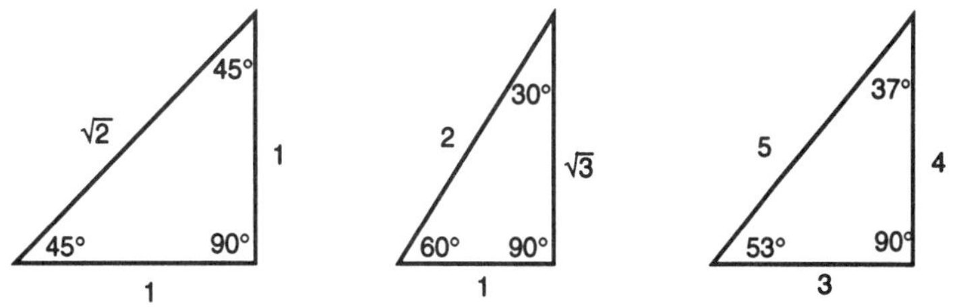

Figure 3.11 — Trigonometric Elements for 45°- 45°- 90°, 30°- 60°- 90°, and 37°- 53°- 90° Triangles

Problem 4: Using the right triangles above, find sin θ , cos θ, and tan θ for θ = 30°, 45°, and 60° (these should be memorized).

Problem 5: Find x:

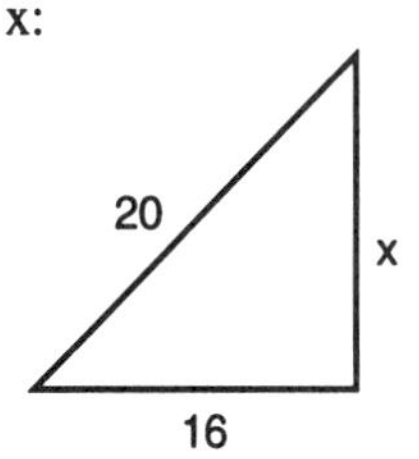

Problem 6: Find x and y:

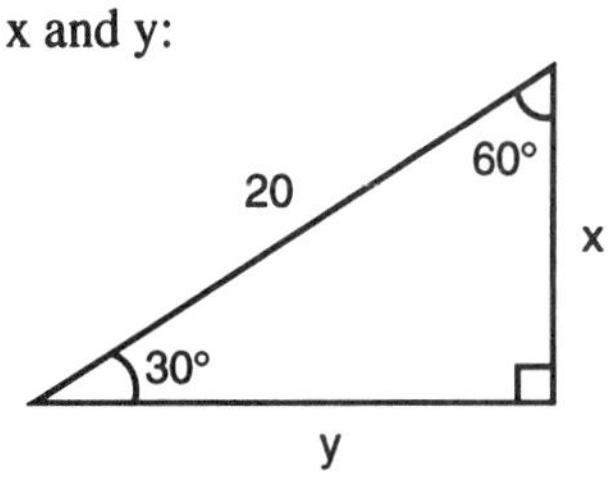

Up to this point, we have used degrees to measure angles; an alternative angular measure that you should be familiar with is the radian. A complete revolution about a point, it should be recalled, is 360°; the same revolution is alternatively represented by 2π radians (normally it is written as just 2π; the units of radians is assumed). The 2π to 360° equivalence determines the proportionality of the two angular measures, e.g., 180° = π, 90° = $\frac{\pi}{2}$, 720° = 4π; etc. (1 radian = 57.3°).

Problem 7: What are 30°, 45°, and 60° in radian units?

The Pythagorean Theorem finds many applications in solving problems on the OAT as well:

$$a^2 + b^2 = c^2$$

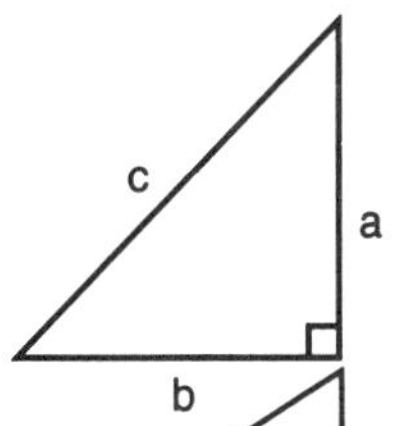

Problem 8: Find b:

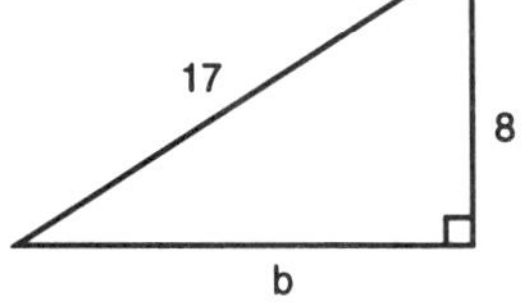

Problem 9: Evaluate $\sin^2 \theta + \cos^2 \theta$, giving the answer in its simplest form.

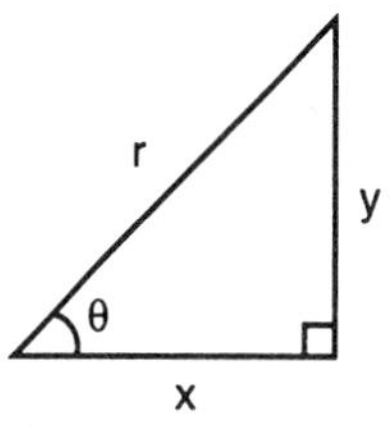

3.9.2 Solutions to Trigonometry Problems

(1) Using the right triangle definitions of the trigonometric functions:

$$\sin A = \frac{7}{25}, \cos A = \frac{24}{25}, \text{ and } \tan A = \frac{7}{24}$$

(2) As in (1), using the right triangle definitions:

$$\sin B = \frac{7}{8.6}, \cos B = \frac{5}{8.6}, \text{ and } \tan B = \frac{7}{5}$$

(3) Reading values directly from the graph, the following table can be constructed:

	θ			
Function	0°	90°	180°	270°
sin θ	0	1	0	−1
cosθ	1	0	−1	0
tan θ	0	∞ (undefined)	0	∞ (undefined)

(4) Using the right triangles shown, the following table can be constructed:

	θ		
Function	30°	45°	60°
sin θ	$\frac{\sqrt{1}}{2}$	$\frac{\sqrt{2}}{2}$	$\frac{\sqrt{3}}{2}$
cos θ	$\frac{\sqrt{3}}{2}$	$\frac{\sqrt{2}}{2}$	$\frac{\sqrt{1}}{2}$
tan θ	$\frac{\sqrt{1}}{\sqrt{3}}$	$\frac{\sqrt{3}}{\sqrt{3}}$	$\sqrt{3}$

(5) This should be recognized as a 3-4-5 right triangle. A 3-4-5 right triangle is recognized by noting some combination of any two sides in the ratio 3:4, 4:5, or 3:5; the third is the missing side. The triangle in this problem corresponds to the known triangle:

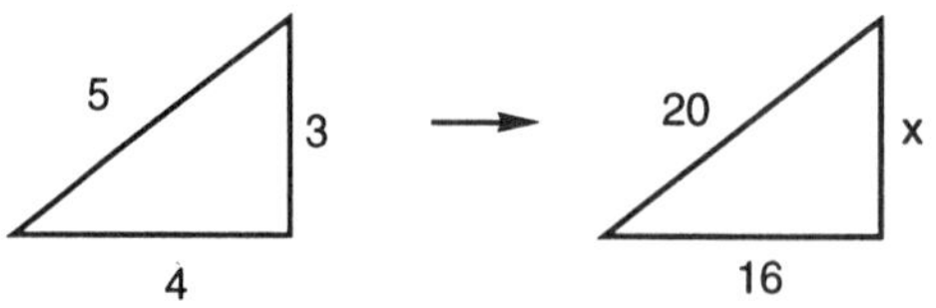

Since these are similar triangles, the corresponding sides are proportional, i.e.,

$$\frac{x}{3} = \frac{20}{5} \text{ or } \frac{x}{3} = \frac{16}{4}$$

In either case, x = 12

(6) $\sin 30° = \frac{x}{20}$; $x = 20\sin 30° = 20\left(\frac{1}{2}\right) = 10$

$\cos 30° = \frac{y}{20}$; $y = 20\cos 30° = 20\left(\frac{\sqrt{3}}{2}\right) = 10\sqrt{3}$

(7) Using the proportionality based on the equivalence of 360° and 2π:

$$\frac{30°}{360°} = \frac{x}{2\pi} \quad \rightarrow \quad x = \frac{\pi}{6};\ 30° \quad \rightarrow \quad \frac{\pi}{6}$$

$$\frac{45°}{360°} = \frac{x}{2\pi} \quad \rightarrow \quad x = \frac{\pi}{4};\ 45° \quad \rightarrow \quad \frac{\pi}{4}$$

$$\frac{60°}{360°} = \frac{x}{2\pi} \quad \rightarrow \quad x = \frac{\pi}{3};\ 60° \quad \rightarrow \quad \frac{\pi}{3}$$

(8) Using the Pythagorean Theorem:

$$b^2 + 8^2 = 17^2$$

$$b^2 + 64 = 289$$

$$b^2 = 225$$

$$b = 15$$

(9) $\sin\theta = \frac{y}{r}$ and $\cos\theta = \frac{x}{r}$

$$\sin^2\theta + \cos^2\theta = \frac{y^2}{r^2} + \frac{x^2}{r^2} = \frac{x^2 + y^2}{r^2} = \frac{r^2}{r^2} = 1$$

($x^2 + y^2 = r^2$ by the Pythagorean Theorem)

3.10 APPLIED MATHEMATICS PROBLEMS

When word problems or applications are used on standardized tests such as the OAT, they often introduce an element of anxiety. The diversity and depth of appropriate applications generate a feeling of uneasiness for many students. Applied problems can be particularly difficult because they are often more difficult and require multiple steps. You must understand more than just the mathematics related to a problem situation; you must also understand certain facts about the situation. To solve science-related problems, you must know certain basic ideas about force, weight, measures, or other concepts of science.

There are many different types of applied word problems such as percents, ratio and proportion, distance problems, and motion problems. Each of these types are discussed later in this section.

Enough theory! Time now for a little practice. Do the following problem NOW and complete it before you read further. As you work the problem, write out ALL the steps.

Problem: A man 2 meters tall stands 3 meters from an intense source of light at the level of his feet. The man's shadow appears on a wall 15 meters from the source of light. How tall is the shadow?

A. 6 meters
B. 10 meters
C. 12.5 meters
D. 17.5 meters
E. 22.5 meters

A FORMULA FOR PROBLEM SOLVING

1. Fully understand the problem, including both the *question asked* and the *situation described* (context). Most students spend too little time making sense of the problem situation. Here it is often helpful to draw a rough diagram. When complex data are presented you will need to use the techniques described in section 3.6.1 on data analysis.
2. Decide what things YOU must bring to the problem. These may include facts you have learned, mathematical formulas, or patterns of reasoning. These are the tools you will need to get from the situation that has been described to a point from which you can answer the questions that have been asked.
3. Use the tools you selected in step 2 above to manipulate the problem situation and thereby produce answers to the questions asked. Here you may find that your tools are inadequate and your knowledge of the problem is inaccurate or vague. Care and attention to steps 1 and 2 can stop you from wasting time on a series of dead ends.
4. Check everything. Is your answer reasonable within the scope of the problem?

In the above problem, if you recognize that you had two similar triangles, solving the problem becomes easy because you can *carefully* make a ratio according to the rule that allows you to compare similar triangles: 3/15 = 2/x.

We underlined the word *carefully* in the paragraph above because the test-maker, who knows that some students will do this step carelessly, has included a distracter that fits. For example, if your answer was 6, you probably put 12 in place of the 15 in the ratio.

Many students don't have the patience or confidence to work through all the steps to solve the problem; they take short-cuts and make errors. For example, some students draw the picture accurately and then try to solve for the hypotenuse—a complicated and time-consuming task that fails to yield the correct answer, although, once again, the test-maker included a distracter that fits.

The third step, solving the problem, is elementary only if you have correctly completed the first two steps. This problem is not especially difficult either in content or mathematics, but in order to solve it correctly you must think carefully and be precise. These are the qualities of a good problem solver. If you think about it, these are the qualities we want in our optometrists as well.

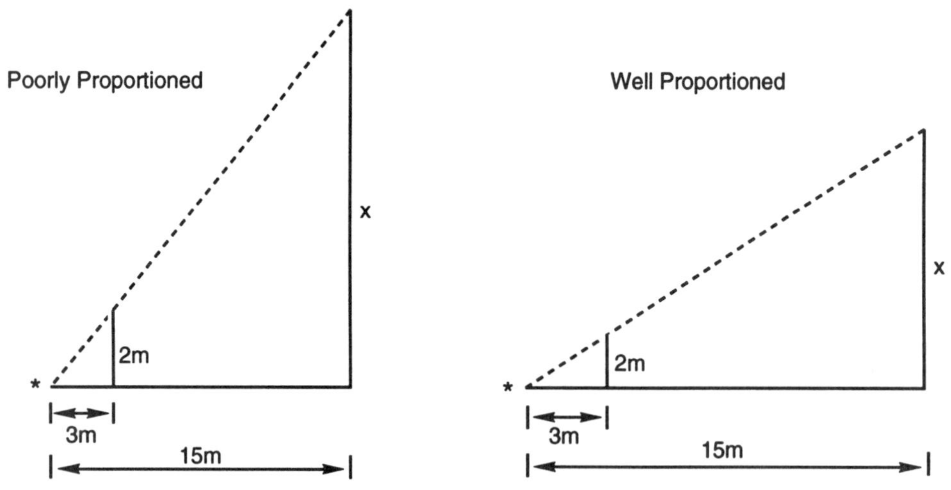

Figure 3.12— Sketching Problem Data

3.10.1 Word Problems Using Percents

Problems involving percents were explained and illustrated in a previous section (section 3.4) and therefore will not be discussed here.

3.10.2 Word Problems Using Ratios and Proportions

A *ratio* is the comparison by division of two quantities expressed in the same units. For example, the heights of two poles may be in the ratio of 3 to 7, which means that the height of the first pole could be 3 feet and the height of the second could be 7 feet. The colon (:) is used to indicate ratio and is written 3:7, which means 3 to 7. The ratio is often written as a fraction, 3/7.

Example: Ann has $300. Bob has $1,200. Compare Ann's amount to Bob's amount.

$$\frac{\text{Ann}}{\text{Bob}} = \frac{3}{12} = \frac{1}{4}$$

A *proportion* states that two ratios are equal. For example, the ratios 2:3 and 4:6 are equal and form a proportion, which may be written as 2:3 = 4:6, or 2:3::4:6.

The proportion 2:3::4:6 is read "2 is to 3 as 4 is to 6." The inside numbers 3 and 4 are called the means, and the outside numbers 2 and 6 are called the extremes.

Any proportion can be written in fractional form: 2/3 = 4/6.

In any proportion, the product of the means is equal to the product of the extremes, i.e., 3:4 = 6:8 is a proportion and the product of the means (4) (6) = 24 and the product of the extremes (3) (8) = 24.

Example: Determine a if 3:5 = a:15

$$\begin{aligned} \frac{3}{5} &= \frac{a}{15} \\ 5a &= 3(15) \\ a &= \frac{45}{5} \\ a &= 9 \end{aligned}$$

Example: If 3 cups of beans will serve 12 people, how many people will 6 cups serve (assuming equal serving size)?

Solution:
$$\begin{aligned} \frac{3 \text{ cups}}{12 \text{ people}} &= \frac{6 \text{ cups}}{x \text{ people}} \\ 3x &= 6(12) \\ 3x &= 72 \\ x &= 24 \end{aligned}$$

Answer: 6 cups will serve 24 people.

3.10.3 Word Problems Using Distance, Rate, and Time

The solution of distance problems is based on the equation d = rt, where d is the distance traveled, r is the rate of travel, and t is the time spent traveling.

(a) Distance determination skill
Example: A car travels an average speed of 60 miles per hour for 5 hours. How far does it travel in that time?
The distance traveled is the rate multiplied by the time.
60 miles per hour × 5 hours = 300 miles.

(b) Rate determination skill
Example: A train travels 400 miles in 8 hours. What is the train's average speed?
The rate is the distance traveled divided by the time.
400 miles ÷ 8 hours = 50 miles per hour.

3.10.3.1 RELATING MOTION OF TWO OBJECTS

Combined quantities involve more than one distance, rate, or time.

Example: The rate at which two objects approach each other when traveling toward each other or in directly opposite directions, and the rate at which they separate, is the sum of their respective rates.

Skills involved in solving a combined quantity problem:

Example: A car leaves a town traveling 30 miles per hour. Two hours later, a second car leaves the same town, on the same road, traveling at 50 miles per hour. In how many hours will the second car be passing the first car?

(a) Draw a diagram to illustrate

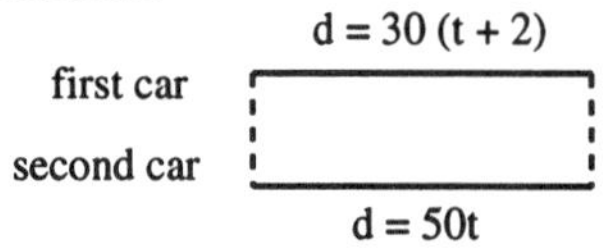

(b) For each object, write a numerical or variable expression for the distance, rate, and time. The results can be recorded in a table.

The first car traveled two hours longer than the second car.

	Rate,r	×	Time,t	=	Distance,d
First car	30	×	t + 2	=	30 (t + 2)
Second car	50	×	t	=	60t

(c) Determine how the distances traveled by each object are related.

Example: The total distance traveled by both objects may be known or it may be known that the two objects traveled the same distance.

$$30(t+2) = 50t$$
$$30t + 60 = 50t$$
$$60 = 50t - 30t$$
$$60 = 20t$$
$$3 = t$$

The second car will be passing the first car after 3 hours.

Example: Two long distance runners, Beth and Paul, ran the same course. Paul traveled 2 miles per hour slower than Beth. Beth finishes the course in 4 hours and Paul finishes in 6 hours. What is the speed of each runner and what is the length of the course?

Solution: Let r represent Beth's rate. Then r – 2 represents Paul's rate. Since d = rt, Beth's distance is r•4, and Paul's distance is (r – 2)6.

	Rate	×	Time	=	Distance
Beth	r	×	4	=	4r
Paul	r – 2	×	6	=	6(r – 2)
			4r	=	6r – 12
			12	=	2r
			6	=	r

Beth's rate is 6 miles per hour, and Paul's rate is 4 miles per hour.

The length of the course can be determined by applying d = rt to either runner.

Using Beth's rate, we obtain
d = rt
d = 6.4
d = 24

Therefore, the length of the course is 24 miles.

3.10.3.2 DETERMINING AVERAGE RATE

(a) To average two or more different rates when the time is the same for both rates, add the rates and divide by the number of rates.

Example: If a woman travels for 4 hours at 40 miles per hour, at 50 miles per hour for the next 4 hours, and 60 miles per hour for the next 4 hours, then her average rate for the 12 hours is (40 + 50 + 60) ÷ 3 = 50 miles per hour.

(b) To average two or more different rates when the times are not the same but the distances are the same,
   1. assume the distance to be a convenient length,
   2. find the time at each given rate, and
   3. find the sum of the distances and divide by the total time to find the average rate.

Example: Two boys travel a certain distance at the rate of 40 miles per hour and return at the rate of 20 miles per hour. What is the average rate for both trips?

Solution: Assume the distance is the same for both trips (80 miles).
time for first trip = 80 ÷ 40 = 2 hours.
time for second trip = 80 ÷ 20 = 4 hours
total distance = 160 miles
total time = 6 hours
average rate = 160 ÷ 6 = $26\frac{2}{3}$ miles per hour

Example: A man travels 200 miles at 40 miles per hour, 100 miles at 50 miles per hour, and 60 miles at 20 miles per hour. What is the average rate for the three trips?

Solution: Time for first trip : 200 ÷ 40 = 5 hours
Time for second trip : 100 ÷ 50 = 2 hours
Time for third trip = 60 ÷ 20 = 3 hours
The total distance is 360 miles
The total time is 10 hours
The average rate is 360 ÷ 10 = 36

Example: If a car travels 200 miles using 8 gallons of gas, what is its gas consumption?

Solution: mph = distance in miles ÷ number of gallons
mph = 200 ÷ 8
mph = 25 mph

3.10.4 Ten Steps for Problem Solving

1. Read the word problem at least twice: first to discover what it is all about, then read it carefully in detail (sentence by sentence or sometimes even phrase by phrase) to make sure you are clear about all the elements of the problem and their relationship, and what you are asked to discover.

2. It may be possible to draw a picture representing the elements of the problem. If it is, do so to clarify the details of the situation.

3. Write down in your own words statements of the facts presented in the problem. One way or another, the problem is likely to say that one part of the problem equals something else. Once you have stated the elements you should be able to write an equation (using words, not algebraic symbols) connecting or relating the elements of the problem.

4. When you know what you are asked to find, use an algebraic symbol (variable x, y, or whatever you choose) to represent this element (the unknown) for your developing equation. Clearly state what the symbol represents.

5. See if you can now make algebraic statements of the values of other elements of the problem in terms of the main variable defined in step #4.

6. Now write an equation substituting for step #3 the algebraic expressions (variables) you have worked out in steps #4 and #5.

7. Solve the new algebraic equation for the numerical value of the variable.

8. Use the solution of the equation to determine all answers requested in the problem.

9. Check your answers against the statements and data of the original word problem.

10. Finally, describe with a statement the required answer(s) asked for in the original word problem.

The following sections illustrate special word problems with solutions.

3.10.5 Word Problems Relating Work Rate of Two People

Work problems involve finding the rate at which two or more people working together can do a job. Knowing the rate at which each person works alone, you can find the rate at which they work together.

Steps used to solve work problems are

1. find the fractional part of the job each can do in the time given,
2. multiply each fraction from step 1 by x, and
3. set the sum of the fractions from step 2 equal to the number 1 and solve for x.

The *numerator* represents the time actually spent working. The *denominator* represents the total time needed to do the job alone.

Example: Jane can do house work alone in 3 hours. Sue can do the same job alone in 2 hours. How long will it take the two of them working together to finish the job?

Solution:

1. Express the fraction of the job each can do in 1 hour.
   1/3 = fraction of the job Jane can do in 1 hour. (If she can do the whole job in 3 hours, she can do 1/3 the job in 1 hour.)

   1/2 = fraction of the job Sue can do in 1 hour.

2. Express the fraction of the job each can do in x hours, when x = time it takes to complete the job together.

   1/3 x = fraction of the job Jane can do in x hours.
   1/2 x = fraction of the job Sue can do in x hours.

3. Set the sum of the two fractions equal to 1 and solve for x.

$$\frac{1}{2}x + \frac{1}{3}x = 1$$

$$\frac{5}{6}x = 1$$

$$x = \frac{6}{5}$$

$$x = 1.2 \text{ hours}$$

3.10.6 Word Problems Using Odd and Even Integers

Integers are real numbers. They consist of negative numbers, zero, and positive numbers. The set of integers are (...–4, –3, –2, –1, 0, 1, 2, 3, 4...).

The set of even integers are (...–4, –2, 0, 2, 4...)

The set of odd integers are (...–3, –1, 0, 1, 3...)

All even integers are divisible by 2.

Consecutive integers are integers that *are* listed in consecutive order. If n is even, three consecutive even integers are n, n + 2, n + 4; e.g., if n = 2, the three consecutive even integers are 2, 4, and 6.

If n is an odd integer, three consecutive odd integers are n, n + 2, n + 4; e.g., if n = 1, then the three consecutive odd integers are 3, 5, and 7.

Example: Find five consecutive odd integers that have a sum equal to 45.

Solution: Let n represent the smallest integer. The other four integers will be expressed in terms of n. Consecutive integers differ by one, therefore consecutive odd integers will differ by 2.

Let n = 1st odd integer
n + 2 = 2nd odd integer
n + 4 = 3rd odd integer
n + 6 = 4th odd integer
n + 8 = 5th odd integer

(n) + (n+2) + (n+4) + (n+6) = (n+8) = 45

5n + 20 = 45
5n = 45 – 20
5n = 25
n = 5

Answer: 5, 7, 9, 11, 13

Example: Find three consecutive even integers such that the first equals the sum of the second and third.

A. 0, –2, –4
B. –6, –4, –2
C. 4, 6, 8
D. 8, 10, 12
E. –8, –10, –12

Answer: B

Solution: Let n = first integer
n + 2 = second integer
n + 4 = third integer
n = (n+2) + (n+4)
n = 2n+6
–6 = n

3.10.7 Word Problems Using Coins or Stamps

The best method to solve such problems is to change the value of the money being dealt with to dollars and cents; e.g., the number of nickels should be multiplied by 5 because \$.05 = 1 nickel. The number of dimes should be multiplied by 10 because \$.10 = 1 dime. The number of half dollars should be multiplied by 50 because \$.50 = one half dollar, etc.

Example: A cash register contains \$30.90 in nickels and quarters. If there are 130 coins in all, how many of each coin are in the cash register?

Let x = number of nickels, then
130-x = number of quarters

number of nickels •	value of nickels	= value in cents
x	5	= 5x

number of quarters •	value of quarters	= value in cents
130 – x	25	= 25 (130 – x)

value of nickels + value of quarters = total value in cents

$$5x + 25(130 - x) = 3090$$
$$5x - 25x + 3250 = 3090$$
$$-20x = 3090 - 3250$$
$$20x = 160$$
$$x = 8$$

Answer: x = 8 nickels and
130 – x = 130 – 8 = 122 quarters
Check: 8 (.05) + .25 (122)
= .40 + 30.50 = \$30.90

Example: A person has 100 stamps with a total value of \$18.00. Some stamps are worth 15¢ each and the others are worth 30¢ each. How many stamps of each type does he have?

Solution: Let x = number of 15¢ stamps
100 – x = number of 30¢ stamps

number of stamps	• values of stamps	= value in cents
x	15	= 15x
100 – x	30	= 30 (100 – x)

value of 15¢ stamps	+ value of 30¢ stamps	= total value in cents
15x	+ 30(100 – x)	= 1800

$$15x + 30\,(100-x) = 1800$$
$$15x + 3000 - 30x = 1800$$
$$15x - 30x = 1800 - 3000$$
$$-15x = -1200$$
$$x = 80$$

Answer: x = <u>80 (15¢) stamps</u>
100x = 100-80 = <u>20 (30¢) stamps</u>

3.10.8 Word Problems Using Ages of Relatives

Solving age problems is done by comparing ages of relatives at the present, in the future and in the past. If the present age is represented by x, then the future age is found by adding years to x. If the present age is represented by x, then the past age is found by subtracting years from x.

Example: A mother was 36 years old when her daughter was born. How old will the daughter be when her age is 1/4 of the mother's age? What will the mother's age be?

Let x = daughter's age
Let x + 36 = mother's age

$$x = \frac{1}{4}(x + 36)$$
$$x = \frac{x}{4} + 9$$
$$x - \frac{x}{4} = 9$$

$$4x - x = 36$$
$$3x = 36$$
$$x = 12$$

Daughter's age = x = <u>12</u> years
Mother's age = x + 36 = <u>48</u> years

3.11 QUANTITATIVE REASONING SAMPLE TEST

1. If $\frac{1}{3}(x - 2) \leq \frac{x + 2}{6}$, then

A. $x \geq 6$
B. $x \leq 6$
C. $x \leq 4$
D. $x \geq 3$
E. $x \leq -4$

2. Simplify: $\frac{-3}{4} + \frac{1}{6} - \frac{5}{8}$

A. $\frac{5}{4}$

B. $1\frac{5}{24}$

C. $\frac{-5}{4}$

D. $-1\frac{5}{24}$

E. $\frac{4}{5}$

3. $3\frac{1}{3} \times 2\frac{1}{2} = ?$

A. 2
B. 6
C. 3
D. $6\frac{1}{6}$
E. $8\frac{1}{3}$

4. If $(a^3b^{-2})^{-2}$ is simplified to a form in which exponents are positive, the result is

A. $\frac{b^4}{a^6}$

B. $\frac{1}{a^2b}$

C. $\frac{a^6}{b^4}$

D. a^2b

E. $\frac{a}{b^4}$

5. $\frac{\sqrt{12}\sqrt{2}}{\sqrt{18}} = ?$

A. $\frac{2}{5}$

B. $\frac{2\sqrt{5}}{5}$

C. $\frac{\sqrt{3}}{6}$

D. $\frac{2\sqrt{3}}{3}$

E. $\frac{\sqrt{6}}{3}$

6. If $\frac{x-2}{x+2} = \frac{2}{3}$, then x =
A. 12
B. 6
C. no value possible
D. 5
E. 10

7. A car is run until the gas tank is $\frac{1}{6}$ full. The tank is then filled to capacity by putting in 15 gallons. The capacity of the gas tank of the car is
A. 12 gallons.
B. 15 gallons.
C. 18 gallons.
D. 21 gallons.
E. 24 gallons.

8. If John must have a mark of 70% to pass a test of 30 items, the number of items he may miss and still pass the test is
A. 9
B. 8
C. 10
D. 28
E. 30

9. A man insures 60% of his property and pays a $2\frac{1}{2}$% premium amounting to $348.00. What is the total value of his property?
A. $19,000
B. $18,000
C. $18,400
D. $23,200
E. $25,200

10. If the scale of a blue print is $\frac{1}{8}$ inch equals 1 foot, what is to be the actual length of a wall $8\frac{1}{2}$ inches by scale?
A. $5\frac{2}{3}$ feet
B. 7.7 feet
C. 8.5 feet
D. 102 feet
E. 68 feet

11. If cards are lettered as follows: T, H, O, M, E, R, R, M, E, E, T, and if you choose one of the cards above without looking, what is the probability that you will choose E?
A. $\frac{2}{9}$
B. $\frac{3}{11}$
C. $\frac{8}{11}$
D. $\frac{3}{8}$
E. $\frac{11}{9}$

12. Find the perimeter of a roller rink with the following dimensions. Use 3.14 for π.

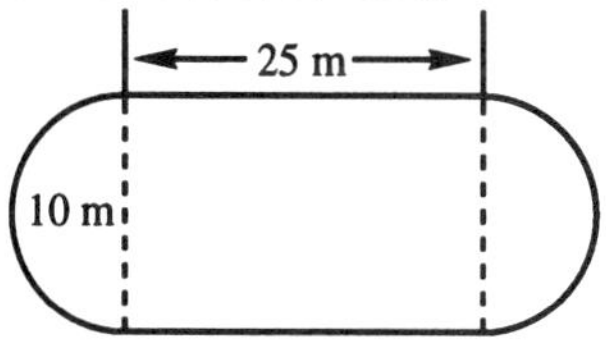

A. 81.4
B. 101.4
C. 112.8
D. 56
E. 120

13. Find the area of the following figure. Use 3.14 for π.

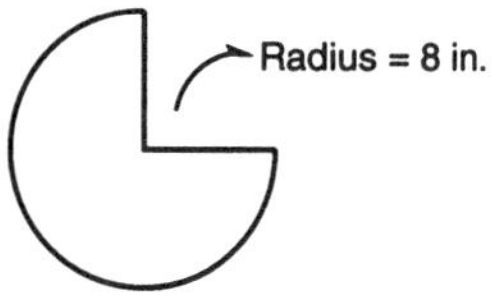

A. 150.72 in^2
B. 200.96 in^2
C. 602.88 in^2
D. 25.12 in^2
E. 45.50 in^2

14. A 25-foot ladder is placed against a building at a point 20 feet from the ground. Find the distance from the base of the building to the base of the ladder.

A. 13 feet
B. 25 feet
C. 30 feet
D. 45 feet
E. 15 feet

15. Triangles ABC and DEF are similar. Find the area of DEF.

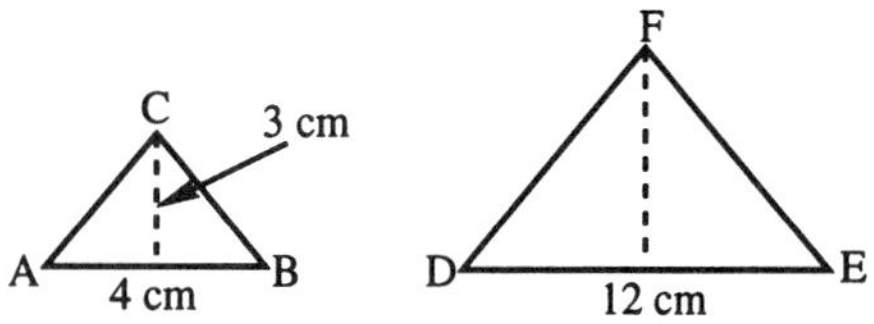

A. 36 cm^2
B. 54 cm^2
C. 48 cm^2
D. 144 cm^2
E. 108 cm^2

16. The slope of the line whose equation is $y = -\frac{1}{4}x - 1$

A. $\frac{1}{4}$
B. -1
C. $-\frac{1}{4}$
D. 1
E. 0

17. The value of cot θ is equal to

A. $\sin\theta / \cos\theta$
B. $1/\sec\theta$
C. $1/\tan\theta$
D. $1/\sin\theta$
E. $1/\cos\theta$

18. Determine the value of cos q if P is a point on the terminal side q and the coordinates of P are P(–3, 4)

A. $\cos q = -\frac{3}{5}$

B. $\cos q = \frac{3}{5}$

C. $\cos q = -\frac{4}{3}$

D. $\cos q = -\frac{5}{3}$

E. $\cos q = -\frac{3}{4}$

19. If 25% of the inhabitants of a town are foreign born, the ratio of native born to foreign born is

A. 4:1
B. 10:40
C. 300:100
D. 3:1
E. 400:100

20. If *a* finishes the job in 3 hours and *b* can finish it in 4 hours, how long will it take both if they work together?

A. $3\frac{1}{2}$ hours

B. 7 hours

C. $1\frac{5}{12}$ hours

D. $1\frac{5}{7}$ hours

E. $\frac{3}{4}$ hours

3.12 ANSWERS TO QUESTIONS IN SECTION 3.11

1. B	**2.** D	**3.** E	**4.** A	**5.** D	**6.** E	**7.** C	**8.** A	**9.** D	**10.** E
11. B	**12.** A	**13.** A	**14.** E	**15.** B	**16.** C	**17.** C	**18.** A	**19.** C	**20.** D

3.13 SOLUTIONS TO QUESTIONS IN SECTION 3.11

Question 1: [B] The answer is found merely be applying routine steps of solving inequalities. First, clear the fraction by multiplying both sides of the inequality by the GCD, which is 6.

$$6[\tfrac{1}{3}(x-2)] \le 6\frac{(x+2)}{6}$$
$$2(x-2) \le x+2$$
$$2x-4 \le x+2$$
$$2x-x \le 4+2$$
$$x \le 6$$

Question 2: [D] Find the LCM of 4, 6, 8

4 = 4, 8, 12, 16, 20, 24
6 = 6, 12, 18, 24
8 = 8, 16, 24
LCM = 24

$$\frac{-3}{4} + \frac{1}{6} - \frac{5}{8} = \frac{-18}{24} + \frac{4}{24} - \frac{15}{24}$$
$$= \frac{-18+4-15}{24}$$
$$= \frac{-29}{24} = -1\frac{5}{24}$$

2	4,6,8
1	2,3,4
2	1,3,2
LCM	2(2)(3)(2) = 24

Question 3: [E] $3\frac{1}{3} \times 2\frac{1}{2}$ Change to improper fraction

$$3\frac{1}{3} = \frac{9}{3} + \frac{1}{3} = \frac{10}{3}$$

$$2\frac{1}{2} = \frac{4}{2} + \frac{1}{2} = \frac{5}{2}$$

$$\frac{10}{3} \times \frac{5}{2} = \frac{2 \times 5}{3} \times \frac{5}{2} = \frac{25}{3} = 8\frac{1}{3}$$

Question 4: [A] $(a^3b^{-2})^{-2}$ =
Use the rule for exponential notation and negative exponent.

$$(a^3b^{-2})^{-2} = (a^3)^{-2}\,(b^{-2})^{-2}$$

$$= a^{-6}b^4 = \frac{b^4}{a^6}$$

Question 5: [D]

$$\frac{\sqrt{12}\sqrt{2}}{\sqrt{18}} = \frac{\sqrt{2}\sqrt{6}\sqrt{2}}{\sqrt{2}\,\sqrt{9}}$$

$$= \frac{\sqrt{12}}{3}$$

$$= \frac{\sqrt{3}\,\sqrt{4}}{3}$$

$$= \frac{2\,\sqrt{3}}{3}$$

Question 6: [E] $\frac{x-1}{x+1} = \frac{2}{3}$

$$2(x+2) = 3(x-2)$$

$$2x + 4 = 3x - 6$$

$$2x - 3x = -6 - 4$$

$$-x = -10$$

Question 7: [C] If the gas tank is $\frac{1}{6}$ full, then an additional $\frac{5}{6}$ of capacity is left.

$\frac{5}{6}$ of capacity = 15 gallons, therefore

$$15 \div \frac{5}{6} = \frac{15}{1} \times \frac{6}{5}$$

$$= \frac{3 \times 5}{1} \times \frac{2 \times 3}{5} = 18$$

Question 8: [A] Using the formula R/100 = P/B, he must answer 70% of 30 correctly. Therefore, he may miss 30% of 30.

R = 30
P = Unknown
B = 30

$$\frac{30}{100} = \frac{P}{30}$$

$$100P = 30(30)$$

$$P = \frac{30(30)}{100}$$

$$P = \frac{3(30)}{10}$$

$$P = 9$$

Question 9: [D] Find the solution in 2 steps. $2\frac{1}{2}$ % of insured value = \$348

1. First find the insured value using the formula $\frac{R}{100} = \frac{P}{B}$

$$R = 2\frac{1}{2}\% \qquad \frac{2\frac{1}{2}}{100} = \frac{348}{B}$$

$$P = \$348$$

Find B $\quad 2\frac{1}{2}B = 348\ (100)$

$$B = \frac{34800}{5/2}$$

$$B = \frac{34800}{1} \times \frac{2}{5} = 13{,}920$$

Therefore the insured value = \$13,920

2. The insured value (\$13,920) is 60% of the total value. Find the total value:

$$R = 60\% \qquad \frac{60}{100} = \frac{13920}{B}$$

$$P = 13{,}920$$

Find B $\quad 60B = 13{,}920 \times 100$

$$B = \frac{13920 \times (10)\ (10)}{(6)\ (10)}$$

$$B = \frac{139200}{6} = 23{,}200$$

Therefore the total value of the property is \$23,200.

Question 10: [E] Since $\frac{1}{8}$ inch = 1 foot

$$8\frac{1}{2} \text{ inches} \div \frac{1}{8} \text{ inch} = \frac{17}{2} \times 8 = 68 \text{ feet.}$$

Question 11: [B] Each card has an equally likely chance of being chosen. There are three outcomes that are **E**. There are 11 possible outcomes.

Probability of **E** = $\frac{\text{number of E outcomes}}{\text{number of possible outcomes}}$

$$P(M) = \frac{3}{11}.$$

Question 12: [A] Perimeter = 2(circumference of semi-circle) + (perimeter of rectangle) – 2(width)

$$P = 2\frac{(\pi d)}{2} + 2(L + W) - 2W$$

$$P = 2\frac{[3.14(10)]}{2} + 2(25 + 10) - 2(10)$$

$$P = 3.14\ (10) + 70 - 20$$

$$P = 31.4 + 50$$

$$P = 81.4 \text{ m}$$

Question 13: [A] To find the area of the figure in this example, use the formula area = πr^2. Notice the figure is $\frac{3}{4}$ of a circle. To find the area of $\frac{3}{4}$ of the circle, take $\frac{3}{4}$ of the area. Therefore,

$$A = \frac{3}{4} \text{ of } \pi r^2$$

$$A = \frac{3}{4} \text{ of } 3.14(8)^2$$

$$A = \frac{3}{4} \times 200.96 = \frac{602.88}{4}$$

$$A = 150.72 \text{ in}^2$$

Question 14: [E] To find the distance from the base of the building to the base of the ladder, draw a figure, then

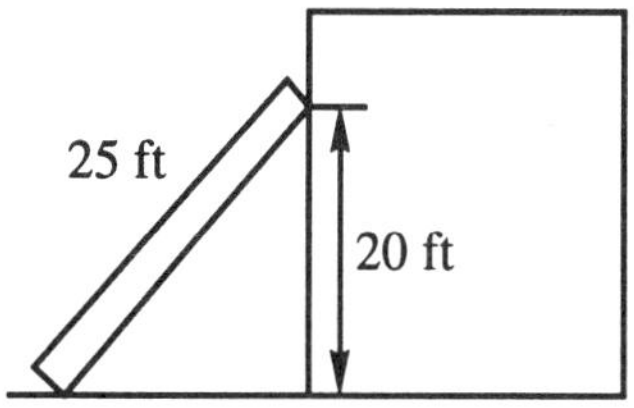

use the Pythagorean theorem. The hypotenuse is the length of the ladder (25 feet). One leg is the distance along the building from the ground to the top of the ladder. The distance from the base of the building to the base of the ladder is the unknown leg. Using the Pythagorean theorem, $a^2 + b^2 = c^2$ find b.

$$\begin{aligned} a^2 + b^2 &= c^2 \\ (20\text{ ft})^2 + b^2 &= (25\text{ ft})^2 \\ 400\text{ ft}^2 + b^2 &= 625\text{ ft}^2 \\ b^2 &= 625\text{ ft}^2 - 400\text{ ft}^2 \\ b^2 &= \sqrt{225\text{ ft}^2} \\ b &= 15\text{ ft} \end{aligned}$$

The distance from the base of the building to the base of the ladder is 15 feet.

Question 15: [B] To find the area of triangle DEF, (a) solve a proportion to find the height of triangle DFE, and (b) use the formula area $= \frac{1}{2} \times$ base $\times$ height.

$$\begin{aligned} \frac{AB}{DE} &= \frac{\text{height of triangle ABC}}{\text{height of triangle DEF}} \\ \frac{4\text{cm}}{12\text{cm}} &= \frac{3\text{cm}}{\text{height}} \\ 4\text{x height} &= 12 \times 3\text{ cm} \\ 4\text{x height} &= 36\text{ cm} \\ \text{height} &= \frac{36\text{ cm}}{4} \\ \text{height} &= 9\text{ cm} \end{aligned}$$

$$\begin{aligned} \text{Area} &= \frac{1}{2} \times \text{base} \times \text{height} \\ A &= \frac{1}{2}BH \\ &= \frac{1}{2} \times 12\text{ cm} \times 9\text{ cm} \\ &= 54\text{ cm}^2 \end{aligned}$$

The area is 54 cm^2.

Question 16: [C] Find two ordered pairs that are solutions of the equation,

$$y = -\frac{1}{4}x - 1$$

$$P_1 = (0, -1)$$

$$P_2 = (1, -1\tfrac{1}{4})$$

Using the slope formula, $M = \dfrac{y_2 - y_1}{x_2 - x_1}$

$$M = \frac{(-1\frac{1}{4}) - (-1)}{1 - 0} = \frac{-1\frac{1}{4} + 1}{1} = \frac{-1}{4}$$

A quick method is to inspect $y = -\frac{1}{4}x - 1$ ($y = mx + b$) and determine m as $-\frac{1}{4}$.

Question 17: [C] $\cot\theta = 1/\tan\theta$, which is a reciprocal relationship.

Question 18: [A] $\cos\theta = \frac{-3}{5}$

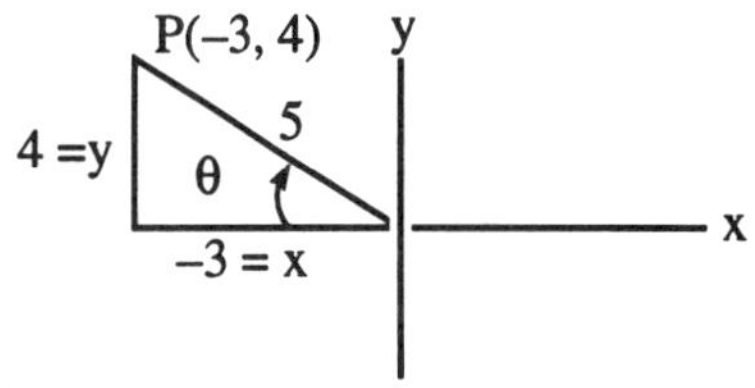

$$\begin{aligned} r &= \sqrt{(-3)^2 + 4^2} \\ &= \sqrt{9 + 16} \\ &= \sqrt{25} \\ &= 5 \end{aligned}$$

$$\cos\theta = \frac{\text{abscissa}}{\text{distance}} = \frac{x}{r} = \frac{-3}{5}$$

Question 19: [C] If 25% of the inhabitants are foreign born, then 75% are native born. The ratio of native born to foreign born would have to be 3:1, which is equivalent to 300:100.

Question 20: [D] Since multiple choice answers are given, the correct answer is smaller than the shortest time given. No matter how slow a worker is, he does part of the job and therefore it will be completed in less time.

Let $A = \frac{x}{3}$ The sum of all individual fractions should be 1.

Let $B = \frac{x}{4}$

	A		B	
$\frac{\text{Time spent}}{\text{Total time needed to do job}}$	$\frac{x}{3}$	+	$\frac{x}{4}$	= 1

Solve the equation $\frac{x}{3} + \frac{x}{4} = 1$

Find the LCD.

Multiply by 12 to eliminate fraction

$$\begin{aligned} 4x + 3x &= 12 \\ 7x &= 12 \\ x &= \frac{12}{7} \\ x &= 1\tfrac{5}{7} \text{ hours} \end{aligned}$$

3.14 REFERENCES

1. Aufmann, Richard N., and Vernon C. Barker, *Introductory Algebra: An Applied Approach,* 1st Edition. Houghton Mifflin, 1983. Used with permission.
2. Aufmann, Richard N., and Vernon C. Barker, *Basic College Mathematics: An Applied Approach,* 1st Edition. Houghton Mifflin Company, 1985. Used with permission.
3. *A Complete Preparation for the MCAT*, 6th edition. Betz Publishing Company, 1992.
4. Whimbey, Arthur, and Jack Lochhead, *Problem Solving & Comprehension,* 5th Edition. Lawrence Erlbaum Associates, 1991.
5. Whimbey, Arthur and Jack Lochhead, *Beyond Problem Solving and Comprehension: An Exploration of Quantitative Reasoning.* Lawrence Erlbaum Associates, 1984.

PART 2

OAT Physics and Natural Sciences

4.0 DEVELOPING REASONING AND PROBLEM-SOLVING SKILLS IN THE SCIENCES: PREOPTOMETRY

You need a solid foundation from college to take you into optometry school, and the OAT attempts to test your level of mastery. That is, on a specific topic such as optics, do you really understand or have you merely memorized what you need in order to pass? Applying something you learned in one way, can you solve a problem that is unlike anything you have seen before? In your own words, can you explain a concept to a colleague who is having trouble understanding it? If you find yourself saying: "I know that material, but I just can't put it into words" you know you have not mastered the information.

The OAT is designed to help optometry schools choose the best possible candidates. The best students tend to be those who can effectively and efficiently analyze information and then integrate it (synthesis). Thus academic learning can be thought of as having two steps: analysis and synthesis.

Content mastery can be tested by asking you to use skills developed throughout your academic life in analytical reading, logical reasoning, quantitative reasoning, perceptual reasoning and problem solving. These skills are like tools in a toolbox. You need to be able to use them all, and it is better to do so consciously than to fumble around in a hit-or-miss fashion.

A conscious awareness of reasoning skills can improve your understanding of the material you study and result in improved test performance. Anticipate how test questions could be formulated to assess particular reasoning skills and how test items are structured around different patterns in reasoning.

ANALYTICAL REASONING

Review Section 2.3.2 in Chapter 2.

Analytical Reasoning Exercises

Exercise 1: Four doctors—Harry, Louise, Kate and Bob—collect automobiles. Among them are owned 20 cars of which 12 are vintage. Harry has three new cars and Louise has the same number of vintage autos. Louise has 1 more car than Harry, who has 5. Kate has three more vintage cars than new ones and the same number of new ones as Bob. How many vintage cars does Bob have?

Exercise 2: Make a Venn Diagram to illustrate the relationship between the following words:
• dogwood trees • dogs • cats • dead animals • caterpillars

As with any skill, it is important to practice the process of visually representing and summarizing concepts. While relational maps condense and integrate classroom information, they can also be used on the OAT as a "sorting" tool to organize and analyze content.

Exercise 3: Read the following biological sciences passage and develop a relational map.

"The eye is a layer of photoreceptor cells and associated neurons packaged within a fibrous, rubber-like protective globe that is transparent in front. The eyeball is almost spherical in shape, about 2.5 centimeters in diameter, with three concentric coats or tunics surrounding the refractive media. These coats are the fibrous coat, the vascular coat, and the nervous coat.

The fibrous tunic is the outermost coat and consists of the sclera and the cornea. The sclera, meaning "hard", is a tough, white supporting tunic. It covers the posterior five-sixths of the eye. The cornea, meaning "horny", covers the anterior one-sixth and is continuous with the sclera. The radius of the cornea is less than that of the sclera—that is, it has a greater curvature, so it bulges somewhat. In addition to transmitting light, the cornea also is a refractive medium and focuses the light rays.

The middle coat, or vascular tunic, is divided into the iris, the ciliary body, and the choroid. The iris forms a diaphragm between the cornea and the lens and is like a curtain with a central perforation—the pupil. The diameter of the pupil may be altered by the muscles in the iris that are oriented in two directions. One set of muscles pulls the iris back toward the ciliary body to dilate the pupil. The other muscle draws the iris down around the front of the lens to constrict the pupil. The color of the iris is largely a function of the amount of pigment within. The ciliary body is ring-shaped with protrusions or folds on the internal surface that are responsible for the secretion of aqueous humor. The choroid, chiefly composed of blood vessels and pigment, lines the posterior part of the sclera. This vascular, highly pigmented layer absorbs the light and prevents scattering.

The innermost coat, or tunic, is the retina which is the light-sensitive layer of the eye. It consists of several layers of cell bodies and fibers. One of these layers consists of photoreceptor neurons called rods and cones. The rods are highly sensitive to light and insensitive to color, whereas the cones are sensitive to color and provide the highest visual acuity."

Make sure your map contains the following elements:

- main concept in modified sentence form
- organizational pattern
- details represented relative to main idea
- summary statement

Exercise 4: Read the biological sciences passage below and construct a Venn diagram.

Review of Cellular Metabolism

The four key processes of energy production are glycolysis, the citric acid cycle (Kreb's cycle, Tricarboxylic Acid Cycle or TCA cycle), the electron transport system (ETS), and oxidative phosphorylation. Glycolysis takes glucose (C_6) and converts it to two pyruvates (C_3). This produces 2ATPs and 2NADHs. If no oxygen is around, the NADH converts pyruvate to lactic acid, which may be converted to alcohol (as in a type of fermentation). The latter process (to pyruvate) is anaerobic glycolysis. In the presence of oxygen, the pyruvate (C_3) is converted to acetyl CoA (C_2) and CO_2 with 2NADHs produced per original glucose. CoA (Coenzyme A) is an acyl carrier and the vitamin pantothenic acid is a key component. Acetyl CoA may also arise from fatty acid and amino acid breakdown. The acetyl CoA (C_2) enters the citric acid cycle by combining with oxaloacetic acid (C_4) to form citrate (C_6). This is degraded step-wise to oxaloacetic acid again producing 3NADHs, 1$FADH_2$, and 1ATP (from GTP) for each cycle (must double to get production per original glucose) as well as CO_2 and H_2O. The NADH and $FADH_2$ enter the ETS in a special sequence. Each intermediate is first reduced (receives electrons from) by the preceding and oxidized (gives electrons to) by the following, with oxygen as the final acceptor being converted to water. ATPs are produced at 1, 2, and 3 by the process called oxidative phosphorylation. Each NADH produces 3ATPs and each $FADH_2$ produces 2ATPs. Malonate is a potent inhibitor of the citric acid cycle. Cyanide is a potent inhibitor of the ETS at Cyt a. An exception is the NADH produced outside the mitochondria from glycolysis. The electrons of NADH are transported by a shuttle to ubiquinone and only 2ATPs per NADH (of glycolysis) are produced. Anaerobic glycolysis yields a net of 2ATPs per glucose. Aerobic glycolysis (because it proceeds to the citric acid cycle and ETS) yields a total of 38ATPs per glucose.

Using the information above, make an association diagram to compare and contrast characteristics of various biochemical processes. Use the following words: citric acid, glucose, anaerobic glycolysis, ATP, NADH, lactic acid, CoA, $FADH_2$.

<u>COMPARATIVE REASONING</u>

Comparative Reasoning Exercises:

Exercise 5: Compare and contrast the two figures below. How are they similar; how are they different? List ten similarities and ten differences.

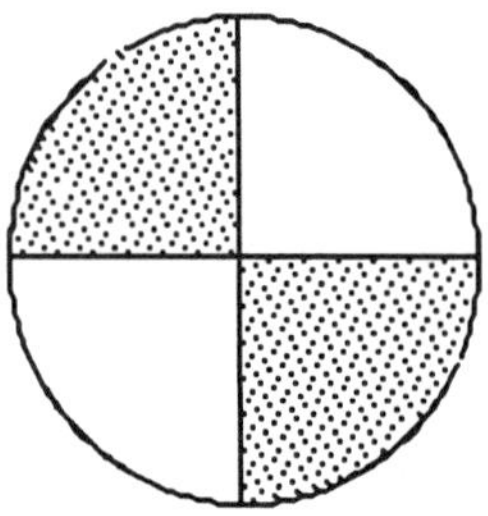

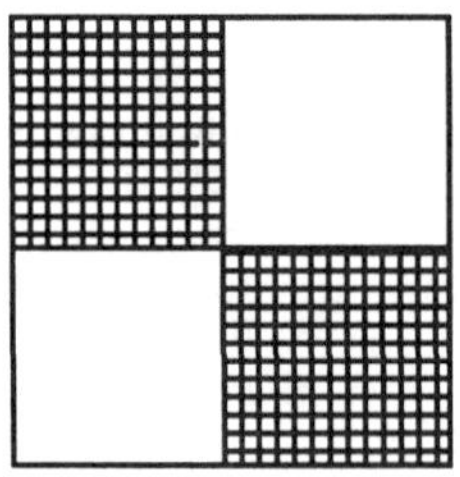

Exercise 6: For the following comparison-contrast exercises, list aspects that are shared or are not shared and make a yes/no list for each. Then check your list against information in your text book or other references.

(a) Electrolytic, galvanic, and concentration cells.
(b) Heterozygous and homozygous genes.
(c) Period and group for the atomic table.
(d) Entropy and enthalpy.
(e) Capacitors and resistors.

INTUITIVE REASONING

Review Section 2.3.2 in Chapter 2.

Intuitive Reasoning Exercises:

Exercise 7: The electric knife and electric spoon exist. How could an electric fork be used?
Exercise 8: How long would it take to skateboard from Seattle to Maine?
Exercise 9: You are a passenger on a train. How could you calculate its speed? Repeat this problem for a subway and an airplane.
Exercise 10: Prove that light travels in straight lines without using any equipment.

VISUAL REASONING

Review Section 2.3.2 in Chapter 2.

Visual Reasoning Exercises

Notice that in addition to picturing objects you must also be able to imagine how they move.

Exercise 11: A box is set on a series of rollers with a circumference of 3 feet. The rollers lie on level ground. If the box is pushed causing the rollers to make one revolution, how far does the box travel with respect to the ground? (Assume no slippage occurs.)

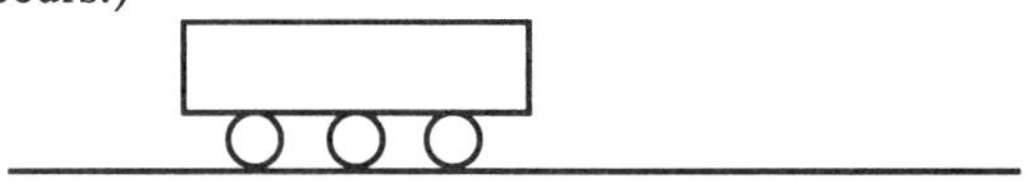

Exercise 12: In the following science exercises draw a schematic or a clear sketch which demonstrates your mastery of the concept:

(a) Visualize the Doppler effect. Can you explain in one sentence what causes it?
(b) Draw the molecules of epimers and anomers to help you conceptualize them in your mind. (Use straight lines.)
(c) Sketch the filtration process that takes place in the glomerulus and nephron of a human kidney.

Exercise 13: Describe the trace of corner **A** as the illustrated square turns end-over-end along level ground.

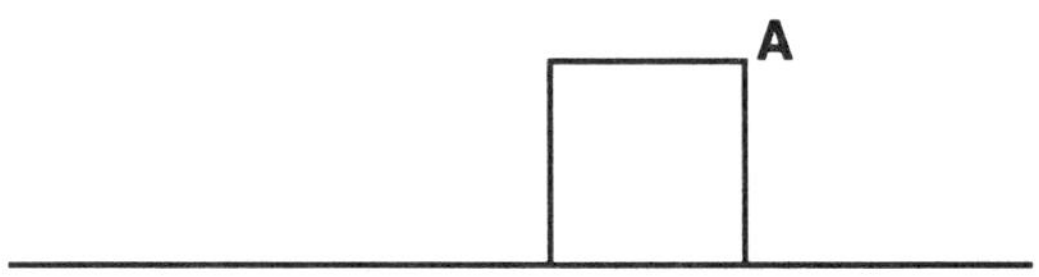

4.0.1 Solutions to Reasoning Exercises

Analytical Reasoning

1. For this type of problem it is useful to make a table. The table below shows information that is given directly for the problem.

	new	**vintage**	**total**
Harry	3		5
Louise		3	5 + 1
Kate	n	n + 3	
Bob	n	?	
	8	12	20

Next, work with the rows and columns to figure the missing elements.

	new	vintage	total
Harry	3		5
Louise	3	3	5 + 1
Kate	n	n + 3	
Bob	n	?	
	8	12	20

It is clear that n = 1, hence Kate has 5 cars; therefore Bob must have 4 cars of which only 1 is new. Bob owns 3 vintage cars.

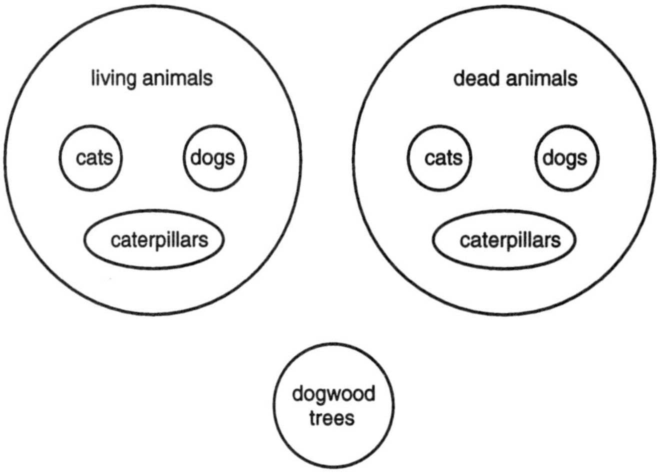

3. Instructions for this exercise include a statement of the main idea, which is physical description; the organizational pattern, which is spatial; and representation of details relative to the main idea, which is in drawing the parts of the eye. The summary statement is "physical characteristics and functions."

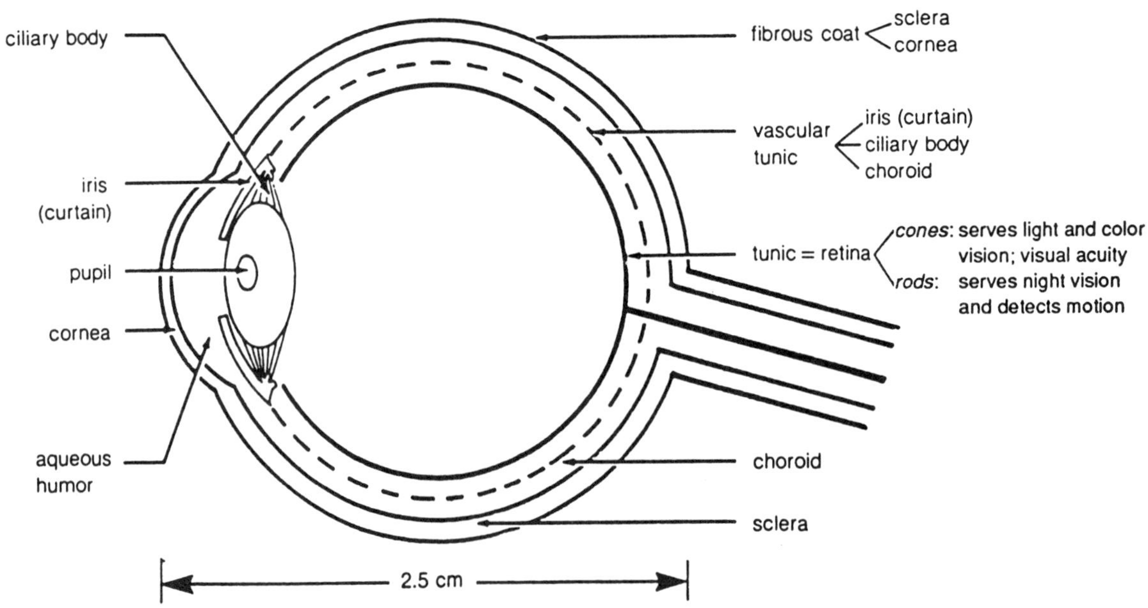

4.

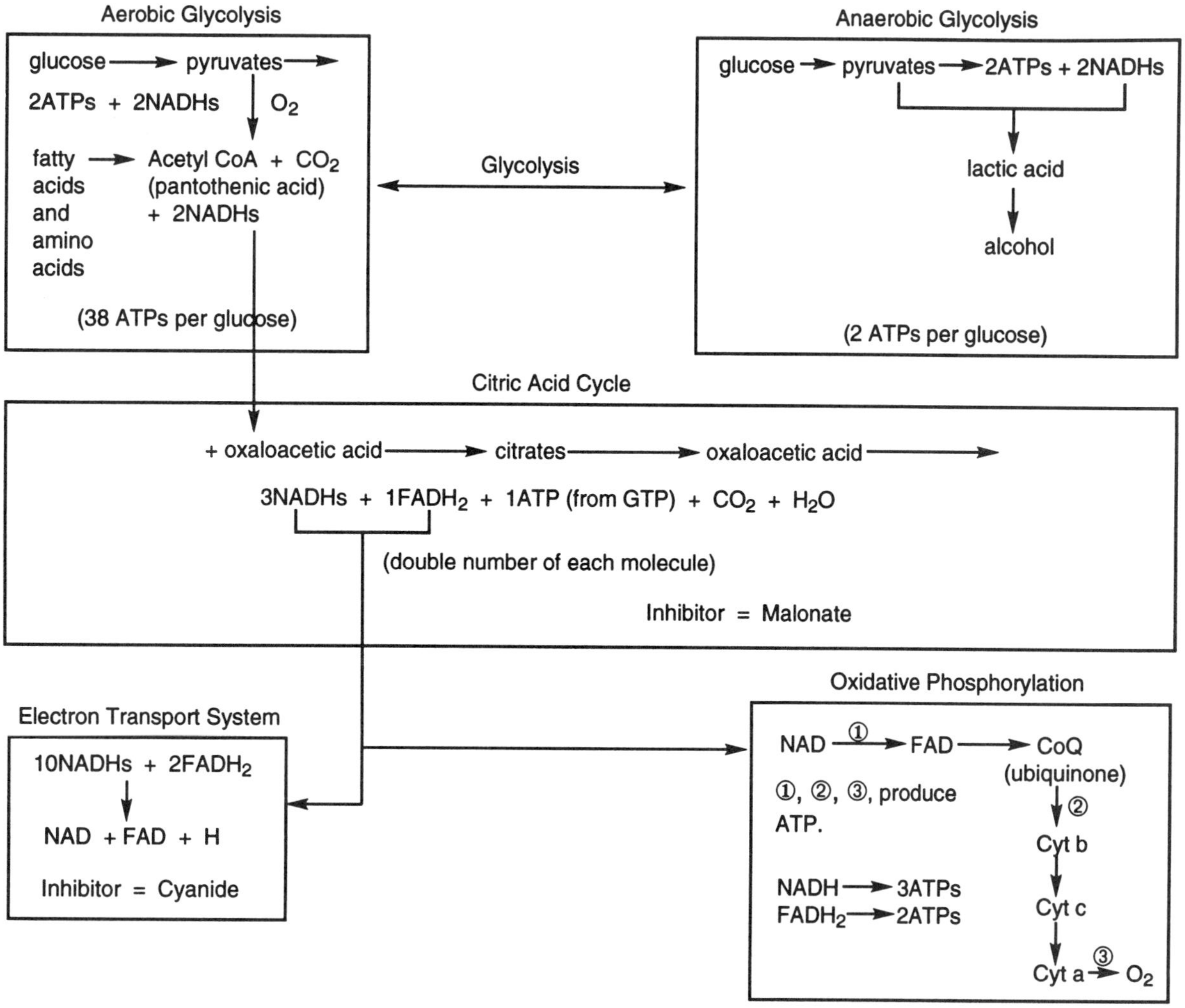

Comparative Reasoning

5. • Both figures are divided into quarters with half of the area shaded.
• The left figure is round while the right figure is square.
• The first and third quadrants of the right figure are shaded, while on the left figure these quadrants are clear...., etc.

6. The comparison-contrast exercises should be done using the text in Chapters 5 and 7.

Intuitive/Creative or Abstract Reasoning

7. Electric fork problem. Answers will vary depending on how an electric spoon and knife are used by you.

8. Estimate the distance, perhaps 4,000 miles. Try to think how far one can skateboard in an hour, remembering that some roads may not be as easy to skateboard on. It is probably quicker than a fast walk, maybe 6 miles per hour. If you cover 40 miles per day it will take 100 days.

9. For the train, measure how many seconds between the telephone poles, and then estimate the spacing of the poles. For the subway it is much harder to find a repetitive object with an even spacing that you can estimate, but there may be one if you look for it. For the plane, you may be able to use the wing edge to measure how long it takes to cross a field, but estimating the field size could prove difficult. If you cannot see the ground, the problem is much harder; you might find the average speed for the trip using the flight time and estimating the distance using the map in the flight magazine.

10. The phenomenon that "light travels in straight lines" can be demonstrated by holding a book in front of a light source. No equipment is allowed, though! Watch sunrise and sunset and how sun rays filter in straight paths through branches of trees. On a partially sunny day the sun rays travel through clouds in straight lines.

Visual Reasoning

11. This may require that you actually try the problem with a model. The box will move forward one circumference with respect to the roller and the roller will move forward one circumference with respect to the ground. The box therefore moves two circumferences by 6 feet.

12. Use your science knowledge to answer this question.

13.

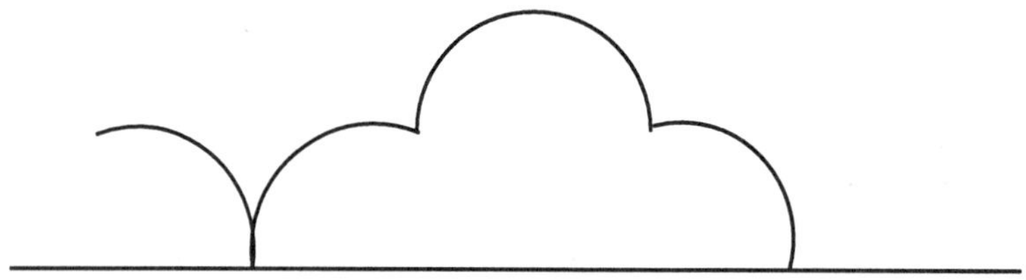

4.0.2 Problem-Solving Exercises in Physics

No problem can involve only one kind of reasoning, nor is it possible to solve a problem using only reasoning and no facts. The OAT problems are designed to see how well you can coordinate several different kinds of reasoning while working with the knowledge you gained from your undergraduate science courses. Try to identify the types of reasoning you use in solving the wheelchair and ladder problems that follow:

Wheelchair

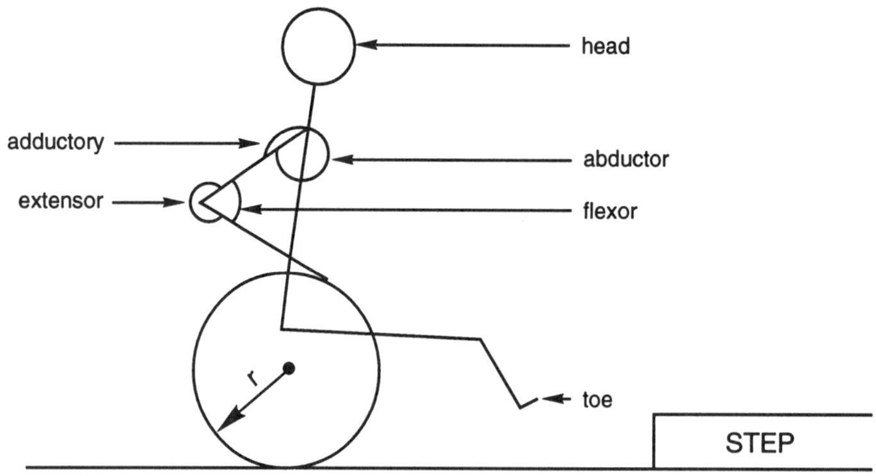

1. Which pattern of muscle activity will have the effect of moving the wheelchair forward?

   A. Stimulate the extensor and abductor, inhibit the flexor and adductor
   B. Stimulate the abductor and adductor, inhibit the flexor and extensor
   C. Inhibit the flexor and abductor, stimulate the extensor and adductor
   D. Inhibit the extensor and abductor, stimulate the flexor and adductor

2. The maximum technical advantage is found in:

   A. the adductor or the abductor.
   B. the flexor or the adductor.
   C. the extensor.
   D. the wheel.

3. In the diagram above, the force applied to the wheel is directed along a tangent to the wheel at an angle of about 45 degrees in the horizontal. In which of the following directions could the force be applied to obtain an equally efficient or a more efficient effect? There may be more than one correct answer.

A. Tangential to the wheel applied closer to the hub
B. Tangential to the wheel applied horizontally
C. Any horizontal force whether or not it is tangential
D. A force applied at 30 degrees to the horizontal plane

4. When the wheelchair reaches the step indicated in the diagram the extra force needed will be

A. W (the weight of the chair and the occupant)
B. W/r (W divided by the radius of the wheel)
C. $W/2\pi r$
D. W/2

5. The wheelchair comes to a smooth up-ramp with railing which it can negotiate without having the wheels slip. Will more force need to be applied pulling on the railings or pushing on the top rim of the wheel?

A. More on the railings
B. More on the wheels
C. The same on each
D. Depends on the slope of the ramp

Ladder

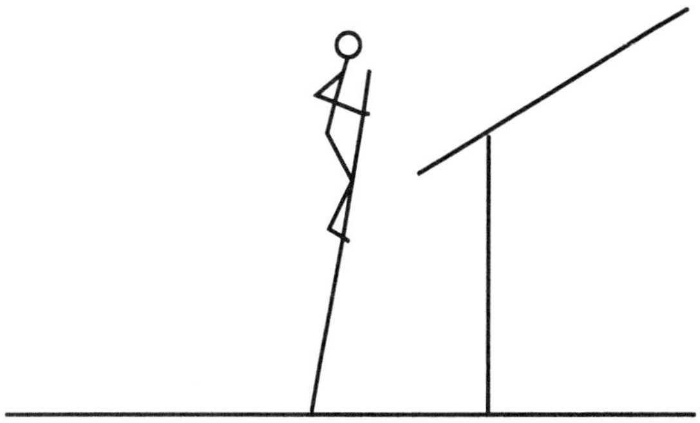

6. The ladder in the diagram above starts to swing out to the left. In order to return to the house, which of the following actions should the man take? More than one way may be correct.

A. Swing his arms clockwise
B. Swing his arms counter-clockwise
C. Lean forward
D. Lean backward

7. The man will have less leeway in time to react if (indicate all correct responses):

A. the ladder is long.
B. the ladder is short.
C. he recently had two shots of alcoholic beverages.
D. he is over 40 years old.

8. As the ladder continues to swing left (indicate all correct responses):

A. the man's heart rate will increase and he will begin to lose heat rapidly.
B. the man's vision will blur.
C. the man's angular momentum will be conserved.
D. the concentration of CO_2 in his exhaled breath will decrease.

4.0.3 Solutions to Problem-Solving Exercises in Physics

Wheelchair Problems

1. A Extensor increases the angle at joint, abductor moves bone away toward midline

2. D All muscles work at a fractional mechanical advantage

3. B Tangential to the wheel applied at rim

4. D The wheel will act as a lever of length 2r with the weight concentrated at its center

5. A You can think of the wheel as a lever or consider the distance through which the forces are applied. When the rail is pulled, the force is applied through the same distance as the chair moves. But when pushing on the rim of the wheel, the force is applied through twice the distance as the chair moves. This is not easy to see. One revolution of the wheel produces a forward movement of one revolution. The point of force application at the top of the wheel moves forward both by the forward motion of the entire chair and by the rotation of the wheel.

Ladder problems

6. A and **C** Swinging the arms and leaning forward will produce counter torques on the ladder. The counter torques should resist the counter-clock-wise torque of the falling ladder.

7. A, C, and **D** The period of swing decreases with length: therefore, the longer the ladder the longer it will take the ladder to move, giving the man more time to respond. Age and alcohol both increase human reaction times making it much harder to respond in time.

8. A, C, and **D** The fright response includes an increased heart rate, sharper vision, faster blood flow, increased rate of breathing. Faster blood flow and rapid movement through the air would increase heat loss. Faster breathing without strenuous exercise would decrease the concentration of CO_2 in each breath.

4.0.4 Problem-Solving Models

The following problem-solving steps should be used as a guide to solve problems in Physics, Biology, General and Organic Chemistry.

STEP I: Understanding the Given in the Problem Statement (What is Given?)

STEP II: Organizing and Assembling Pertinent Information (How Can the Given Be Used?)

STEP III: Understanding the Problem: What is the Question?

This step is critical before you solve the problem. Ask yourself, "What question is really being asked?" The following substeps will help you:

Substep 1 — Try to condense the question as much as possible, to really comprehend the nature of the question.

- Check to see if the question is complete and directly stated. A word of caution! Do not try to rephrase the question according to a simpler or easier version that you have seen before.
- Do not assume or pretend that if you can answer a simpler question, you also know this problem equally well. In order to test you, the test-maker may have considered the simpler option and included a response to check your precision in understanding the question

Substep 2 — The limitations and assumptions inherent in the question stem should be isolated and examined.

- The process of elimination used to delete wrong answers (from the four multiple-choice responses) will prove to be successful if the limitations of the question are properly examined

STEP IV: Finding the Appropriate Problem Solving Method: How do You Solve It?

This step is time consuming because it integrates the earlier steps of given information, organizing the given information and the nature of the question asked. You could waste time in this step if you do not know which way to go. It is important to mention here that OAT problems are not mechanical--you should not plug any numbers in any equation unless you are sure. Each calculation that you carry out uses up precious time. It is always worthwhile to break a complex or long problem into simpler and easily manageable units. A few fundamental approaches are suggested to help you pick up the right one. Do not be discouraged if the answer is not obvious. You should not sacrifice a systematic approach in problem solving for any other short cuts. Use one or more of the following approaches as you need them:

(1) You should apply already-learned concepts to fill in the gaps from information provided in the passage. Only use principles, definitions, equations, theories and laws to fill in the gaps. Information given in problems should be integrated with the solution.

(2) When working with mathematic problems watch for consistency in units and conventions, and always start from the given data (see Step II)

(3) Use all the relevant facts, only

(4) Do not erase or write over your calculations. Performing mathematical operations in small spaces can be a frustrating experience. Write carefully and clearly.

(5) Do not expect formulas and equations to be provided during the test. You have to learn to memorize important formulas.

(6) Use proportional reasoning as and when required to compare various options.

(7) Always try to get the answer in the form presented, especially in data analysis problems. Organize and interpret your data so it is directly linked to the format of the answers presented.

(8) You should learn how to test the five responses against your answer and make sure to follow basic logic.

(9) Pick up various strategies and approaches to solve the problem in any order as long as they are well connected and sequential in solving the problem.

STEP V: Evaluating the Given Answers and Your Solution (Is Your Solution Accurate?)

4.1 PHYSICS

This section outlines the subject of physics for the OAT. The material is subdivided into content groups with a brief introduction to major concepts. A physics review test is included to illustrate the level of difficulty of OAT questions. Use these sample questions to gauge your understanding of OAT physics and to identify specific topics requiring more independent study and comprehensive review. Use the GRE subject book in Physics (without the calculus problems).

4.1.1 Physics Outline

A. Units of Measurement
- **1.** Length
- **2.** Mass
- **3.** Time
- **4.** Derived Units
- **5.** Conversions

B. Vector Operations and Rules
- **1.** Vectors and Scalars
- **2.** Graphical Addition of Vectors
- **3.** Resolution of Vectors

C. Kinematics (Translation and Rotation)
- **1.** Equations of Translational Motion
- **2.** Angular Velocity
- **3.** Angular Acceleration

D. Dynamics
- **1.** Force, Weight
- **2.** Momentum
  - **a.** Linear
  - **b.** Angular
- **3.** Gravitation, Gravity
- **4.** Newton's Laws of Motion
- **5.** Dynamic Equilibrium

E. Statics
   1. Equilibrium
   2. Moment of a Force
   3. Center of Mass
   4. Types of Levers
F. Work and Energy
   1. Work and Power
   2. Energy
      a. Potential
      b. Kinetic
   3. Impulse-Momentum Equation
   4. Colliding Objects
      a. Elastic
      b. Inelastic
G. Wave Characteristics and Periodic Motion
   1. Oscillations, Vibrations
   2. Characteristics of Waves
      a. Wave length
      b. Wave period
      c. Wave amplitude
      d. Wave period, frequency
      e. Wave velocity
   3. Simple Harmonic Motion
      a. Pendulum
      b. Resonance
H. Solid and Fluid Properties
   1. Properties of Solids
   2. Fluid Statics
   3. Fluid Dynamics (Optional)
I. Sound
   1. The Human Ear
   2. Speed of Sound
   3. Sound Intensity
   4. Doppler Effect
   5. Ultrasonics
J. Thermal Energy and Heat Transfer
   1. Heat and Temperature
   2. Temperature Scales and Conversions
   3. Heat Transfer
      a. Conduction
      b. Convection
      c. Radiation
   4. Calorie, BTU
   5. Laws of Thermodynamics
      a. First law
      b. Second law
   6. Entropy
   7. Enthalpy
K. Electrostatics and D.C. Circuits
   1. Electric Charge
   2. Coulomb Definition
   3. Conductors/Insulators
   4. Coulomb's Law
   5. Electric Resistance
   6. Electric Current
   7. Electric Potential
   8. Ohm's Law
   9. Capacitance
   10. Single-Loop Circuits
L. Magnetism
   1. Magnetic Field
   2. Units of Measurement
   3. Electromagnetism

4. Magnetic Properties of Materials
    a. Paramagnetic
    b. Diamagnetic
    c. Ferromagnetic

M. Optics
  1. The Human Eye
  2. Reflection and Mirrors
  3. Refraction and Lenses
  4. The Lens Equation
  5. Optical Instruments
    a. Microscope
    b. Telescope
    c. Colonfiberscope
    d. Periscope
    e. Modern optical instruments

N. Nuclear and Atomic Structure
  1. Fission
  2. Fusion
  3. Half-life
  4. Radioactivity

4.2 PHYSICAL MEASUREMENTS IN OPTOMETRY

Units of measurement are important in optometry. High precision and accuracy are required in physical measurements of the eye, e.g., pupilometer is used to measure the center to center distance between the left and the right eye. An inaccuracy in measurement will result in wrong design of optical devices such as glasses, lenses, etc.

4.2.1 Measurements Using Metric and British Unit Systems

Basic Units and Conversions

The **metric system** is based on the decimal system. There are three basic units:

length: meter (m)

mass: gram (g)

volume: liter (l)

All other units of the metric system depend on using the following prefixes:

pico - (p)............. 10^{-12}	deca .... 10^{1}
nano - (n)............. 10^{-9}	kilo - (k) .... 10^{3}
micro - (μ) .... 10^{-6}	mega - (M) .... 10^{6}
milli - (m)............ 10^{-3}	giga................... 10^{9}
centi - (c) .... 10^{-2}	tera .... 10^{12}
deci - (d)............. 10^{-1}	

Examples are:

kilometer = 1000 m

centimeter = $\frac{1}{100}$ meter

kilogram	=	1000 g
milligram	=	$\frac{1}{1000}$ g
deciliter	=	$\frac{1}{10}$ liter

The English System has no rational basis. The basic units of it can be said to be:

length: foot (ft)

mass: pound (lb)

volume: gallon (gal)

But multiples of these are used just as often:

1 foot (ft)	=	12 in		
1 yard (yd)	=	3 ft	=	36 in
1 mile	=	1,760 yds	=	5,280 ft
1 pound (lb)	=	16 oz		
1 ton	=	2,000 lbs		
1 quart	=	2 pts		
1 gallon (gal)	=	4 qts		
1 pt	=	16 fluid ounces		

The key **conversions** between the metric and English systems are:

length:	2.54 cm	=	1 inch
mass:	454 g	=	1 pound
volume:	0.95 liters	=	1 quart.

Converting Units and Balancing Units in Equations

The OAT requires: (1) the ability to convert units (conversion factors between metric and English systems being provided where needed), and (2) the ability to balance physical units in equations.

Problem 1.
Convert 20 kg to ounces.

Problem 2.
Convert 40 km to miles.

Problem 3.
Convert 10 liters to pints

Problem 4.
Since the electric field $E = \frac{F}{q}$, where F = force = (mass × acceleration) and q = charge, what are the units of E in terms of mass (m), length (l), time (t), and charge (q)?

Solutions to Unit Conversion Problems

(1) $$(20\text{ kg})\left(\frac{1000\text{ g}}{1\text{ km}}\right)\left(\frac{1\text{ lb}}{454\text{ g}}\right)\left(\frac{16\text{ oz}}{1\text{ lb}}\right) = \frac{(20)(1000)(16)}{454}\text{ oz} = 705\text{ oz}$$

(2) $$(40\text{ km})\left(\frac{1000\text{ m}}{1\text{ km}}\right)\left(\frac{100\text{ cm}}{1\text{ m}}\right)\left(\frac{1\text{ in}}{2.54\text{ cm}}\right)\left(\frac{1\text{ ft.}}{12\text{ in}}\right)\left(\frac{1\text{ mi}}{5280\text{ ft}}\right)$$

$$= \frac{(40)(1000)(100)}{(2.54)(12)(5280)}\text{ mi} = 24.9\text{ mi}$$

(3) $$(10\text{ liters})\left(\frac{1\text{ qt}}{0.95\text{ liters}}\right)\left(\frac{2\text{ pt}}{1\text{ qt}}\right) = \frac{(10)(2)}{(0.95)}\text{ pts} = 21\text{ pints}$$

(4) $$E = \frac{F}{q} = \frac{ma}{q} = \frac{(m)\left(\frac{1}{t^2}\right)}{q} = \frac{m \bullet 1}{q \bullet t^2}$$

4.2.2 Precision and Accuracy in Measurements

So far, we have been concerned with characterizing various units of measurement. When analyzing data or solving problems, we are also interested in examining the nature of (e.g., the limitations of) the measurements that a set of data comprises. These considerations lead to the notion of measurement error which stems from a desire to know the possible difference between the exact, true value of a quantity and our measured (or calculated) value of it. Review Section 3.1 to understand how "rounding" of numbers is related to significant digits.

Before embarking on a discussion of precision and accuracy, the **significant digits** of a number must be understood. A digit is significant when it has been measured exactly. Examples of determining the number of significant digits are:

(1) 7.000 4 significant digits; digits listed after a decimal point are assumed to be accurately measured.

(2) 7000 1 significant digit; no decimal point—see (3) below.

(3) 7000. 4 significant digits; the decimal point implies that all zeros are accurately measured.

(4) 7001 4 significant digits; all zeros between nonzero digits are significant.

When adding, multiplying, etc., the number of significant digits in the result cannot be such that it is any more precise than the least precise number involved in its calculation (see discussion of precision below). Consider as examples:

Each piece of data in a certain experiment has 2 (e.g., 8.3) or 3 (e.g., 10.3) significant digits. When the mean for these data is calculated, it comes out initially as 9.65 but is rounded off to 9.7 because some of the numbers used to calculate this mean have only two significant digits. Likewise, the variance of these data is initially calculated as 3.643 but has to be rounded off to 3.6 (2 significant digits).

Measurement errors occur in data because it is not possible to get exact numbers from experiments. In any experiment, there is a limit to how close we can get to knowing the true value of the quantity being measured. Consequently, there are several definitions/concepts with which you should be familiar that are used to describe and assess the error in a measurement or calculation.

The **precision** of a number or an experimental value is the smallest unit of measurement and is therefore closely related to the significant digits in a measured number. For example, times for rats running a maze are recorded to the nearest 0.1 seconds; therefore, the precision of these time measurements is 0.1 seconds. It is also called the "least count" of the measuring instrument.

The **accuracy** of a number is how far the measured value of a variable may be from its true value. The true value is normally considered as an "average" obtained from a large set of data values. For example, the precision of the watch used to measure each rat maze solution time is 0.1 seconds. Neglecting any other possible sources of error, the accuracy of each time measurement is ± 0.05 seconds. Specifically, when a rat's measured solution time is

8.8 seconds, the true solution time is 8.8 ± 0.05 seconds, i.e., it is known to be between 8.75 and 8.85 seconds. Another example is to determine the precision in the blood cholesterol level experiments as 1 mg/100 ml; therefore, the accuracy is ± 0.5 mg/100 ml. A measured value of 196 corresponds to a true value that is somewhere between 195.5 and 196.5.

However, when error results from sources other than the limitations of the measuring device, the accuracy and the precision are not usually so simply related. In many experiments, there may be factors other than the precision of the measurements involved which decrease the accuracy of results. Measurement errors can be classified under three headings: mistakes, systematic errors, and random errors. **Mistakes** are usually nonrepetitive errors that might result from human errors, such as misreading an instrument or occasions of performing a step wrong in an experimental procedure. The error that results from a mistake is largely unpredictable and unless caught will probably affect the data in some unknown way.

A **systematic error** is a repetitive error caused by human error, instrument error, or experimental design error. It is repeated in every measurement, usually, to the same extent. If a systematic error is detected, there is a possibility that it can be corrected to some extent. An example of a systematic error would be a case where we are measuring a series of temperatures in an experiment and the thermometer being used to make these measurements is miscalibrated 2°C too high. In this case, the set of temperature measurements would have a systematic error of 2°C (too high).

We always attempt to do experiments under uniform conditions. Nevertheless, in practice, there is always some variability in these "uniform" conditions that cannot be removed. Thus, even if all human, instrument, and experimental design errors are corrected in an experiment, a variability that is called **random error** will still probably exist in its measurements. Consider as an example of random error:

Example: We perform an experiment to determine the temperature dependence of the solubility of a particular organic salt in water. Our experimental apparatus is capable of maintaining a constant temperature of ± 1°C. Say we are particularly interested in measuring the salt's solubility at 37°C. Although we take it to be 37°C, each time we take a solubility measurement the true temperature is actually somewhere between 36°C and 38°C. Since the salt's solubility is temperature dependent, this variability in the true temperature results in a random error in the solubility measurements at 37°C. This random error, of course, directly affects the accuracy of these solubility measurements.

4.2.3 Vector Operations and Rules

A **vector quantity** is one that is completely specified by a magnitude and a direction. A **scalar quantity** is one that is completely specified by its magnitude, there being no sense of direction. A vector is graphically symbolized by an arrow—the tail being the origin point, the head being the finish point, the length being proportional to the magnitude, and its angle (in relation to a reference) being indicative of its direction.

Problem 1.

What is the x-component of the vector $\vec{F}$?

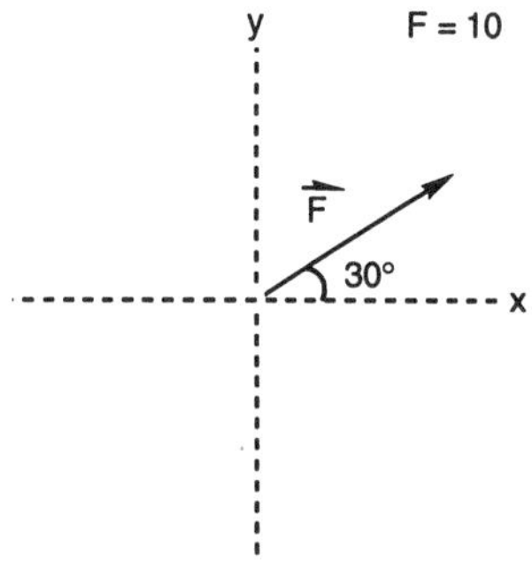

Problem 2.

What is the y-component of the vector $\vec{H}$?

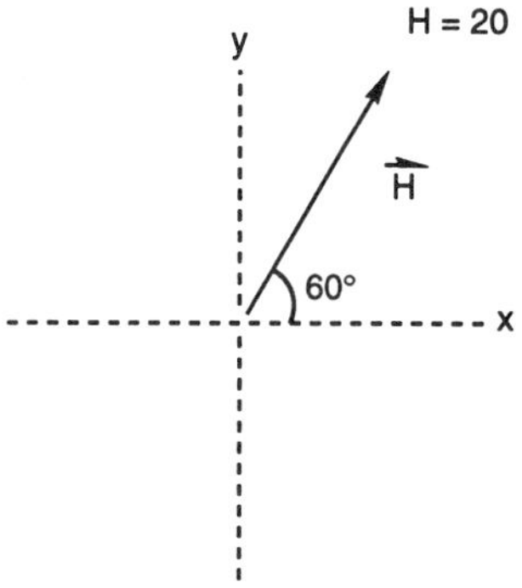

Solutions to Vector Problems

(1) Resolving the vector $\vec{F}$:

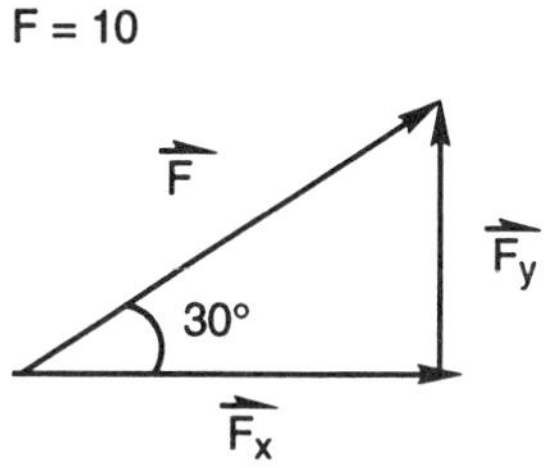

$$F_x = F \cos \theta = 10 \cos 30° = 10\left(\frac{\sqrt{3}}{2}\right) = 5\sqrt{3}$$

(2) Resolving the vector $\vec{H}$:

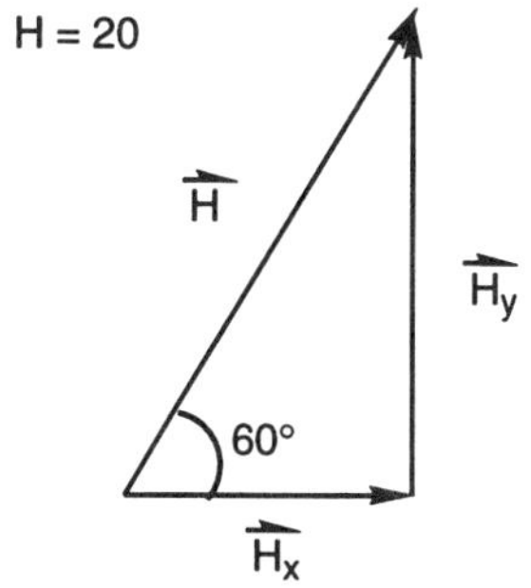

$$H_y = H \sin \theta = 20 \sin 60° = 20\left(\frac{\sqrt{3}}{2}\right) = 10\sqrt{3}$$

4.3 TRANSLATIONAL MOTION (KINEMATICS)

An important branch of physics is Newtonian Mechanics. Mechanics is divided into two categories: Statics (study of forces and couples acting on a body at rest, e.g., a magnifying glass sitting on a table), and Dynamics (study of forces, couples, acceleration of a body in motion, e.g., a hot air balloon rising vertically).

Dynamics is further divided into kinematics and kinetics. Kinematics is the study of the geometry of motion of a particle or body. Forces are usually *not* studied in kinematic analysis, e.g., calculating the lift velocity and the drag velocity of the hot air balloon as they relate to displacement and time without considering forces. The forces *causing* the balloon to rise are not considered in kinematics.

Distance depends on the path taken, has no fixed direction, and has magnitude only. *Speed* is the distance traveled divided by the change in time. Both speed and distance are scalar quantities—have magnitude but no fixed direction. They have positive values only. *Displacement* is independent of the path taken (i.e., depends only on initial and final positions of the object) and has a constant direction and magnitude. *Velocity* is the displacement divided by the change in time. Both velocity and displacement are vector quantities (i.e., have direction and magnitude). *Acceleration* is the change in velocity divided by the change in time, and it is a vector.

The units of distance and displacement are length such as feet (ft), meters (m) miles, and kilometers (km). *Force* is defined as the *action* of one particle on another, e.g., pushing a book with your hand. Forces act upon objects to cause an acceleration. A constant force produces a constant (unchanging) acceleration. The motion produced in this case is called *uniform accelerated motion. Translational motion,* also known as linear motion, is the movement of an object in a straight line. The above equations illustrate uniform accelerated motion along a straight line. *Free fall motion* is vertical motion (in reference to the earth), that is, upward or downward in a straight line. *Projectile motion* is conveniently thought of as having vertical (affected by g) and horizontal (independent of g) components.

4.3.1 Questions to Review Translational Motion

1. Which of the following depends on direction?
- **A.** distance
- **B.** displacement
- **C.** both
- **D.** neither

2. A constant acceleration is caused by a
- **A.** constant force.
- **B.** changing force.
- **C.** constant displacement.
- **D.** either **A** or **B**
- **E.** both **A** and **B**

3. An object starts 5 m from a reference point with an initial velocity of 10 m/sec and an acceleration of 5 m/sec^2. How far is the object from the reference point after 5 secs?
- **A.** 75m
- **B.** 80m
- **C.** 117.5m
- **D.** 180.5m
- **E.** 211 m

4. The analysis of projectile motion is greatly simplified by
- **A.** using the formula for describing the motion as a parabola.
- **B.** realizing that the time of ascent is one-half the time of descent.
- **C.** neglecting the effect of gravity if the object is considered a point mass.
- **D.** separating the motion into vertical (free fall) and horizontal (uniform accelerated motion) components.

5. An unbalanced force acting upon an object causes
- **A.** a change in the mass of the object.
- **B.** an acceleration of the object.
- **C.** the object to maintain a constant velocity.
- **D.** none of the above.

6. An object dropped from the edge of a cliff will fall how far in 10 seconds?
- **A.** cannot be determined without the mass of the object.
- **B.** 98m
- **C.** 980m
- **D.** 490m
- **E.** 49m

4.3.2 Answers to Questions in Section 4.3.1

(1) B (2) A (3) C (4) D (5) B (6) D

4.4 FORCE AND MOTION, GRAVITATION (DYNAMICS)

"Body" and "object" are used interchangeably in Physics. A body generally refers to a rigid body. A body consists of a large number of particles.

The *center of mass* (COM) of a body is that point whose motion can be described like a particle (e.g., as linear, circular, parabolic) even if the motion of the object cannot be so described. In collisions, the COM velocity (of the system) is not changed. The *center of gravity* (COG) is the COM but is conceptualized as that point where the sum of gravitational forces acting on an object can be represented by a summation force (action at the COM). An object is in *stable equilibrium* if the COG is as low as possible, and any change in orientation will lead to an elevation of the COG. *Unstable equilibrium* is when the COG is high (e.g., relative to a surface supporting it), and any change in orientation would lead to a lowering of the COG. *Neutral equilibrium* is an intermediate location of the COG and a change in orientation would not change the level of the COG. *Mass* is a dimension that cannot be broken down into simpler units. This is to be contrasted with *weight,* which is a force. Units of mass are slugs (weight in pounds divided by $g = 32\ ft/sec^2$), kilograms, grams, etc. Units of weight are pounds (defined differently from the pounds of mass), dynes ($gms \bullet cm/sec^2$) and newtons ($kg \bullet m/sec^2$).

Newton's Second Law relates an unbalanced force acting upon an object, producing an acceleration in the direction of the force that is directly proportional to the force and inversely proportional to the mass of the body: $a = F/m$, or, $F = ma$.

Newton's Second Law of Motion is considered to be the *most* important one for the OAT student. Applications and uses of the *Second Law* include driving a nail into the wall, putting your foot on the accelerator of your car while driving, freely falling objects, inclined plane motion with friction, running compared to jogging, the movement of blood and drugs in your arteries and veins.

Newton also formulated the *Law of Gravitation* as:

$$F = K_G(m_1 m_2/r^2),\ K_G = G = \text{Gravitational constant (do not confuse with Gibbs Free energy, } \Delta G)$$

Frictional forces are illustrated in Fig. 4.1.

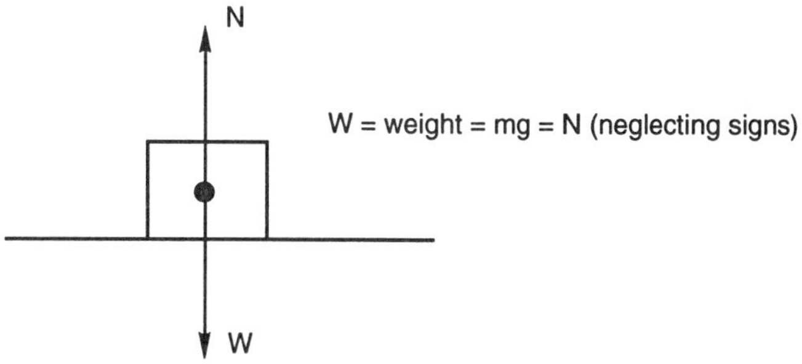

Figure 4.1 — Frictional Forces Related to Normal Forces

Friction is the resistance offered to the motion of a body and is mostly caused by the roughness (ups and downs or indentations) between two rough bodies. Friction depends on the texture of the contact surface of two bodies.

4.4.1 Questions to Review Force and Motion, Gravitation

1. One of Newton's laws of motion states that
A. an unbalanced force acting upon an object produces an acceleration of that object.
B. objects moving in circles at constant tangential velocity have no force acting upon them.
C. the square of the period of revolution is proportional to the cube of the radius of revolution.
D. objects falling to earth describe a hyperbolic projectory.

2. Frictional forces exist between an object and the surface it is on, and they
A. are proportional to the normal force to the surface that the object rests on.
B. are dependent on the area of contact between the surfaces.
C. always augment the motion of the object.
D. are conservative forces.
E. are dependent on the density of the object.

3. The force of gravitation between two objects is
A. inversely proportional to the products of the masses.
B. inversely proportional to the distance between them.
C. directly proportional to the square of the radius.
D. inversely proportional to the square of the distance between them.

4. If F = force, ΔU = potential energy change, Δx = displacement over which ΔU occurs, then
   A. $F = \Delta U \Delta x$
   B. $F = 1/\Delta U \Delta x$
   C. $F = -\Delta x/\Delta U$
   D. $F = -\Delta U/\Delta x$

5. What value of weight (W_1) is required such that the object (A) does not move down the incline (assume no friction)?

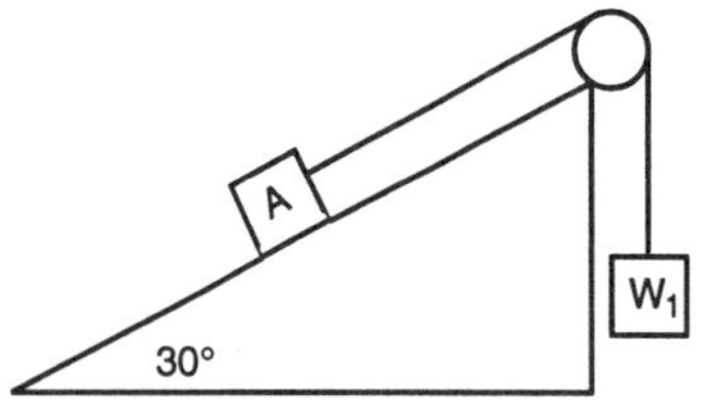

   A. 5 newtons
   B. 10 newtons
   C. 49 newtons
   D. 98 newtons
   E. none of the above.

4.4.2 Answers to Questions in Section 4.4.1

(1) A (2) A (3) D (4) D (5) C

4.5 EQUILIBRIUM, MOMENTUM, AND ROTATIONAL MOTION

When a force acts upon an object, the object will undergo translational motion or rotational motion. Translational motion is the motion of the object through space when the force is acting along an axis and/or the center of mass (that point whose motion can be described like a particle). Rotational motion is the rotation of an object about an axis caused by a force not directed along that axis. The effective force causing rotation about an axis is the *torque.*

Newton's First Law states that objects at rest or in motion tend to remain as such unless acted upon by an outside force. That is, objects have inertia (resistance to motion). *Momentum* (M) is a vector quantity. Its formulation for magnitude is, M = mv, m = mass, v = velocity.

Linear momentum is a measure of the tendency of an object to maintain motion in a straight line. *Impulse* is a measure of the force required to impart or change momentum of an object. Impulse is also a vector, given by: $I = F\Delta t = M = mv$. Review the laws of conservation of momentum and conservation of energy.

4.5.1 Questions to Review Equilibrium, Momentum, and Rotational Motion

1. Rotational motion represents
   A. movement of an object along a curved line.
   B. movement of an object through space.
   C. motion of an object about a fixed point.
   D. motion of an object about an axis.

2. The product of two unlike parallel forces times the perpendicular moment arm is called the
   A. energy.
   B. work.
   C. torque.
   D. couple.

3. What is the net torque acting about the axis through the center **A** (perpendicular to the paper) of the square with sides equal to 4m?

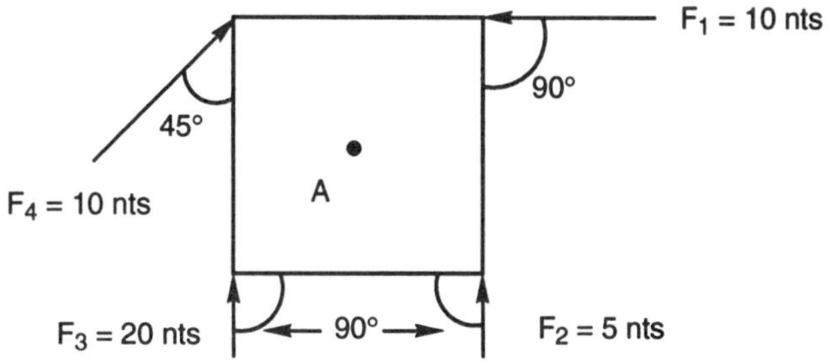

A. 38.2 nt – m counterclockwise
B. 76.4 nt – m clockwise
C. 38.2 nt – m clockwise
D. none of the above.

4. What is the net force on the following object?

A. 15 nts
B. 5 nts to the right
C. 5 nts compressive force
D. none of the above

4.5.2 Answers to Questions in Section 4.5.1

(1) D (2) D (3) C (4) B

4.6 WORK AND ENERGY

Mechanical energy is divided into kinetic energy (K) and potential energy (U). *Kinetic energy* is the energy associated with the motion of objects. *Potential energy* is the energy that results by position or configuration (of a system); there is no motion. When motion begins, potential energy is converted into kinetic energy. The formulation of potential energy depends on the system.

$U = mgh$ = gravitational potential energy
m = mass
h = height above earth's surface
$k = \left(\frac{1}{2}\right)mv^2$ = kinetic energy
v = speed of object

Additional features of potential energy are: (1) potential energy *cannot* be defined for frictional forces, and (2) the potential energy of a system is independent (in contrast to work) of the path to reach that system.

Potential energy can be of many types such as: magnetic, electric, chemical. Always remember potential energy is a *field* that exists around molecules.

The *Law of Conservation of Mechanical Energy* is:
Total Energy (TE) = kinetic energy (K) + potential energy (U) + energy due to dissipative forces (e.g., friction).

Work can also be defined in terms of the change in mechanical energy of an object. Remember that the potential energy between two points (or positions) is the amount of work that would be required to move an object between those two points. The change in kinetic energy of an object is the work performed by the object assuming all the energy goes into work. To summarize:

$W = E_f - E_i = \Delta E$
$E = K + U$ = mechanical energy
f = final, i = initial, Δ = change

This means work and energy have the same units:

$$W = (\text{force})(\text{distance}) = \text{newtons-meters} = \text{joules}$$
$$= \text{dynes-cms} = \text{ergs}$$

Joules and ergs are units of work or energy.
Pressure (P) times volume (V) also yields work (W), W = (P)(V).
This is used to study heat engines.

Power (P) is a scalar and is the rate at which work is done:

$$P = \text{work/time} = \text{joules/secs} \equiv \text{watts}.$$

4.6.1 Questions to Review Work and Energy

1. The law of conservation of energy takes into account all of the following, except

A. conversion of mass into energy
B. potential energy
C. kinetic energy
D. energy loss due to dissipative forces

2. If W = work and t = time, the power (P) is

A. P = W/t
B. P = t/W
C. P = Wt
D. P = 1/Wt

3. If a 5 kg object is 20 meters above the earth's surface and it falls to 10 meters above the surface, what is the change in potential energy (U)?

A. gains 490 joules
B. loses 490 joules
C. loses 50 joules
D. The potential energy does not change, only the kinetic energy changes.

4. A force of 10 newtons pushes a 5 kg object 20 meters. The work performed is

A. 200 joules
B. 40 joules
C. 10 joules
D. 2.5 joules

4.6.2 Answers to Questions in Section 4.6.1

(1) A (2) A (3) B (4) A

4.7 WAVE CHARACTERISTICS AND PERIODIC MOTION

A *wave* is a disturbance that transfers energy in a medium. Each particle in the medium vibrates about an equilibrium point which defines simple harmonic motion (below). If the direction of vibration is perpendicular to the direction of propagation of the wave, the wave is called a *transverse wave* (e.g., light). If the direction of vibration is in the same direction as propagation of the wave, the wave is called a *longitudinal wave* (e.g., sound). Longitudinal waves are characterized by condensations (regions of crowding of particles) and rarefactions (regions where particles are far apart) along the wave in the medium. See Fig. 4.2 on the following page.

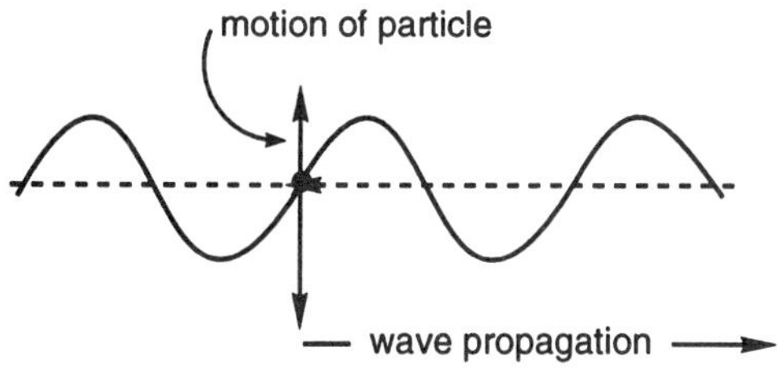

Figure 4.2(a) — Transverse Wave

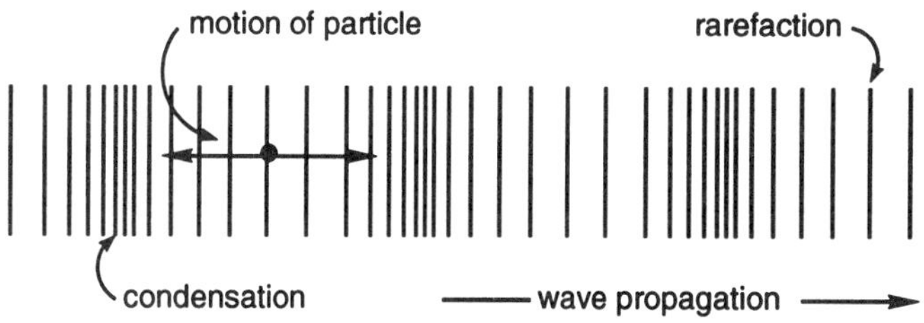

Figure 4.2(b) — Longitudinal Wave

The *wavelength* (λ) is the distance from crest to crest (or valley to valley) of a transverse wave. It may also be defined as the distance between two particles with the same displacement and direction of displacement. The *amplitude* (A) is the maximum displacement of a particle in one direction from its equilibrium point. *Frequency* (f) is the number of wavelengths (cycles) that pass a point per unit time. *Period* (T) is the time required for one wavelength to pass a point. *Speed* (v) of a wave refers to its propagation through the medium. *Phase* (ϕ) is the difference in displacement and direction of a particle due to two different waves.

The *superposition principle* states that the effect of two or more waves on the displacement of a particle are independent. *Interference* is the summation of the displacements of different waves in a medium. *Constructive interference* is when the waves add to a larger resultant wave than either original. *Destructive interference* is when the waves add to a smaller resultant wave than either original wave.

The particles that are undergoing displacement when a wave passes through a medium undergo motion called simple harmonic motion (SHM) and are acted upon by a force described by Hooke's Law. SHM is caused by an inconstant force (called a restoring force) and as a result has an inconstant acceleration. Hooke's law is expressed as $F = -kx$.

Features of Hooke's Law and SHM are
(1) Force and acceleration are always in the same direction.
(2) Force and acceleration are always in the opposite direction of the displacement.
(3) Force and acceleration have their maximal values at + A and – A; they are zero at the equilibrium point.
(4) Velocity direction has no constant relation to displacement or acceleration.
(5) Velocity is a maximum at equilibrium and zero at A and – A.

The *electromagnetic spectrum* has the sequence below from long wavelength (λ) and low frequency (f) to short wavelength and high frequency. The visible light is broken down into colors remembered by the mnemonic ROY G. BIV; Red, Orange, Yellow, Green, Blue, Indigo, Violet.

Planck developed the relation between energy (E) and the frequency (f) of electromagnetic radiation, $E = hf$; h = Planck's Constant.

4.7.1 Questions to Review Wave Characteristics and Periodic Motion

1. If the direction of vibration of particles of a medium is in the direction of propagation of a wave, the wave is called
A. longitudinal.
B. transverse.
C. both.
D. neither.

2. At the node of a wave,
A. the displacement is maximal.
B. there is no displacement.
C. there may be an open or a free point.
D. both **A** and **B**.
E. neither **A** nor **B**.

3. All of the following are true about simple harmonic motion *except*
A. force and acceleration have their maximum values at the equilibrium point
B. force and acceleration are always in the same direction
C. velocity direction has no constant relation to displacement or acceleration direction
D. velocity is maximal at the equilibrium point

4. If f = frequency and λ = wavelength of light, then the speed of light (c) is
   A. $c = 1/f$
   B. $c = \lambda/f$
   C. $c = f/\lambda$
   D. $c = f\lambda$
   E. $c = f + \lambda$

5. If the frequency of a wave is 10,000 hertz and it is traveling at 5000 m/sec, then its wavelength is
   A. 5 m
   B. 2 m
   C. 0.5 m
   D. 0.2 m

6. In a vibrating column of air
   A. open ends can only have nodes.
   B. nodes can occur at open or closed ends.
   C. open ends can only have antinodes.
   D. antinodes may only occur at closed ends.

4.7.2 Answers to Questions in Section 4.7.1

(1) A (2) B (3) A (4) D (5) C (6) C

4.8 SOUND

4.8.1 Review of Sound

Sound is a longitudinal mechanical wave that travels through an elastic medium. Sound is thus produced by vibrating matter. There is no sound in a vacuum (because there is no matter). Compressions (condensations) are regions where particles (of matter) are close together and are high pressure regions. Rarefactions are regions where particles are sparse and are low pressure regions of sound waves.

The *speed* (v) of sound is proportional to the square root of the elastic restoring force and inversely proportional to the square root of the inertia of the particles (e.g., density, ρ, is a measure of inertia),

$$v \propto \sqrt{F}$$
$$v \propto 1/\sqrt{\text{inertia}}$$

The speed in various substances is as follows:

wire or rod	$v = \sqrt{Y/\rho}$	Y = Young's modulus
fluid (gas or liquid)	$v = \sqrt{B/\rho}$	B = bulk modulus

The speed of sound also increases with temperature.

Forced vibrations occur when a series of waves impinge upon an object and cause it to vibrate. Natural frequencies are the intrinsic frequencies of vibration of a system. If the forced vibration causes the object to vibrate at one of its natural frequencies, the body will vibrate at maximal amplitude. This situation is called *resonance.*

The *quality* depends on the number and the relative intensity of the overtones of the waveforms. Frequency, and therefore *pitch*, are perceived by the ear from 20 to 20,000 Hz (Hertz = cycles/second). Frequencies below 20 Hz are called infrasonic. Frequencies above 20,000 Hz are called ultrasonic. *Sound* intensity (I) is the rate of energy (power) propagation through space.

4.8.1.1 THE HUMAN EAR

The human ear is devided into an *external ear* (pinna and auditory canal), the *middle ear* (the tympanic membrane and the three bones—malleus or hammer, incus, or anvil, and stapes or stirrup), and the *internal ear* (the cochlea, the semicircular canals, and the origin of the vestibulocochlear nerve). The *tympanic membrane* (eardrum) is attached to the *malleus*, which attaches to the *incus*, which attaches to the *stapes,* which attaches to the *oval window* of the cochlea. The outer and middle ear function to match the impedance of the air outside and the fluid of the cochlea inside. This mechanism results in more efficient transmission of sound. Sound waves are transmitted from the stapes via the oval window to the fluid in the *cochlea.* This fluid sets up vibrations in the *basilar membrane*, which causes special hair cells to send impulses to the auditory part of the vestibulocochlear (VIII) nerve, which transmits them to the auditory cortex in the temporal lobe of the cerebrum. The basilar membrane, tectoral membrane, and hair cells run the full length of the cochlea and together constitute the *organ of Corti.* The distance from the oval window that the vibration of the basilar membrane is at maximum determines the *frequency (pitch)* of the sound—highest frequencies are closest to the oval window. The *round window,* at the other end of the cochlea, serves as a release of pressure imparted to the cochlear fluid by the stapes.

The *vestibular system* is continuous anatomically but not functionally with the cochlea. The system is filled with fluid (endolymph) and contains the sacculus, the utricle, and three perpendicular *semicircular* canals. Each *semicircular canal* has an *ampulla* region that contains hair cells sensitive to changes in angular acceleration. The *utricle* and *sacculus* contain a special sensory region called the *macula,* which has crystals of calcium carbonate on it. These regions are sensitive to changes in gravity (position) and linear acceleration. Impulses travel from these special regions via the vestibular portions of the vestibulocochlear nerve (Cranial Nerve VIII) to the central nervous system. The vestibular system helps maintain posture, balance, spatial orientation, and stabilization of eye movements. This section should also be used in solving Biological Sciences problems.

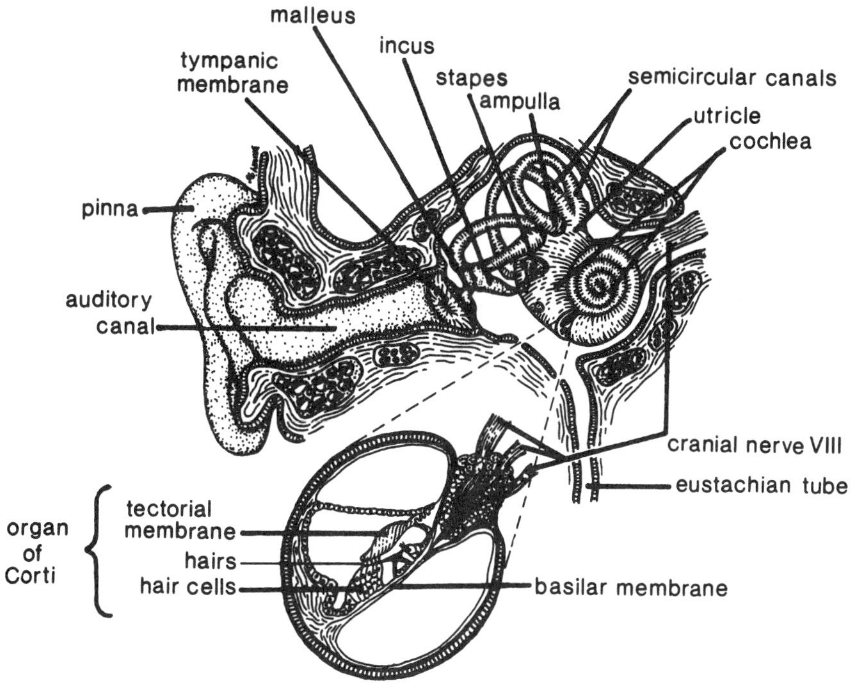

Figure 4.3 — The Human Ear

The *loudness* varies with the amplitude. The ears are most sensitive (hear sound of lowest frequency) at approximately 2,000 to 4,000 Hz. I_0, taken to be 10^{-12} watts/m^2, is barely audible and is assigned a value of 0 (zero) dB (decibels).

The *Doppler Effect* is the effect upon the observed frequency caused by the relative motion of the observer (o) and the source (s). If the distance is decreasing between them, there is a shift to higher frequencies and shorter wavelengths (to higher pitch for sound and toward the blue-violet for light). If the distance is increasing between them, there is a shift to longer wavelengths and lower frequencies (to lower pitch for sound and toward red for light).

4.8.2 Questions to Review Sound

1. Sound waves
   A. are transverse waves.
   B. are produced by vibrating matter.
   C. may be transmitted in a vacuum.
   D. are all of the above.

2. When an object is forced to vibrate at one of its natural frequencies of vibration,
   A. resonance exists.
   B. energy is a minimum.
   C. work is a minimum.
   D. the amplitude of vibration is a minimum.

3. The intensity (power per unit area) of a sound is
   A. inversely proportional to the square of the frequency.
   B. directly proportional to the square of the frequency.
   C. inversely proportional to the frequency.
   D. directly proportional to the frequency.

4. The threshold of human hearing lies between
   A. 20 Hz - 20,000 Hz
   B. 10 Hz - 10,000 Hz
   C. 18 Hz - 8,000 Hz
   D. 12 Hz - 1,200 Hz

5. An ambulance, traveling 24 m/sec, is moving toward an approaching car, which is traveling at a speed of 14 m/sec. The siren emits a frequency of 1,000 Hz, what is the frequency heard by the driver of the car? Speed of sound = 350 m/sec.
   A. 1,000 Hz
   B. 1,116 Hz
   C. 1,350 Hz
   D. 1,038 Hz

6. Semicircular canals are sensitive to
   A. semicircular canals.
   B. changes in angular acceleration.
   C. organ of Corti.
   D. utricle.

4.8.3 Answers to Question in Section 4.8.2

(1) B (2) A (3) B (4) A (5) B (6) B

4.9 SOLID AND FLUID PROPERTIES

4.9.1 Static and Dynamic Properties of Fluids

Density represents the packing of material in a certain volume.

Mass density $\rho = \dfrac{\text{mass}}{\text{volume}}$

Weight density $\gamma = \dfrac{\text{weight}}{\text{volume}}$

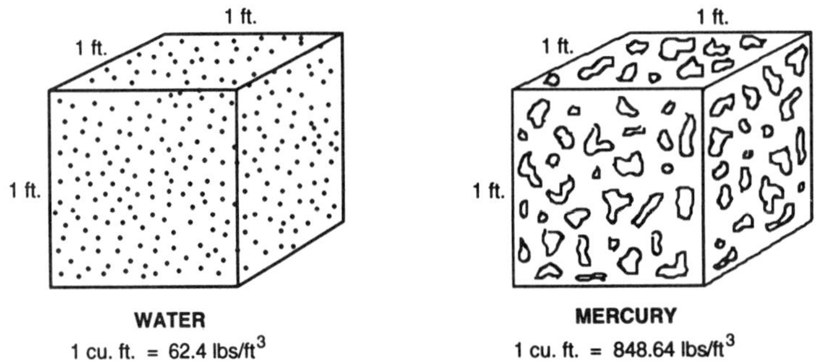

Figure 4.4 — Illustration of the Concept of Density

As an example, an average human being weighing 150 lbs. with 90% water is like a container of water about the same weight:

$150 \times 0.90 = 135$ lbs. The weight density of water = 62.4 lbs/ft^3.

Using: $$\text{weight density} = \frac{\text{weight}}{\text{volume}}$$

$$62.4 = \frac{135}{\text{volume}}$$

This results in the average volume of the human body at 2.16 ft^3.

Generally, solids are more dense than liquids, which are more dense than gases. The *specific gravity* (SG) of a substance is defined as:

$$SG = \left(\frac{\text{density of a substance}}{\text{density of water}}\right) \text{ at a given temperature.}$$

The density of water is about 1 gm/ml over most common temperatures. *In most instances the specific gravity of a substance is the same as its density.* Note that the units of density are mass/volume, whereas SG has no units.

Density is one of the key properties of fluids (liquids or gases) and the other is pressure. Pressure (P) is defined as force (F) per unit area (A):

$$P = F/A$$

F is the normal (perpendicular) force. Fluids can only exert P at an enclosed surface or body. Otherwise, fluids will flow under a shearing stress instead of being deformed elastically as solids would. Pressure is also formulated as potential energy per unit volume as follows:

$$P = F/A = mg/A = (mg/A)(h/h) = mgh/V = \rho gh$$

where, ρ = density
h = depth below liquid surface.

Physical characteristics of force and pressure of fluids are:

(1) Forces exerted by fluids are always perpendicular to the container.
(2) The fluid pressure (hydrostatic) is directly proportional to the depth of the fluid and to its density:
$$P \propto \rho h.$$
(3) At any particular depth, the fluid pressure is the same in all directions.
(4) Fluid pressure is independent of the shape or area of its container.
(5) An external pressure applied to an enclosed fluid is transmitted uniformly throughout the volume of the liquid (*Pascal's law*).
(6) An object that is completely or partially submerged in a fluid experiences an upward force equal to the weight of the fluid displaced (Archimedes' principle). This *buoyant force* (F_B) is:
$$F = V\rho g = mg$$
buoyant force = weight of displaced fluid.
An object that floats must displace its own weight (not volume) in fluid.

If p_1 and p_2 are the pressures at elevations y_1 and y_2 above the same reference level and when ρ and g are constant,

$$p_1 - p_2 = -\rho g\,(y_2 - y_1).$$

Apply this equation to a liquid in an open vessel, as in Figure 4.5 below. Take point 1 at any level and let p represent that pressure at this point. Take point 2 at the top surface where the pressure is atmospheric pressure, p_a. Use the pressure-elevation equation to obtain:

$$p - p_a = \rho g\,(y_2 - y_1),$$
$$p = p_a + \rho gh.$$

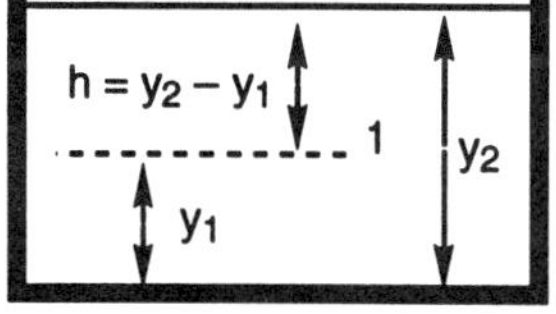

Figure 4.5 — Hydrostatic Pressure

Note that the shape of the fluid container does not affect the hydrostatic pressure. *The pressure is the same at all points at the same depth.*

Concept of Mass Flux (this information may not *be tested on the OAT)*

Mass flux can be defined as the rate of change of mass of a fluid. It represents mass flow per unit time. It is an extremely important parameter to measure flow of blood from the heart, flow of substances into the kidneys, and also the flow of air into the lungs.

Fluids in motion are described by two equations, the continuity equation and Bernoulli's Equation. Fluids are assumed to have streamlined flow that means that the motion of every particle in the fluid follows the same path as the particle that preceded it. Turbulent flow occurs when one path is not followed, molecules collide, energy is dissipated and frictional drag is increased.

Bernoulli's Equation is an application of the Law of Conservation of Energy and is:

$$P + \rho gh + 1/2\rho v^2 = \text{constant}$$

$$\text{pressure energy} + \text{potential energy} + \text{kinetic energy} = \text{constant}$$

Another important property of fluids is *viscosity*. Viscosity is analogous to friction between moving solids. It may, therefore, be viewed as the resistance to flow between layers of fluid (as in streamline or laminar flow) sliding relative to each other. This also means that viscosity, as friction, results in dissipation of mechanical energy.

Surface Tension

Molecules of a liquid exert attractive forces toward each other (*cohesive forces*), and exert attractive forces toward surfaces they touch (*adhesive forces*). As an example, mercury has no adhesion for glass (does not stick to glass), whereas water has adhesion for glass (does stick to glass in droplets).

4.9.2 Questions to Review Fluid Properties

1. All are characteristics of forces and pressures exerted by fluids *except*
A. forces are always perpendicular to the container walls
B. pressure is directly proportional to the product of depth and fluid density
C. pressure depends on the shape and size of the container
D. buoyant force of submerged object equals the weight of the displaced fluid

2. Bernoulli's Equation is an application of
A. the 2nd Law of Thermodynamics.
B. the Law of Conservation of Momentum.
C. the Law of Conservation of Mass.
D. the Law of Conservation of Energy.

3. A fluid has a density (d) of 5 gms/ml and fills a container up to a height (h) of 10 cms. The pressure (P) on the floor of the container is
A. 49,000 dynes/cm^2.
B. 50 nts/m^2.
C. 50 V dynes/cm^2 where V = volume in ml.
D. unknown and cannot be calculated.

4. In order for an object to float in a fluid, it must
A. be made of a substance more dense than the fluid.
B. be made of a substance less dense than the fluid.
C. displace its own weight in the fluid.
D. displace its own volume in the fluid.

5. The relative diameters of the blood vessels of the body and the relative flows are:
arteries > arterioles > capillaries
In which of the above is turbulent flow most likely?
A. artery
B. arteriole
C. capillary
D. all equal

4.9.3 Answers to Questions in Section 4.9.2

(1) C (2) D (3) A (4) C (5) A

4.10 THERMAL ENERGY, HEAT TRANSFER, AND THERMODYNAMICS

Thermodynamics deals with the physical laws that determine transfer and flow of heat.

4.10.1 Thermal Energy

Heat is a form of energy. Bodies *do not contain* heat; they either emit or absorb energy as heat. *Thermal equilibrium* results when the average kinetic energies per molecule of two bodies are equal. This is also the case when the heat flow between the bodies is zero, the when the temperatures of the two bodies are equal. *Temperature* is taken to be a measure of the average thermal energy of a body; it is also a measure of the amount of energy absorbed or emitted as heat by a body. *Measurement of temperature* is by thermometers. A *thermometer* has (1) a thermometric property (e.g., pressure, density, linear expansion, resistance) that varies directly as temperature; (2) a lower fixed point (e.g., freezing point (FP) of water); (3) a higher fixed point (e.g., boiling point (BP) of water); and (4) a scale calibrated between these two points and extrapolated beyond them. Relative temperature scales are the *Celsius* or *Centigrade* (FP of water = 0°C, BP of water = 100°C) and the *Fahrenheit* (FP of water = 32°F, BP of water = 212°F). Absolute scales (the zero point of the scale is the true absolute zero) are the *Rankine* (°R) calibrated in °F units and the *Kelvin* (°K) calibrated in °C units.

Heat capacity is a measure of the amount of heat a body can gain (or lose) per change in temperature (Δt),

heat capacity = heat gained/temperature change = $Q/\Delta t$.

Specific heat capacity (C) is the heat capacity per unit mass of substance:

$C = (Q/\Delta t)/m = Q/m\Delta t$.

The units of heat most commonly used are calories. A calorie is the amount of heat required to raise the temperature of 1 gram of water one degree Celsius.

A kilocalorie is 1000 calories. Since heat is a form of energy, its units must be equivalent to the unit of other energies (kinetic or potential) or work that is the Joule (or other similar units). *The interconversion of calories and joules is:*

4.184 joules = 1 calorie
4.2 joules = 1 calorie

The *specific heat of water is then:*

1 (calorie/gm – °C).

Heat Transfer Map

It is in the understanding of *phase transitions* that specific heat, heat of fusion and heat of vaporization have particular value. Below are the important features of phase transitions:

Phase Transition	Conditions	Heat Associated
(1) solid $\underset{\text{freeze}}{\overset{\text{melt}}{\rightleftharpoons}}$ liquid	Solid and liquid vapor pressure in equilibrium. Temperature called melting (or freezing) point (MP or FP).	heat of fusion (H_f) H_f = Q/m at MP or $Q = m\,H_f$ Q = heat transferred m = mass
liquid $\underset{\text{condense}}{\overset{\text{evaporate (boil)}}{\rightleftharpoons}}$ gas	Gas and liquid vapor pressure in equilibrium. Temperature called the boiling point (BP)	Heat of evaporation (H_v) H_v = Q/m at BP or $Q = H_v\,m$

Note that $H_V > H_f$ because usually more kinetic energy per molecule is required to separate liquid molecules to become gaseous than to separate solid molecules to become liquid. As a substance gains or loses energy as heat, it passes through the various phases. A scheme for substances gaining heat is:

Phases & Temps	Solid Below MP (1) →	Solid at MP (2) →	Liquid at MP (3) →	Liquid at BP (4) →	Gas at BP (5) Gas above BP
Heat changes	(1) Heat is absorbed to raise the temperature as the specific heat of the solid: $Q = C\,m\Delta t$	(2) Heat is absorbed as heat of fusion to cause solid to melt to the liquid. Note that the temperature does not change: $Q = H_f\,m$	(3) Heat is absorbed as the specific heat of the liquid to raise its temperature: $Q = C\,m\Delta t$	(4) Heat is absorbed as heat of vaporization to cause the liquid to be converted to gas. The temperature does not change. $Q = H_v\,m$	(5) Heat is absorbed as the specific heat of the gas to raise its temperature: $Q = C\,m\Delta t$

Note: C represents specific heat constant for a solid, liquid, or gas.

Figure 4.6 — Phase Transitions and Heat Transfer Map

Heat flows between substances by three mechanisms: conduction, convection and radiation. *Conduction* is a process in which heat energy is transferred by adjacent molecular collisions throughout a material medium—the medium does not move.

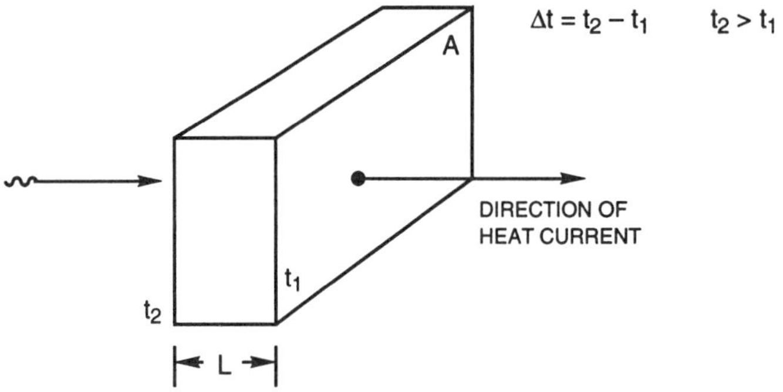

$H = Q/T = kA(\Delta t/L)$
Q = heat exchanged
T = time elapsed
A = cross-sectional area
L = length over which transfer occurs
Δt = temperature difference
k = thermal conductivity of the material.

Figure 4.7 — Heat Conduction

Convection is a process in which heat energy is transferred by the actual mass motion of a fluid (gas or liquid). Convection currents are set up which may be natural (caused by density differences, e.g., wind) or forced (as in a house ventilation system). The rate of energy transfer (H) is:

$H = A/T = hA\Delta t$ (note the relations shown)

The convection coefficient h is not a property of the substance.

Radiation is a process in which heat energy is transferred by electromagnetic waves absorbed or emitted at the atomic level. All substances radiate heat regardless of the temperature. The rate of radiation (heat) emitted per unit area (R) is:

$R = e\sigma T^4$ (Stefan-Boltzmann Law)
T = absolute temperature
e = emissivity = the ability to absorb or emit thermal radiation
σ = Stefan-Boltzmann's constant.

4.10.2 Thermodynamics

Thermodynamics is concerned with physical laws governing the energy states of molecules and chemical reactions. A system is comprised of a large number of molecules, the so-called "object" under study. It is the reference point. When the system gains energy, the (energy) change is positive.

Energy is a property of a system and not a process (like heat exchange or work done). Specifically, the internal energy change (ΔE) of a system depends on the work done and heat exchanged as follows:

$\Delta E = q - W$ *First Law of Thermodynamics*
q = + if heat is added to the system
q = – if heat is lost from the system
$W = +p\Delta V$ is work is done by the system
p = external pressure
$\Delta V = V_f - V_i$ change in volume of the system (this gives the sign to the work done by the system)

The internal energy depends on the kinetic energies of the molecules, on the potential energies of forces between molecules, and the kinetic and potential energies of the electrons and nuclei. The First Law of Thermodynamics is a restatement of the law of conservation of energy. ΔE of a reaction is determined by running the reaction at constant volume and measuring the amount of heat exchanged:

$\Delta E = q - W = q - p\Delta V = q_v$
$\Delta V = 0$
q_v = heat at a constant volume.

A reversible process is one that occurs in such small increments that it can be reversed at any point. An irreversible process is one that cannot be easily reversed. As a concrete example, if you walked down a flight of stairs one step at a time, it would be fairly easy to reverse your direction at any step—this would be a reversible process. But if you jumped out of a window, equivalent to going down a flight of stairs, you could not reverse yourself—this would be an irreversible process. For reversible (rev) and irreversible (irrev) processes, the following are true:

$W_{rev} > W_{irrev}$
$q_{rev} > q_{irrev}$

Entropy (S) and the Second Law of Thermodynamics are based on these concepts.

$\Delta S = (q_{rev}/T)$ for a reversible path = change in entropy

Note: (1) ΔS is still independent of a particular reversible path
(2) $\Delta S = \Delta S$ system + ΔS environment = 0
(3) ΔS exists for an irreversible path but it is not equal to (q_{rev}/T)
(4) ΔS is increasing for an irreversible path.

4.10.3 Questions to Review Thermal Energy, Heat Transfer, and Thermodynamics

1. A measure of the heat of a chemical reaction is
A. entropy.
B. enthalpy.
C. free energy.
D. none of these.

2. Heat
A. is energy contained by an object.
B. is absorbed or emitted by an object.
C. both **A** and **B**.
D. neither **A** nor **B**.
E. is an indirect measure of temperature

3. Heat capacity is
A. the amount of heat a body contains per degree of temperature.
B. the amount of heat a body can gain or lose per degree change in temperature.
C. represented as: temperature/heat.
D. both **A** and **C**.

4. Heat flows between substances by all the following processes *except*
   A. conjugation.
   B. conduction.
   C. convection.
   D. radiation.

5. If C = specific heat capacity, Δt = change in temperature and m = mass, then the amount of heat (Q) exchanged is
   A. $Q = C/m\Delta t$
   B. $Q = C\ m\Delta t$
   C. $Q = Cm/\Delta t$
   D. $Q = C\Delta t/m$

6. In heat transfer in a substance (e.g., a heat-conducting rod), the rate of heat transfer is
   A. directly proportional to the length of the conductor.
   B. indirectly proportional to the temperature difference.
   C. directly proportional to the cross-sectional area of the conductor.
   D. independent of the nature of the substance.

7. A statement of the First Law of Thermodynamics is
   A. $\Delta S = q_{rev}/T$
   B. $\Delta G = \Delta H - T\Delta S$
   C. $\Delta E = q - W$
   D. none of these.

8. An object weighing 10 gms has a specific heat of 2 cals/gm/°C. To raise its temperature from 10°C to 60°C would require how many calories?
   A. 10 cals
   B. 100 cals
   C. 1000 cals
   D. 5000 cals

4.10.4 Answers to Questions in Section 4.10.3

(1) B (2) B (3) B (4) A (5) B (6) C (7) C (8) C

4.11 ELECTROSTATICS AND ELECTROMAGNETISM

4.11.1 Electrostatics

The elementary charges are called positive (+) or negative (–). Each has a charge of 1.6×10^{-19} coulombs but differ in sign. The electron is the negative charge carrier, and the proton is the positive charge carrier. Substances with an excess of electrons have a net negative charge. Substances with a deficiency of electrons have a net positive charge. *Conductors* transmit charge readily. *Insulators* resist the flow of charge.

Charges exert *forces* upon each other. Like charges repel each other; the unlike charges attract. For two charges the force is given by *Coulomb's Law:*

$$F = k(q_1q_2/r^2) = (1/4\pi\varepsilon_0)(q_1q_2/r^2)$$

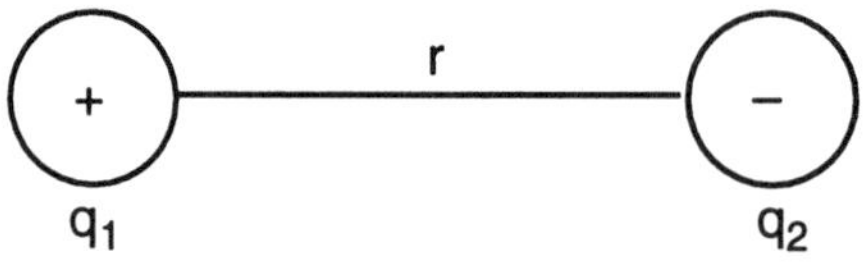

Figure 4.8 — Illustration of Coulomb's Law

q_1, q_2 = charges
k = constant = 9.0×10^9 nt-m²/coul²
ε_0 = permittivity of air to the forces = 8.85×10^{-12} coul²/nt-m²
r = distance between the charges

A charge generates an *electric field (E)* in the space around it. Fields (force fields) are vectors (have direction and magnitude). Charges exert forces upon each other through fields. The direction of a field is the direction a positive charge would move if placed in it. *Electric field lines* are imaginary lines that are in the same direction as E at that point. The direction is away from positive charges and toward negative charges. The *potential energy (PE)* of a charged object in a field would equal the work done on that object to bring it from infinity to a distance (r) from the charge setting up the electric field, or

$$PE = work = Fr = (qE)r = kQq/r$$

Q = charge setting up field

q = charge brought in to a distance r.

The *electric potential (V)* is a scalar, and it is defined at each distance (r) from a charge (Q) generating an electric field. The *potential difference (PD)* is the difference in V between two points, or it is the work per unit positive charge done by electric forces moving a small test charge from the point of higher potential to the point of lower potential (Fig. 4.9).

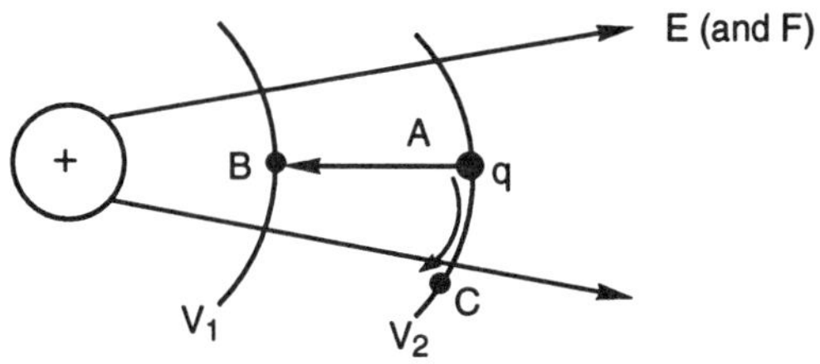

Figure 4.9 — Electrical Potential

An *electric dipole* consists of two charges separated by some finite distance (d). Usually the charges are equal and opposite. A dipole is characterized by its *dipole moment (D.M.)*, which is the product of the charge (q) and d. Dipoles tend to line up with the electric field.

4.11.2 Electromagnetism

This section will enable the student to link magnetism and its numerous applications to electronic structure and the periodic properties of elements; interaction of mechanical, electrical, and magnetic fields; and finally electromagnetic wave spectrum related to accelerating electric charges.

Definition of magnetism and its applications: a magnet has two poles, similar to an electric dipole. Unlike an isolated resting electron that can exist as a monopole, the simplest magnetic structure that can exist is the magnetic dipole. Magnetism is caused by the arrangement of individual atoms in a substance. The applications of magnetism range from stick-on refrigerator magnets to the design of highly sophisticated particle accelerators. As Blackmore discovered, bacteria are guided by the north-end of the magnetic compass, which allows the bacteria to orient themselves in chaotic waters. These *magnetotactic* bacteria have led to advanced research in microbiology.

Types of magnetic materials: Common household magnets are made of Fe_3O_4 molecules. Magnetic materials are of three types: *Diamagnetic.* These are the weakest magnetic materials. The atoms of these materials *do not* have inherent magnetic dipoles. *Paramagnetic.* These substances are relatively stronger than diamagnetic materials. Paramagnetism is the tendency of individual atoms (each with a magnetic dipole) to align along the magnetic field. *Ferromagnetic.* These substances are highly magnetic even without an external magnetic field. These substances have strong inherent magnetic dipoles.

Dimensions of common electromagnetic properties: Electromagnetic properties are represented by a combination of electrical and magnetic variables and constants, e.g., Tesla, Gauss, Weber.

Fundamental rules and laws in Electromagnetism: (1) Opposite magnetic poles attract each other and like magnetic poles repel each other. (2) A moving electric charge or current rearranges the atoms/molecules in a substance. This leads to magnetic fields and a conceptual development of a magnetic charge. (3) If a test charge q is moving at right angles to the magnetic field with $\phi = 90°$, for no deflection,

$$\text{electric force} = \text{magnetic force}$$

$$qE = qvB \sin 90°$$

$$v = \frac{E}{B} \text{ speed of particles in an electron tube}$$

(4) *Biot and Savart law* states that in a long straight wire conducting current I, the magnetic field is proportional to the current and inversely proportional to the perpendicular distance r. (5) *Right-Hand Rule* helps you

determine the direction of the magnetic field set up due to electric current in a wire. (6) *Faraday's law of electromagnetic induction* states that the induced electromotive force in an electric circuit is equal in magnitude to the time rate of change of magnetic flux. (7) *Gauss' law for magnetism* states that isolated magnetic poles (monopoles) do *not* exist.

Electromagnetic Wave Spectrum: It is important to realize that electric fields and magnetic fields are further interrelated. If a magnetic field changes, an electrical field is produced. From the principle of symmetry the reverse is true. An electrical field produced by a changing magnetic field is expressed by Faraday's Law, and a magnetic field produced by a changing electrical field (or by a current, or both) is expressed by the Ampere-Maxwell Law.

4.11.3 Questions to Review Electrostatics and Electromagnetism

1. Concerning fields, which is *incorrect*?
A. They exist in space and are generated by objects (e.g., mass).
B. Gravitational and electrical fields are examples.
C. They are vectors.
D. They exist independently of other objects.
E. Electromagnetic fields are always weaker than electrostatic fields.

2. Electric field lines are
A. directed away from negative charges.
B. directed away from positive charges.
C. directed toward positive charges.
D. directed toward negative charges.
E. none of the above.

3. The potential difference as used in electrostatics is
A. the difference in potential energy between two points.
B. the difference in electric potential between two points.
C. the difference in work between two points.
D. both A and C.
E. A, B, and C.

4. All are true about electric dipoles *except*
A. they consist of two charges separated by a finite distance.
B. the dipole moment is a product of the charge and the distance between them.
C. the motion of dipoles against an electric field requires no energy.
D. the positive end of the dipole points in the direction of the electric field.

5. The electric field (E) generated by a charge
A. is constant at all distances from the charge.
B. decreases directly as distance from the charge increases.
C. decreases proportional to the inverse square of the distance from the charge.
D. decreases proportional to the inverse distance from the charge.

6. Using Gauss' Law of Magnetism, which of the following statements is true:
A. The simplest magnetic structure is a dipole.
B. Magnetic flux varies with the charge.
C. Magnetic flux is not related to change in surface area of the magnetic field.
D. Magnetic flux varies with the velocity of the charge.

4.11.4 Answers to Questions in Section 4.11.3

(1) E (2) B (3) B (4) C (5) C (6) C

4.12 ELECTRIC CIRCUITS

The main elements in an electric (DC = direct current) circuit are the emf source (V) and the resistors (R). The current (I) results from their interaction. These three quantities are interrelated in *Ohm's Law* as:

$$V = IR.$$

V, I, and R are the total of each in the circuit. Capacitors may also be used in electronic circuits. Circuit elements may be in series, in parallel, or in combinations of both. Two components are in *series* when they have only one point in common; that is, the current traveling from one of them back to the emf source *must* pass through the other. Two components are in *parallel* when they are connected to two common points in the circuit; that is, the current traveling from one such element back to the source of emf (assume current started at source of emf) need not pass through the second component because there is an alternate path.

Electromotive force (V) maintains a constant potential difference and thereby maintains a continuous current. The emf source replaces energy lost by the moving electrons. The *units of emf (E)* are volts. The actual voltage delivered to a circuit is not equal to the V_T value of the source. V_T represents the total potential difference across the external source terminals. It is also called the EMF of the source. Generally $V_T = V$ unless otherwise specified.

Resistance (R) is the opposition to the flow of electrons in a substance. *Resistivity (ρ)* is an inherent property of a substance and is directly related to resistance. Resistivity varies directly as resistance and cross-sectional area, and indirectly as length. Resistance increases with temperature because the thermal motion of atoms (molecules) increases and results in more collisions with electrons that impede their flow. The units of resistance are ohms symbolized by Ω (omega).

Resistance in a series circuit is

$$R = R_1 + R_2 + R_3 + \dots$$

Resistance in a parallel circuit is

$$1/R = 1/R_1 + 1/R_2 + 1/R_3 + \dots$$

Capacitance (C) is an inherent property of a conductor and is formulated as

$$C = \text{charge/electric potential} = Q/V = \text{farad} = \text{coulomb/volt}.$$

This means that C is the number of coulombs that must be transferred to a conductor to raise its potential by one volt. The amount of charge that can be stored is determined by the size, shape, and surroundings of the conductor. A *capacitor* is two or more conductors with opposite but equal charges placed near each other. The *dielectric substances* set up an opposing electric field to that of the capacitor, which decreases the net electric field and allows the capacitance of the capacitor to increase (C = Q/Ed).

The *energy associated with each charged capacitor* is

$$V_{avg} = 1/2V$$

$$\text{Potential Energy (PE)} = W = (1/2V)(Q) = 1/2QV = 1/2(CV)(V) = 1/2CV^2$$

$$= 1/2\ Q(Q/C) = 1/2Q^2/C.$$

The *symbol for a capacitor* is

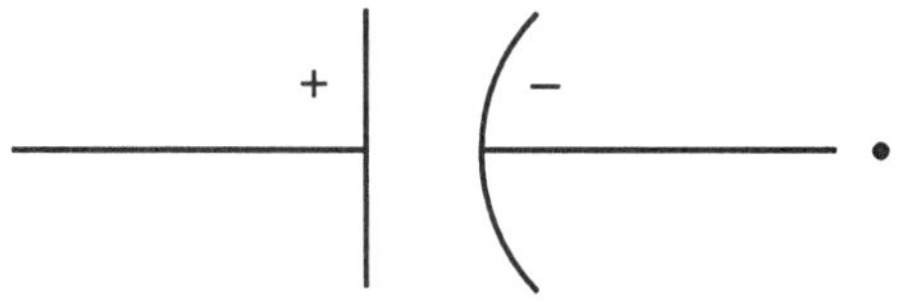

Figure 4.10 — Symbol for a Capacitor

In an *electric circuit, the capacitor* charges up until the charge (Q_{max}) equals V_tC and then the current stops. In an *alternating electric circuit (AC))*, there is an alternating surge of charge onto and off the capacitor, and a current exists there even though there is no transfer of charge between the plates.

4.12.1 Questions to Review Electric Circuits

1. In a DC circuit:
   A. if series, the currents are different for each component (e.g., resistors, capacitors)
   B. if series, the voltages are the same for each component.
   C. if parallel, the currents are equal for all paths (of the circuit)
   D. if parallel, the voltages are equal for all paths

2. The actual voltage output of an electromotive source
   A. may be equal to, less than, or greater than the expected voltage of the source.
   B. is always equal to the expected voltage.
   C. is always more than the expected voltage.
   D. is always less than the expected voltage.

3. Normally, a charge gains energy as it moves through a source of emf, but it can lose energy if
   A. the emf source has an internal resistance.
   B. the emf source has a reversed polarity.
   C. the emf source is a generator.
   D. the emf source is of low voltage.

4. The resistance of a substance can be expected to increase for all the following situations *except*
   A. increasing cross-sectional area
   B. increasing length
   C. increasing temperature
   D. increasing resistivity of materials

5. Current is
   A. caused by the movement of positive charge.
   B. increased by the thermal motion of atoms.
   C. decreased by impurities in the conductor.
   D. all of the above.

4.12.2 Answers to Questions in Section 4.12.1

(1) D (2) D (3) B (4) A (5) C

4.13 OPTICS

4.13.1 The Human Eye

Anatomically, the eye is separated by the *lens* into an anterior region filled by the *aqueous humor* and a posterior region filled by the *vitreous humor.* There are three layers in the eye. The *sclera* (dense connective tissue) is the outermost. It is covered anteriorly by the conjunctiva (whites of the eyes). It is continuous with the clear portion called the *cornea*, which is important in focusing light. Inside the sclera is the *choroid*, which contains the blood vessels and black pigment to prevent light scattering. Continuous with the choroid in front are the *iris* (which gives the eye its color and opens and shuts to let light in through the *pupil*) and the *ciliary muscle* (which controls the shape of the lens and helps to focus or accommodate the eye to distance). The innermost layer is the *retina*, which is the light sensitive layer containing a mixture of rods and cones. *Rods* are concentrated more peripherally in the eye, are concerned with vision in dim light and peripheral vision, and contain *rhodopsin* (retinal from Vit A and a protein called opsin). Light converts retinal from a *cis* to a *trans* form, which causes rhodopsin to fall apart and somehow sets up an impulse that is eventually transmitted to the optic nerve (Cranial Nerve II). Cones are concentrated more centrally, are more sensitive to bright light and are responsible for color vision, contain *iodopsin* (light sensitive substance) and are maximally concentrated at the *fovea* (or macula area) which has the highest visual acuity (ability to see clearly points that are close together).

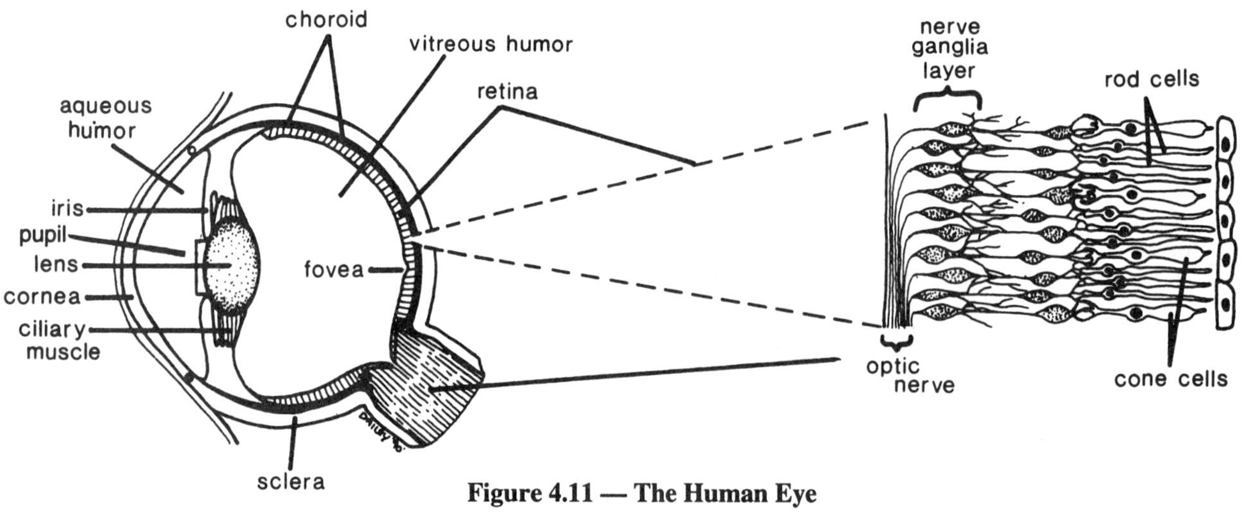

Figure 4.11 — The Human Eye

Light passes through the cornea where it is refracted (bent). It then passes through the aqueous humor and then through the pupil. The pupil size is regulated by the iris, which is regulated by the parasympathetic (causes pupil to get smaller) and the sympathetic (causes pupil to get larger) systems. Next, the light passes through the lens where it is refracted further and focused upon the retina (after it passes through the vitreous humor). The lens is flat for objects far away (ciliary muscle relaxed), and it is rounded for objects nearby (ciliary muscle contracted—parasympathetic). Light then stimulates the cones and rods of the retina. From here nerve impulses are transmitted via the Ocular nerve (II) to the visual center in the occipital cortex of the cerebrum.

Emmetropia means that light is focused on the retina (by the cornea-lens system) when objects are near or far. *Myopia* (near-sightedness) means light is focused on the retina only when objects are near but not when objects are far away. *Hypermetropia* (far-sightedness) means light is focused on the retina when objects are far away and not when they are near.

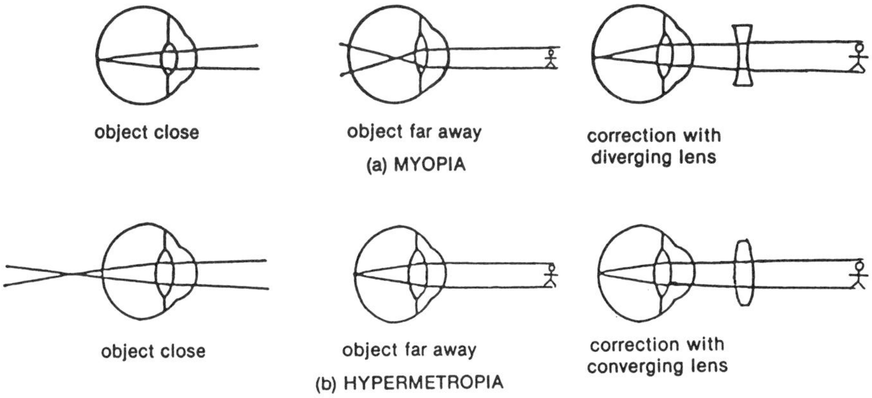

Figure 4.12 — (a) Myopia and (b) Hypermetropia

4.13.2 Reflection

Reflection is the process by which light rays (imaginary lines drawn perpendicular to advancing wave fronts) bounce back into a medium from a surface with another medium (versus being refracted or absorbed). The *Laws of Reflection* are (1) the angle of incidence (I) equals the angle of reflection (R) at the normal (N, perpendicular to surface), and (2) the I, R, N all lie on the same plane.

Mirrors may have a plane surface or a curved surface; only spherical curved mirrors will be discussed. A *virtual image* has no light rays passing through it and cannot be projected on a screen. A *real image* has light rays passing through it and can be projected on a screen. *Spherical mirrors* may have the reflecting surface convex (diverges light) or concave (converges light). Note the images formed by a converging mirror (concave) are like those for a converging lens (convex); and diverging mirrors (convex) and diverging lens (concave) also form similar images.

With *concave mirrors (spherical)* the incident light is converged (toward the axis). With *convex (spherical) mirrors,* the incident light is diverged (from the axis) after reflection. The *mirror equation* and derivations from it allow the relations between object and image to be calculated instead of memorized. The equation is valid for convex and concave mirrors:

$$1/i + 1/o = 1/f$$
$$f = R/2$$
$$M = \text{magnification} = -i/o$$

conventions: for i and o, positive values mean real, negative values mean virtual,
for R and f, positive means converging, negative is diverging,
for M, positive means erect, negative is inverted.

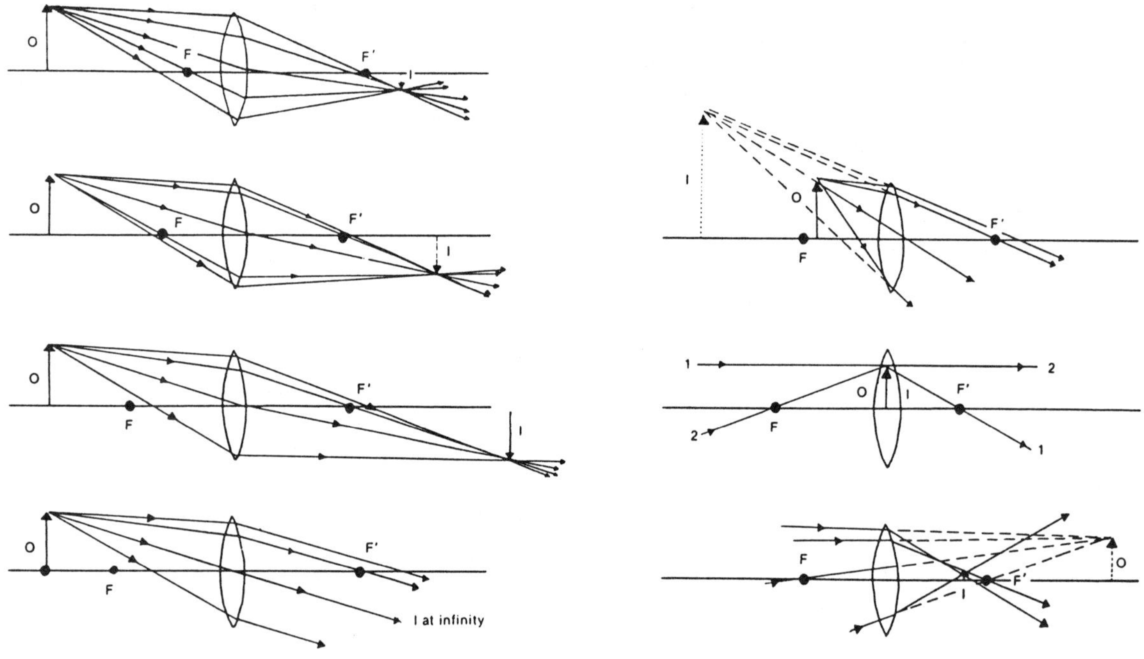

Figure 4.13 — Refraction through Convex Lens

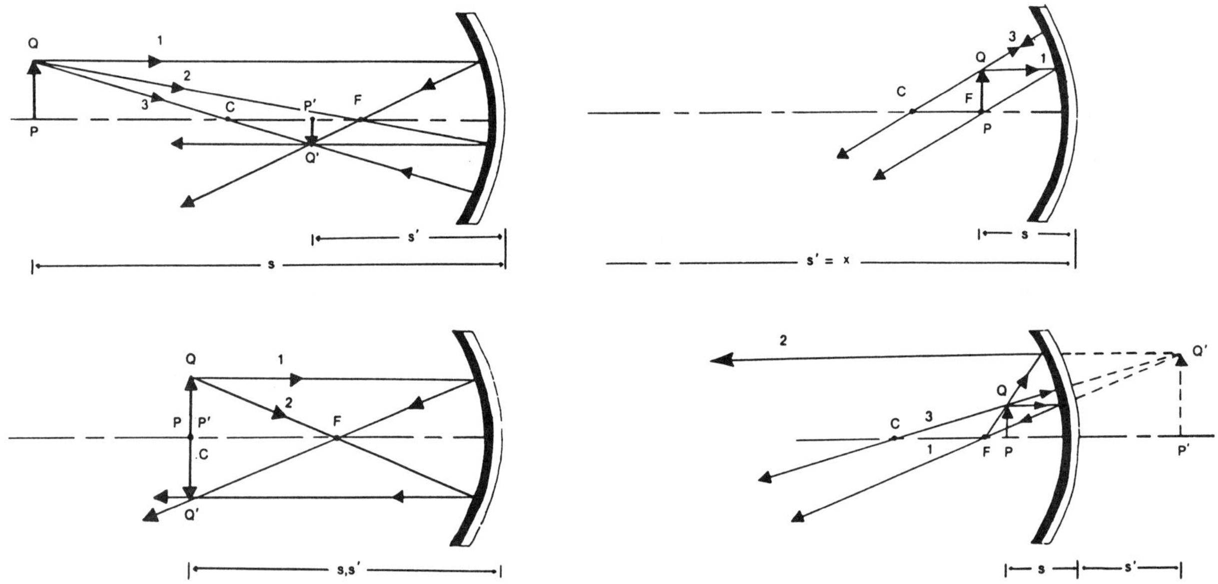

Figure 4.14 — Reflection from Concave Mirrors

4.13.3 Refraction

Refraction is the bending of light as it passes from one transparent medium to another and is caused by the different speeds of light in the two media. The *Laws of Refraction* are (1) The incident ray, the refracted ray, and the normal ray all lie in the same plane. (2) The path of the ray (incident and refracted parts) is reversible.

A *lens* is a transparent material that refracts light. Converging lenses refract light toward the axis, and diverging lenses refract light away from the axis. A converging lens is wider at the middle than at the ends, and a diverging lens is thinner at the middle than at the ends.

For a *converging lens* (biconvex, e.g.) the image formed depends on the object distance relative to the focal length (f). For a *diverging lens* (biconcave, e.g.) the image is always virtual, erect, and reduced in size as for a diverging mirror.

4.13.4 Questions to Review Optics

1. All are true of images seen in plane (flat) mirrors *except*
A. they are always virtual.
B. they appear at a distance behind the mirror equal to the distance (perpendicular) of the object in front of the mirror.
C. they are right-left reversed.
D. they are inverted.

2. The reflected rays from a convex mirror
A. diverge.
B. converge.
C. are parallel.
D. are diffused.

3. The mirror equation is
(f = focal length, o = object distance, i = image distance)
A. f = o + i
B. f = 1/o + 1/i
C. 1/f = o + i
D. 1/f = 1/o + 1/i

4. The index of refraction of a medium is
A. the speed of light in free space divided by the speed of light in that medium.
B. the density of the medium divided by the density of air.
C. the absorption of light in the medium divided by the absorption of light in water.
D. none of the above.

5. A concave lens
A. diverges light.
B. converges light.
C. both.
D. neither.

6. Which structure is anterior to the lens in the human eye?
A. aqueous humor
B. vitreous humor
C. retina
D. choroid

7. All are functions or properties of cones of the eye *except*
A. provide for high visual acuity.
B. peripheral vision.
C. color vision.
D. vision in bright lights.

4.13.5 Answers to Questions in Section 4.13.4

(1) B (2) A (3) D (4) A (5) A (6) A (7) B

4.14 NUCLEAR AND ATOMIC STRUCTURE

4.14.1 Review of Nuclear Structure

An atom is made of a *nucleus* containing protons (mass = 1 a.m.u., charge + 1) and neutrons (mass = 1 a.m.u., charge = 0). The *atomic number (AN)* is the number of protons in the nucleus of an atom. An *element* is a group of atoms with the same AN; i.e., it is the number of protons that make elements different from each other. The *mass number (MN)* is the sum of protons and neutrons in a given atom (not element!). *Isotopes* are atoms of the same elements with different MNs, i.e., they have the same number of protons but different numbers of neutrons. The *atomic weight (AW)* is the weighted average of all naturally occurring isotopes of an element.

Coulomb repulsive forces (between protons) in the nuclei are overcome by *nuclear forces.* The nuclear force is a nonelectrical type of force that binds nuclei together and is equal for protons and neutrons. The *nuclear binding energy (E_b)* is a result of the Coulomb and nuclear binding forces. Einstein derived the relation between energy and mass changes associated with nuclear reactions,

$\Delta E = \Delta mc^2$ = ergs if m = grams and c = cm/sec
ΔE = energy released or absorbed
Δm = mass lost (*mass deficit*) or gained, respectively
c = speed of light = 3.0×10^{10} cm/sec

conversions:

1 gram = 9×10^{20} ergs
1 amu (atomic mass unit) = 931.4 MeV
1 amu = 1/12 the mass of $_6C^{12}$

The above is a statement of the *Law of Conservation of Mass and Energy.*

Not all combinations of protons are equally likely or stable. an even number of protons or an even number of neutrons, in general, means the nuclei are more stable. The *most stable* nuclei are those with an even number of protons and an even number of neutrons. The *least stable* nuclei are those with an odd number of protons and an odd number of neutrons.

Unstable nuclei can become stable nuclei by fission (splitting) to smaller nuclei or by absorbing or emitting small particles. Spontaneous fission is rare. *Spontaneous radioactivity* (emitting particles) is common. The common particles are (1) *alpha (α) particle* ^4_2He (helium nucleus); (2) *beta (β) particle* -1^{e° (an electron); (3) a *positron* $+1^{e^\circ}$; (4) *gamma (γ) ray*—no mass, just energy; and (5) *orbital electron capture*—nucleus takes electrons from K shell and converts a proton to a neutron.

Nuclear reactions are reactions in which changes in nuclear composition occur.

4.14.2 Review of Electron Energy Levels

The energy that an electron contains is not continuous over the whole range of possible energies. Rather, electrons in an atom may contain only discrete energies and occupy certain orbits. Electrons of each atom are restricted to these discrete energy levels. These levels have an energy below zero. This means energy is released when an electron moves from infinity into these energy levels. A representative set of energy levels of an electron in an atom may be:

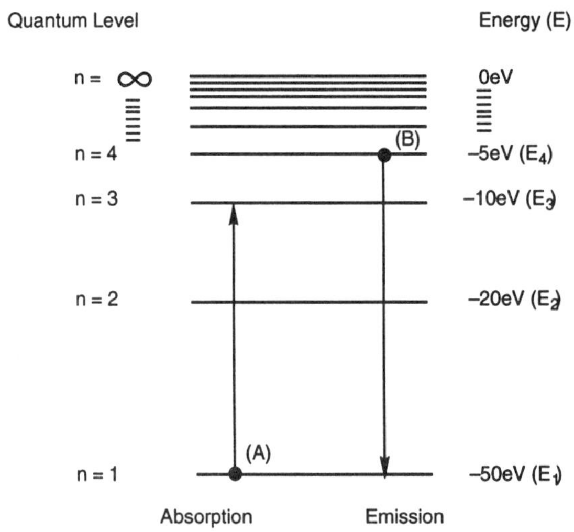

Figure 4.15 — Absorption and Emission Spectra

If there is one electron in the atom above, its *ground state* will be in the n = 1, or lowest energy level available. Any other energy level, n = 2 or n = 3, e.g., is considered an *excited state* for that electron. The difference in energies (E) between the levels gives the energy and, hence, frequency (f) of light necessary to cause the excitation (absorption, electron A):

$$E_3 - E_1 = hf$$

E_1 = energy level one
E_3 = energy level three
h = Planck's Constant
f = frequency of light absorbed.

An *emission spectrum* results when an electron is excited to a higher level by another particle or by an electric discharge, for example. Then, as the electron falls from the excited state to lower states, light is emitted that has wavelength (frequency) corresponding to the energy difference between the levels.

Fluorescence is an emission process that occurs after light absorption excites electrons to higher electronic and vibrational levels. The electrons spontaneously lose excited vibrational energy to the electronic level and then emit light as they fall to the ground vibrational and electronic states.

4.14.3 Questions to Review Nuclear and Atomic Structure

1. A proton is _______ charged and has a mass of _______ amu(s).
A. positively, one
B. negatively, 1/1845
C. neutral, one
D. none of the above

2. The particles that distinguish one element from another are the
A. neutrons.
B. protons.
C. electrons.
D. mesons.

3. Which of the following particles is emitted by nuclei in spontaneous radioactivity?
A. α-particle
B. β-particle
C. γ-ray
D. all of the above

4. The atomic weight of an element is
A. the weighted average of naturally occurring isotopes.
B. the sum of protons and neutrons.
C. twice the number of protons.
D. none of the above.

4.14.4 Answers to Questions in Section 4.14.3

(1) A (2) B (3) D (4) A

4.15 EXPLANATORY SOLUTIONS TO PROBLEMS IN PHYSICS

Discussion of Answers to Questions in Section 4.3.1

Questions #1, #2: Use your physics textbook or the Penguin dictionary of physics.

Question #3 (Answer: C) Use the formula for distance:

$$d = d_o + v_o t + \frac{1}{2}at^2 = 5 + (10)(5) + \frac{1}{2}(5)(5)^2$$
$$= 5 + 50 + \left(\frac{1}{2}\right)(5)(25) = 55 + \frac{1}{2}(125)$$
$$= 55 + 62.5 = 117.5$$

Question #4, #5: Use your physics textbook or the Penguin dictionary of physics.

Question #6 (Answer: D) Using the equations for accelerated motion and g = gravitational acceleration:

$$d = d_o + v_o t + \frac{1}{2}gt^2$$
$$d = 0 + (0)(10) + \left(\frac{1}{2}\right)(-9.8)(10)^2 = -490 \text{ m}$$

Discussion of Answers to Questions in Section 4.4.1

Questions #1 to #3: Use your physics textbook or the Penguin dictionary of physics.

Question #4 (Answer: D) If the relationship is not already known to you, it may be determined (in this case) by knowing unit interrelations (i.e., by doing dimensional analysis as shown):

energy = work = Fd
Force = energy/displacement, which is the *form* of answer (4).

Force = newtons and energy = joules = *newtons-meters* and d = meters, the only way to combine the units of energy and displacement to yield the units of force is:

$$\text{newtons (force)} \propto \frac{\text{newtons-meters (energy)}}{\text{meters (displacement)}} = \text{newtons}$$

or

$$\text{Force} \propto \frac{\text{energy}}{\text{displacement}}$$

Force is proportional to energy/displacement.

Question #5 (Answer: C) The schematic showing the forces is:

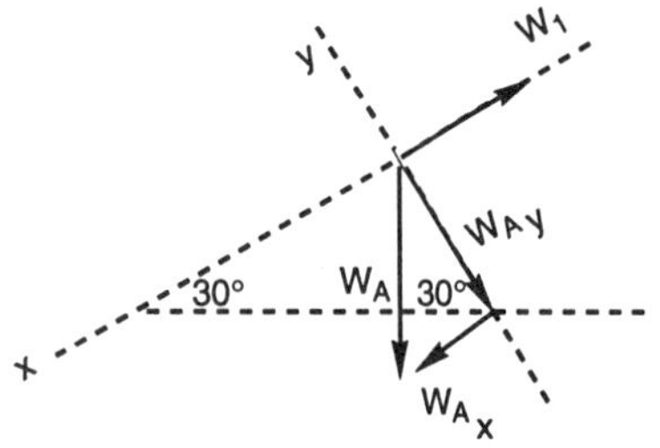

$W_A = mg = (10)(9.8) = 98$ nts

$W_{A_x} = W_A \sin 30° = (98)(1/2) = 49$nts

Remember:

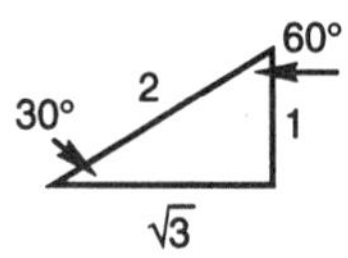

sin 30° = 1/2

Discussion of Answers to Questions in Section 4.5.1

Questions #1, #2: Use your physics textbook or the Penguin dictionary of physics.

Question #3: The forces, their moment arms (r) and directions of rotation (R) are:

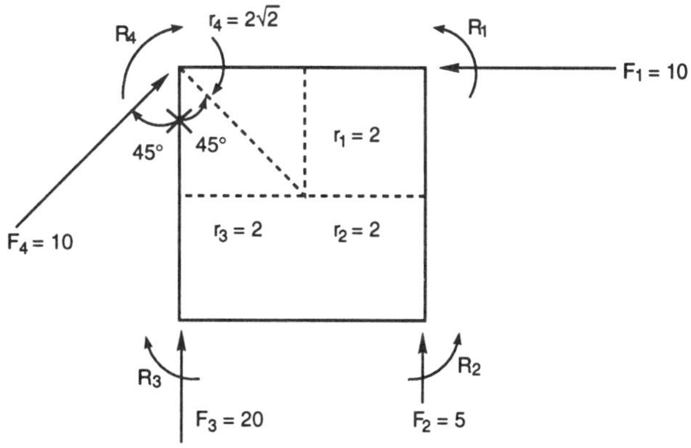

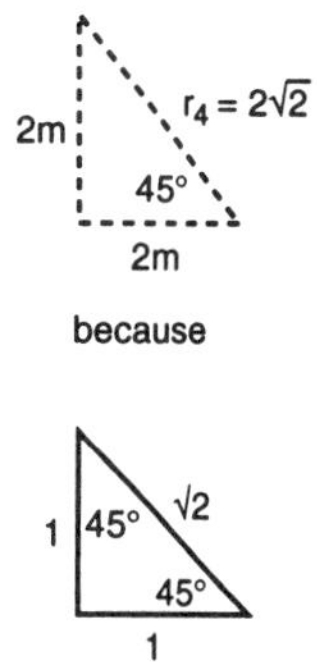

The torques are:

Counterclockwise (+)

$L_1 = F_1 \times r_1 = (10)(2) = +20 \text{ nt} \bullet \text{m}$

$L_2 = F_2 \times r_2 = (5)(2) = +10 \text{ nt} \bullet \text{m}$

Clockwise

$L_3 = F_3 \times r_3 = -(20)(2) = -40 \text{ nt} \bullet \text{m}$

$L_4 = F_4 \times r_4 = -(10)(2\sqrt{2}) = -20\sqrt{2} = -28.2 \text{ nt} \bullet \text{m}$

The net torque (L) is:

$L = L_1 + L_2 + L_3 + L_4 = +20 + 10 - 40 - 28.2 = +30 - 68.2$

$L = -38.2 \text{ nt} \bullet \text{m}$ (which is clockwise).

Question #4: These are opposing forces acting along the same line of action. The net force is the algebraic sum (assume positive is to the right):

net force = +10 nts – 5 nts = + 5 nts.

Discussion of Answers to Questions in Section 4.6.1

Questions #1, #2: Use your physics textbook or the Penguin dictionary of physics.

Question #3 (Answer: B)

$$\Delta U = U_2 - U_1 = mgh_2 - mgh_1 = mg(h_2 - h_1)$$
$$= (5)(9.8)(10 - 20) = (5)(9.8)(-10) = -490 \text{ joules.}$$

Question #4: (Answer: A)

$W = Fd \cos\theta$

For $\theta = 0°, \cos\theta = 1$

$W = Fd = (10)(20) = 200$ joules

Discussion of Answers to Questions in Section 4.7.1

Questions #1, #2, #3, and #6 Use your physics textbook or the Penguin dictionary of physics.

Question #4 (Answer: D)

c = speed of light = λf

Question #5 (Answer: C)

$v = \lambda f$

$\lambda = v/f = 5{,}000/10{,}000 = 0.5$ m

Discussion of Answers to Question in Section 4.8.2

Questions #1 through #4: Use your physics textbook or the Penguin dictionary of physics.

Question #5: (Answer: B) v = sound speed

$$F_o = f_s\left(\frac{v + v_o}{v - v_s}\right) = 1000\frac{(350 + 14)}{(350 - 24)} = 1000\frac{(364)}{(326)} = 1{,}116 \text{ Hz}$$

Question #6: Use your physics textbook or the Penguin dictionary of physics.

Discussion of Answers to Questions in Section 4.9.2

Questions #1 and #2: Use your physics textbook or the Penguin dictionary of physics.

Question #3 (Answer: A)

$$P = F/A = \rho gh$$

$$P = (5 \text{ gms/cm}^3)(980 \text{ cms/sec}^2)(10 \text{ cms}) = 49{,}000 \text{ (gm-cm/sec}^2\text{)/cm}^2$$

$$P = 49{,}000 \text{ dynes/cm}^2$$

$$\text{dyne} = \text{(gm-cm)/sec}^2.$$

Question #4 (Answer: C) If (B) were true, large ships would never float by virtue of their shape, which makes the density of the whole object (not the steel material) less than that of water.

Question #5 (Answer: A) Turbulence is best estimated using Reynolds number (R) or by remembering the relations from R. The viscosity and density of the fluid (i.e., the blood) is constant. Since diameter (d) and velocity (v) are greatest in the arteries and

$$\text{turbulence} \propto (v)(d)$$

they have the highest turbulence. The velocity is greater in the arteries because the total cross-sectional area of the arteries is less than the total cross-sectional area of the capillaries.

Discussion of Answers to Questions in Section 4.10.3

Questions #1 to #7: Use your physics textbook or the Penguin dictionary of physics.

Question #8: (Answer: C)

$$Q = C\,m\Delta t = 2(\text{cals/gm} \cdot {}^\circ\text{C})(10 \text{ gms})(60 - 10^\circ\text{C}) = (2)(10)(50) \text{ cals}$$

$$Q = 1000 \text{ cals}$$

Discussion of Answers to Questions in Section 4.11.3

Questions #1 through #4: Use your physics textbook or the Penguin dictionary of physics.

Question #5: (Answer: C) The formula for the electric field (E) is:

$$E = F/q_o = kq/r^2; \text{ hence } E \propto 1/r^2.$$

Question #6: Use your physics textbook or the Penguin dictionary of physics.

Discussion of Answers to Questions in Section 4.12.1

Questions #1 through #5: Use your physics textbook or the *Penguin Dictionary of Physics..*

Discussion of Answers to Questions in Section 4.13.4

Questions #1 through #7: Use your physics textbook or the Penguin dictionary of physics.

Discussion of Answers to Questions in Section 4.14.2

Question #1 to #4: Use your physics textbook or the Penguin dictionary of physics.

4.16 REFERENCES

1. Tippens, Paul E., *Applied Physics,* 3rd or latest Edition. New York: McGraw-Hill Book Company.
2. Halliday, D., and R. Resnick, *Fundamentals of Physics,* 3rd or latest Edition. New York: John Wiley & Sons, Inc.
3. Harris, N. C., and E. M. Hemmerling, *Introductory Applied Physics,* 4th or latest Edition. New York: McGraw-Hill Book Company.
4. Illingworth, V., (editor), *The Penguin Dictionary of Physics*, 2nd edition. New York: Penguin Books USA, 1991.

Common Instruments Used by Veterinarians

Learn the physical principles which control the working of each instrument.

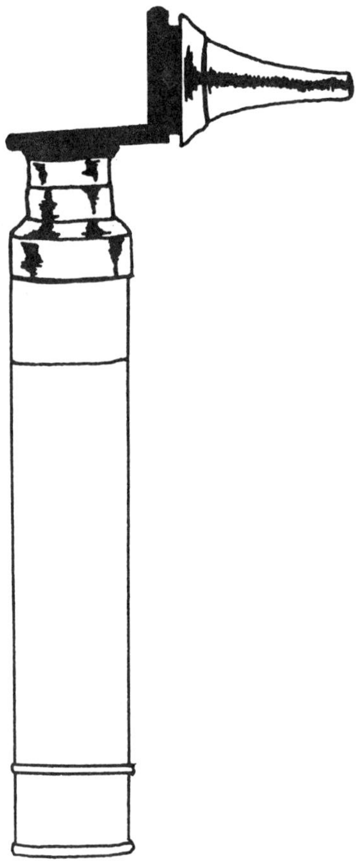

Otoscope

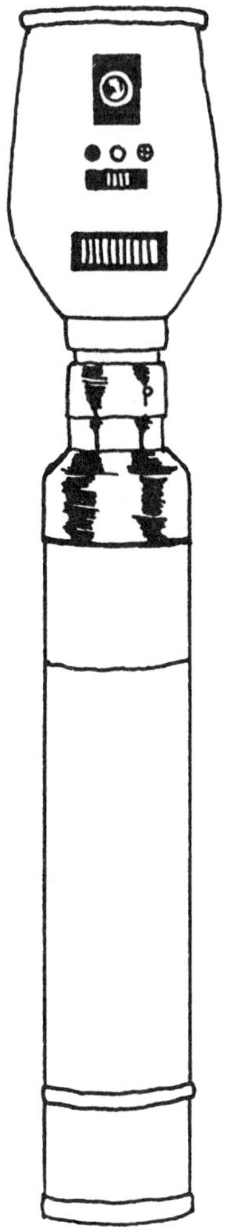

Ophthalmoscope

Otoscope

Otoscopes are used to illuminate and examine the internal ear canal and eardrum in dogs and cats. Each instrument comes with a rechargeable battery in the handle and a selection of plastic speculums in different sizes. Some otoscopes are specially designed to allow passage of a variety of surgical instruments and catheters into the ear canal if needed.

Ophthalmoscope

Ophthalmoscopes have a complex internal structure of lenses that enable the clinician to examine the inner structure of a patient's eye. Through manipulations of these lenses, a veterinarian can measure the size and depth of both normal and abnormal structures within the eye.

Chapter 5

Survey of the Natural Sciences

5.0 INTRODUCTION TO SURVEY OF THE NATURAL SCIENCES

The natural sciences tested on the Optometry Admission Test (OAT) are biology, general chemistry, and organic chemistry. The OAT evaluates a student's scientific ability and aptitude with a total of 100 questions from natural sciences. There are 40 questions in biology, 30 questions in general chemistry, and 30 questions in organic chemistry. Physics is *not* required for the Natural Sciences examination. The questions are sequentially arranged in biology, general chemistry, and organic chemistry, and are not separated by subject matter or content outline. In this chapter, the manual illustrates the types of questions and level of subject matter tested on the OAT. There is no formal review provided in this manual. Biology, general chemistry, and organic chemistry should be reviewed from college textbooks using the detailed subject outline provided below. As mentioned earlier, do *not* forget to blend the various reading comprehension skills, quantitative reasoning skills, and perceptual ability skills in your review of the natural sciences.

In various parts of this chapter, certain salient features of a specific topic are explained briefly to show what subject matter is relatively more important. Do *not* assume that this brief exposure to certain concepts is enough for the OAT review.

5.1 BIOLOGY

This section outlines the subject of biology. The material is divided into content groups with a short listing of the topics that should be mastered. A biology review test is included to illustrate the level of difficulty of OAT questions. Use these questions to gauge your understanding of OAT biology and to identify specific topics requiring more independent study and biology review. To measure your competency, use the book *A Complete Preparation for the MCAT* (the Flowers' Guide) for review and the Graduate Record Examination (GRE) subject books (biology, general, and organic chemistry) to test your aptitude. The GRE special test books are printed by Educational Testing Service and may be purchased from Betz Publishing Company, the publishers of this book.

5.1.1 Biology Outline

A. Origin of Life
- **1.** Introduction
- **2.** Review of Various Theories

B. Cell Metabolism
- **1.** Definition, example
  - **a.** Cellular Respiration
    - **(i)** Aerobic Respiration
    - **(ii)** Anaerobic Respiration
  - **b.** Photosynthesis
    - **(i)** Autotrophs
    - **(ii)** Heterotrophs
    - **(iii)** Definition, equation
  - **c.** Respiration vs. photosynthesis

C. Enzymology
- **1.** Review of enzymes
  - **a.** Definition, function, and example
  - **b.** Coenzymes
  - **c.** Specificity of an enzyme
  - **d.** Enzyme and Substrate (Lock and Key) model
  - **e.** Feedback inhibition
    - **(i)** Definition
    - **(ii)** Graphic Enzyme Reaction
    - **(iii)** Chart of Digestive Enzymes

D. Thermodynamics and Cellular Bioenergetics
- **1.** Definitions
  - **a.** Heat and Internal Energy
  - **b.** Thermal Equilibrium and Temperature
- **2.** Bioenergetics
  - **a.** Basic Definitions
  - **b.** Energy production
    - **(i)** Glycolysis
    - **(ii)** Citric Acid Cycle
    - **(iii)** Electron Transport System
    - **(iv)** Oxidative Phosphorylation

E. Organelle Structure and Function
- **1.** Definition of a Cell, Organelle
  - **a.** Eukaryotic Cell
  - **b.** Prokaryotic Cell
- **2.** Parts of Eukaryotic Cell
  - **a.** Cell Membrane and Transport
    - **(i)** Phospholipids
    - **(ii)** Unit Membrane Model
    - **(iii)** Fluid Mosaic Model
    - **(iv)** Diffusion
    - **(v)** Osmosis
    - **(vi)** Tonicity
    - **(vii)** Facilitated Diffusion
    - **(viii)** Active Transport
    - **(ix)** Phagocytosis
    - **(x)** Pinocytosis
  - **b.** Cytoplasm and Cytoplasm Organelles
    - **(i)** Location of various organelles
    - **(ii)** Function of various organelles
  - **c.** The Nucleus and Cell Mitosis
    - **(i)** Chromatin
    - **(ii)** Chromosomes
    - **(iii)** Cell Division
    - **(iv)** Cell Cycle
      - **(a)** Interphase
      - **(b)** Prophase
      - **(c)** Metaphase
      - **(d)** Telophase
    - **(v)** Centrioles
- **3.** Example of Eukaryotic Cell
  - **a.** Fungus
    - **(i)** Characteristics
    - **(ii)** Life Cycle and Reproduction

F. Biological Organization and Relationship of major Taxa
- **1.** Linnaeus's Classification Chart
  - **a.** Five Kingdom Classification Chart
    - **(i)** Characteristics of Kingdoms
    - **(ii)** Examples of Kingdoms
  - **b.** Kingdom Animalia — Phylum chordata
    - **(i)** Invertebrates (subphylum)
    - **(ii)** Vertebrates (subphylum)
      - **(a)** Class Amphibian
      - **(b)** Class Reptilia
      - **(c)** Class Birds (Aves)
      - **(d)** Class Mammalia
      - **(e)** Class Fish (Osteichthyes)

G. Integumentary System
- **1.** Review of the Skin and Thermodynamics
  - **a.** The Skin Layers
  - **b.** Functions of the Skin
  - **c.** Thermoregulation
    - **(i)** Mechanisms of heat conservation
    - **(ii)** Mechanisms of heat loss

- **H.** Skeletal System
  - **1.** Structure of Bones
    - **a.** Spongy Bone
    - **b.** Compact Bone
    - **c.** Human Bone
      - **(i)** Flat
      - **(ii)** Long
  - **2.** Human Skeleton
- **I.** Muscular System
  - **1.** Types of Muscles
    - **a.** Smooth
    - **b.** Striated
    - **c.** Cardiac
  - **2.** Attachments and Structure of a Muscle
    - **a.** Antagonistic muscle
    - **b.** Synergistic muscle
    - **c.** Muscle Groups
      - **(i)** Flexor and Extensor
      - **(ii)** Abductor and Adductor
    - **d.** Functional Units of Muscle
      - **(i)** Myofibril
        - **(a)** Sarcomeres
        - **(b)** Myosin
        - **(c)** Actin Complex
      - **(ii)** Sarcoplasmic Reticulum
  - **3.** Oxygen Debt and Voluntary Muscle Control
    - **a.** Oxidative Metabolism
    - **b.** Endurance and Cramps
- **J.** Circulatory System
  - **1.** The Heart
    - **a.** Structural Features of Heart
    - **b.** Heart Beats
      - **(i)** Systole
      - **(ii)** Diastole
  - **2.** Circulatory Blood Vessels
    - **a.** Arteries
    - **b.** Veins
    - **c.** Arterioles
    - **d.** Capillaries
  - **3.** The Blood
    - **a.** RBCs
    - **b.** WBCs
    - **c.** Platelets
    - **d.** Lymphocytes
  - **4.** Fundamental Principles of Blood Circulation
    - **a.** Resistance
    - **b.** Ejection Fraction
    - **c.** Critical Velocity
    - **d.** Cardiac Output
- **K.** Immunological System
  - **1.** Review of Bacteria and Viruses
    - **a.** Structure, Shape, Metabolism, and Life Cycle
    - **b.** HIV Virus Life History and AIDS
  - **2.** Characteristics of Bacteriophages and Rickettsiae
  - **3.** Types of Bacterial Classes
    - **a.** Schizomycetes Class
      - **(i)** Order Eubacteriales
        - **(a)** Suborder Eubacteriineae
        - **(b)** Suborder Caulobacteriineae
        - **(c)** Suborder Rhodobacteriineae
      - **(ii)** Order Actinmycetales
      - **(iii)** Order Chlamydobacteriales
      - **(iv)** Order Myxobacteriales
      - **(v)** Order Sphirochaetales

4. Nutritional Grouping of Bacteria
    a. Autotrophic Bacteria
    b. Saphrophytic Bacteria
    c. Parasitic Bacteria
5. Bacteria and Enzyme Relationship
    a. Hydrolytic Enzymes
        (i) Amylolytic Enzymes
            (a) Diastase
            (b) Cellulase
            (c) Disaccharidases
        (ii) Lipolytic Enzymes
        (iii) Proteolytic Enzymes
    b. Oxidizing Enzymes
        (i) Alcoholnidase
        (ii) Zymase
6. Bacterial Respiration
7. The Mechanism of Infection
    a. Virulence of Pathogenic Bacteria
        (i) Virulence of Organism
        (ii) Specificity
    b. Sources of Infection
        (i) Outside the Host
        (ii) Within the Host
        (iii) Transmission of Disease-producing Organisms
8. Kinds of Immunity
    a. Natural
        (i) Racial
        (ii) Individual
    b. Acquired
        (i) Active
        (ii) Passive
9. The Mechanism of Immunity
    a. Opsonins
    b. Bacteriolysins
    c. Agglutinins
    d. Precipitins
    e. Antitoxins
    f. Hypersensitivity
        (i) Anaphylaxis
        (ii) Allergy
10. Viral and Rickettsial Diseases

L. Digestive System
1. Structure and Functional Relationships
2. Digestive Functions of Key Nutrients
3. Origins and Functional Chart for Digestive Enzymes

M. Respiratory System
1. Structure and Functional Characteristics
2. Effects of Smoking

N. Renal Fluid Composition
1. Body Fluid Composition
    a. Extracellular
    b. Intracellular
    c. Acidity of Plasma
2. The Renal System
    a. Structure
    b. Functional Characteristics
3. Homeostasis of Body Fluids
4. Buffers in the Renal System

O. Nervous System
1. Central and Peripheral Systems
    a. Neurons
        (i) Sensory Neurons
        (ii) Motor Neurons
        (iii) Associate Neurons
    b. Neurotransmitters and Impulse Transmission

2. Autonomic System
    a. Sympathetic System
    b. Parasympathetic System
3. Hindbrain
    a. Structure
    b. Functions
4. Spinal Cord
5. Types of Nerves
    a. Cranial Nerves
    b. Spinal Nerves

P. Endocrine System
1. Endocrine Glands (Anatomy and Functions)
2. Major Hormones of Endocrine Glands

Q. Reproductive System
1. Female and Male Anatomy
2. Gametogenesis
    a. Females
    b. Males
3. Meiosis
4. The Menstrual Period

R. Fertilization, Descriptive Embryology, and Developmental Mechanics
1. Fertilization
2. Developmental Mechanics of Embryo
3. Descriptive Embryology
    a. Differentiation
    b. Determination
    c. Induction

S. Mendelian Inheritance, Chromosomal Genetics, Molecular and Human Genetics
1. Nucleic Acids
    a. Nucleotides
    b. Nucleosides
    c. Nucleic Acids
2. RNA Structure
    a. Types of RNA
    b. Differences between DNA and RNA
3. Biosynthesis and Molecular Genetics
    a. Genetic Code
    b. DNA Duplication, Transcription
    c. RNA Translation
    d. Activation of Amino Acid by Activating Enzyme
    e. Protein Synthesis
        (i) Base-Pairing Rule
        (ii) Amino Acids and DNA Codons Chart
4. Chromosomes and Mendelian Genetics
    a. Alleles
        (i) Homozygous
        (ii) Heterozygous
    b. Mendelian Inheritance
        (i) First Law of Segregation
        (ii) Second Law of Independent Assortment
    c. Chromosomal Mutations
    d. Pedigree Charts/Punnet Squares
    e. Hardy-Weinberg Principle and Application

T. Evolution and Adaptation
1. Mechanism of Evolution
    a. Mutations and Hardy-Weinberg Law
2. Consequences of Evolution
    a. Speciation
        (i) Reproductive Isolation
        (ii) Geographic Isolation
    b. Patterns of Evolution
        (i) Convergent
        (ii) Divergent
        (iii) Parallel

3. Population Growth
    a. Growth Curves
    b. Parallel

U. Animal Behavior with Social Behavior
    1. Basic Behavioral Responses (Terms and Graphs)
    2. Effect of Evolution of Neurological Structures on Behavior
    3. Behavioral Modes in Populations
        a. Social Factors
        b. Interspecific Interactions
    4. Communication Between Individuals

5.1.2 Biology Sample Test

Select the one best answer for each question. Eliminate all responses that you know are incorrect and then select an answer from the remaining responses.

1. All autotrophic organisms
   A. must obtain all organic molecules from their environment.
   B. are capable of nitrogen fixation.
   C. belong to the Kingdom Plantae.
   D. can synthesize organic molecules from inorganic raw materials.
   E. are multicellular.

2. Select the substance that is not an electron carrier in cellular energy production.
   A. ATP
   B. NAD+
   C. FAD
   D. Ubiquinone
   E. All of the above

3. The conversion of the code sequence in DNA to a code sequence in mRNA is
   A. secretion.
   B. transcription.
   C. translation.
   D. condensation.
   E. polymerization.

4. The substance(s) below *not* ordinarily found in cell membranes is (are)
   A. globular proteins.
   B. phospholipids.
   C. DNA.
   D. all of the above.
   E. none of the above.

5. The main difference in the outcome of mitosis versus meiosis is
   A. meiosis produces identical daughter cells and mitosis produces different daughter cells.
   B. mitosis occurs only in vertebrates.
   C. meiosis produces somatic cells.
   D. meiosis results in haploid cells and mitosis results in diploid cells when the parents are diploid.
   E. mitosis occurs only in sex cells.

6. Which of the following substances probably would not cross a membrane by simple diffusion?
   A. Ethanol
   B. Chloride ion
   C. Glucose
   D. Water
   E. Urea

7. The function of molecular oxygen in cellular respiration is to
   A. oxidize the fuel molecule.
   B. combine with carbon to form carbon dioxide.
   C. generate ATP.
   D. serve as a final hydrogen acceptor.
   E. form water.

8. All of the following hormones are secreted by the anterior pituitary gland *except*
   A. oxytocin.
   B. prolactin.
   C. luteinizing hormone.
   D. thyroid stimulating hormone.
   E. adrenocorticotropic hormone.

9. Factors important in the differentiation of cells include
   A. cytoplasmic composition and distribution of constituents.
   B. characteristics of neighboring cells.
   C. physical environmental agents.
   D. all of the above.
   E. **A** and **B** only.

10. The control center of respiration is in the
   A. cerebrum.
   B. cerebellum.
   C. diaphragm.
   D. medulla.
   E. thalamus.

11. The secretion of pepsinogen is stimulated by
   A. enterogastrone.
   B. secretin.
   C. gastrin.
   D. enterokinase.
   E. chymotrypsin.

12. The doctrine that living things arise from other living things is
   A. biogenesis.
   B. cellularity.
   C. development.
   D. heredity.
   E. sexuality.

13. The tropic level with the largest biomass in a natural ecosystem is formed by
   A. decomposers.
   B. primary consumers.
   C. producers.
   D. secondary consumers.
   E. tertiary consumers.

14. Below are structures of a typical fatty acid and a hexose.

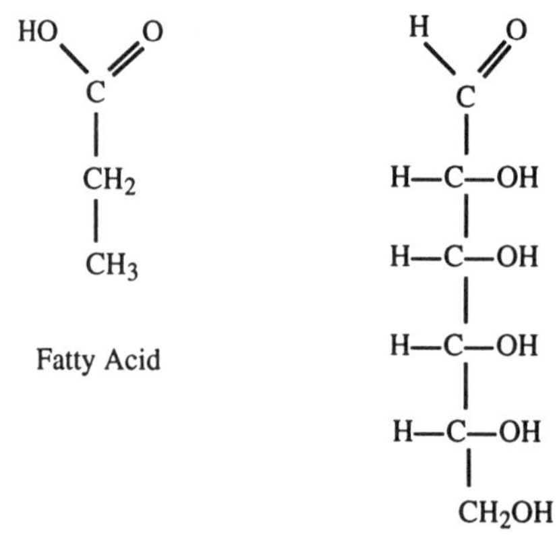

Fatty Acid

Hexose

If both were degraded bioenergetically to CO_2 and H_2O, equal weights of fatty acid would yield
   A. more energy because it is more reduced than hexose.
   B. less energy because it is more reduced than hexose.
   C. less energy because it is more oxidized than hexose.
   D. more energy because it is more oxidized than hexose.
   E. less energy because it has fewer hydroxyl groups than hexose.

15. Sex-linked traits
  A. are found more in females than males.
  B. are not linked to the X and Y chromosomes.
  C. allow recessive alleles to be expressed when one such allele is present in the male.
  D. occur in males who have a 50 percent chance of receiving sex-linked alleles from the father.
  E. will occur only in F_2 generation offspring.

16. Since enzymes are proteins, they are affected by the same factors that affect proteins. An enzyme is "designed" to function under a certain set of conditions. Which of the following conditions would be most conducive to the normal function of a human cellular enzyme?
  A. Temperature = 25°C
  B. Temperature = 37°C
  C. pH = 1.0
  D. pH = 7.0
  E. pH = 10.0

17. Fungi
  A. are prokaryotes.
  B. may be unicellular.
  C. contain chlorophyll.
  D. contain hyphae in unicellular stages.
  E. are not saphrophytic.

18. What probably limits the size a cell may attain?
  A. Surface area
  B. Volume of a cell
  C. Balance of surface area and volume
  D. Specialization of the cell
  E. Osmotic pressure

19. Which type of muscle is a syncytium?
  A. Skeletal
  B. Cardiac
  C. Smooth
  D. All
  E. None

20. Lymph nodes
  A. are found in veins.
  B. contain lymphocytes only.
  C. may contain lymphocytes and macrophages.
  D. are not directly important in protecting the body against disease.
  E. do not swell because of infection.

21. Select the *incorrect* statement concerning bile salts.
  A. Break down (digest) lipids
  B. Emulsify and solubilize lipids
  C. Synthesize in the liver
  D. Are stored in the gall bladder
  E. Are released by the gall bladder

22. During inspiration of air into the lungs
  A. the chest cavity has a positive pressure.
  B. the diaphragm moves upward.
  C. the diaphragm contracts.
  D. all of the above.
  E. none of the above.

23. All are part of the human kidney except
  A. glomerulus.
  B. loop of Henle.
  C. Malpighian tubules.
  D. collecting ducts.
  E. node of Ranvier.

24. All are specifically associated with a neuron except
A. lack of a nucleus.
B. Nissl bodies.
C. dendrite.
D. axon.
E. node of Ranvier.

25. Select the *incorrectly* paired hormone and disease or deranged process associated with an excess/deficiency of it
A. growth hormone — acromegaly
B. insulin — diabetes mellitus
C. cortisol — abnormal calcium/phosphate metabolism
D. thyroxin — altered metabolic rate
E. gonadocorticoids — adrenogenital syndrome

26. One of the scientists who helped the disapproval of spontaneous generation was
A. Leeuwenhock.
B. Redi.
C. Einstein.
D. Miller.
E. Newton.

27. The five major categories to which most living things belong according to Linnaeus are the animalia, plantae, protista, fungi, and monera
A. kingdoms.
B. species.
C. classes.
D. grouped phyla.
E. orders.

28. Diseases such as blights, wilts, and galls are caused by
A. fungi.
B. viroids.
C. rickettsia.
D. bacteria.
E. virions.

29. NAD^+ is a noncovalently bound coenzyme for the enzyme α–glycerol-phosphate dehydrogenase. NAD^+ picks up an H^{-1} (hydride) and becomes NADH; the enzyme is not affected by the reaction. The activation energy is lowered by the system.
A. This is not true catalysis because the NAD^+ is changed in the reaction.
B. This is true catalysis because the NAD^+ is not covalently bonded to the enzyme.
C. This is true catalysis because the activation energy of the reaction is lowered by the enzyme which is unchanged in the reaction.
D. This is true catalysis because the activation energy of the reaction is raised by the enzyme which is unchanged in the reaction.
E. None of the above.

30. What entity of neurons allows for one-way conduction of impulses in the nervous system?
A. Axons
B. Dendrites
C. Synapses
D. Somas
E. Palpebrae

31. Melatonin is produced by the
A. pineal gland.
B. skin.
C. liver.
D. pituitary gland.
E. none of the above.

32. Lymph moves toward the veins due to
- **A.** tissue pressure.
- **B.** muscle action.
- **C.** pumping action of heart.
- **D.** gravity.
- **E.** drainage of lymphocytes.

33. Iron is absorbed in the
- **A.** stomach.
- **B.** jejunum.
- **C.** ileum.
- **D.** duodenum.
- **E.** liver.

34. The autonomic nervous system includes
- **A.** sympathetic system.
- **B.** parasympathetic system.
- **C.** somatic nervous system.
- **D.** both **A** and **B**.
- **E.** both **B** and **C**.

35. Which of the following tissues secrete hormones?
- **A.** Pancreas
- **B.** Ovaries
- **C.** Gastrointestinal tract
- **D.** All of the above
- **E.** None of the above

36. Filtration of blood occurs at which structure in the kidney?
- **A.** Loop of Henle
- **B.** Collecting ducts
- **C.** Tubules
- **D.** Glomerulus
- **E.** Interlobar and interlobular veins

37. Heterotrophs are organisms that
- **A.** feed on inorganic compounds.
- **B.** feed on organic molecules.
- **C.** use aerobic fermentation of glucose.
- **D.** use anaerobic fermentation of nitric acid.
- **E.** use aerobic fermentation of nitric acid.

38. Mollusks are most closely related to
- **A.** roundworms.
- **B.** coelenterates.
- **C.** annelids.
- **D.** flatworms.
- **E.** mollugo.

39. A viral disease is
- **A.** anthrax.
- **B.** syphilis.
- **C.** polio.
- **D.** tuberculosis.
- **E.** cicadidae.

40. All of the following are associated with reproductive functions in fungi except
- **A.** conidia.
- **B.** sporangium.
- **C.** basidium.
- **D.** mesenchymal.
- **E.** chromium.

41. The A-band of striated muscle represents
A. myosin only.
B. actin only.
C. both **A** and **B**.
D. calcium channels.
E. neither **A** nor **B**.

42. An enlarged lymph node may mean
A. infection.
B. inflammation.
C. cancer.
D. metastasis.
E. all of the above.

43. The enzyme responsible for the activation of trypsinogen in the intestine is
A. pepsin.
B. enterokinase.
C. chymotrypsin.
D. carboxypeptidase.
E. succinate dehydrogenase.

44. What structure(s) is(are) used to prevent the bronchi from collapsing?
A. Cartilage rings
B. Bony rings
C. Fibrous tissue
D. All of the above
E. None of the above

45. Select the correct statement concerning the antidiuretic hormone (ADH).
A. Synthesized in the posterior pituitary gland
B. Acts on the collecting duct of the kidney
C. Also called aldosterone
D. All of the above are correct
E. None of the above are correct

46. Reabsorption of most of the water, glucose, amino acids, sodium and other nutrients occurs at
A. loop of Henle.
B. collecting duct.
C. proximal convoluted tubule.
D. distal convoluted tubule.
E. glomerulus.

47. Myelin sheaths are found
A. surrounding tendons.
B. covering the brain.
C. covering muscles.
D. around axons of neurons.
E. around palpebral fissures.

48. All of the following hormones are correctly paired with one of their major functions except
A. thyroxin-increases metabolic rate.
B. glucocorticoids-increases blood sugar levels.
C. aldosterone-role in "fight or flight" sympathetic response.
D. parathyroid hormone-regulation of calcium/phosphorous metabolism.
E. insulin-diabetes mellitus.

49. Ethyl alcohol is converted into lactic acid during the process of
A. aerobic respiration.
B. excretion.
C. autotrophy.
D. coenzyme production.
E. anaerobic respiration.

50. All of the following are vertebrates except
A. sponge.
B. cow.
C. shark.
D. eagle.
E. fish.

51. A fungal disease is
A. influenza.
B. pneumonia.
C. both **A** and **B**.
D. ringworm.
E. **A**, **B** and **D**.

52. Select the correct sequence of filtered blood through the kidney.
A. Bowman's capsule, glomerulus, tubules, collecting duct
B. Glomerulus, Bowman's capsule, collecting ducts, tubules
C. Bowman's capsule, collecting ducts, glomerulus, tubules
D. Glomerulus, Bowman's capsule, tubules, collecting ducts
E. Tubules, glomerulus, collecting ducts, Bowman's capsule

53. In the fungus
A. the haploid phase tends to dominate.
B. the diploid phase tends to dominate.
C. there is only asexual reproduction.
D. spores are sexual structures only.
E. there is only sexual reproduction.

54. Which structure does not play a part in motion of cells?
A. Microvilli
B. Cilia
C. Flagella
D. Pseudopods
E. All of the above

55. The products of triglyceride hydrolysis by lipases in the intestine may include
A. fatty acids.
B. monoglycerides.
C. diglycerides.
D. all of the above.
E. none of the above

56. All of the following may cause an increase in respiratory rate except
A. increased hydrogen ion concentration.
B. increased carbon dioxide tension.
C. increased oxygen tension.
D. decreased oxygen tension.
E. anxiety.

57. The acidity of the plasma is caused by
A. oxidation of glucose and fat.
B. metabolism of sulfur-containing amino acids.
C. production of CO_2 by the tissues.
D. all of the above.
E. none of the above.

58. What ion(s) determine(s) the resting potential of a nerve cell?
A. Sodium
B. Potassium
C. Calcium
D. Both **A** and **B**
E. Both **B** and **C**

59. All of the following are arthropods except
- **A.** jumping spiders.
- **B.** dragonflies.
- **C.** snails.
- **D.** soft shell crabs.
- **E.** water bears.

60. Infectious diseases
- **A.** are inherited.
- **B.** are caused by pathogens.
- **C.** are caused by rickettsias.
- **D.** are caused by bacterial respiration.
- **E.** are never easy to cure.

61. All of the following substances are filtered at the glomerulus except
- **A.** platelets.
- **B.** proteins.
- **C.** glucose.
- **D.** sodium.
- **E.** amino acids.

62. Secretion of bicarbonate and fluid from the pancreas is stimulated by
- **A.** secretin.
- **B.** cholecystokinin.
- **C.** enterokinase.
- **D.** gastrin.
- **E.** chymotrypsin.

63. All are functions of the medulla except
- **A.** voluntary movements.
- **B.** respiratory regulation.
- **C.** circulatory regulation.
- **D.** cough reflex.
- **E.** relaying motor and sensory impulses.

64. In the hypothalamic-pituitary-adrenal axis, if the long feedback loop holds then
- **A.** ACTH inhibits the production of ACTH-RF by the hypothalamus.
- **B.** cortisol inhibits the production of ACTH by the pituitary.
- **C.** cortisol inhibits the ACTH-RF produced by the hypothalamus.
- **D.** all of the above.
- **E.** none of the above.

65. Urea
- **A.** is a product of protein metabolism.
- **B.** contains only carbon, hydrogen, and oxygen.
- **C.** is excreted by the lungs.
- **D.** all of the above.
- **E.** none of the above.

66. During the early phase of the action potential
- **A.** only Na^+ moves.
- **B.** only K^+ moves.
- **C.** only Ca^{++} moves.
- **D.** Na^+ moves into the cell and K^+ moves out.
- **E.** Na^+ moves out of the cell and K^+ moves in.

67. All of the following are types of bacteria except
- **A.** metatrophic.
- **B.** parasitic.
- **C.** autotrophic.
- **D.** tsutsugamuchi.
- **E.** staphylococci.

68. Select the correct sequence of the meninges from outside inward: (A = arachnoid, D = dura, P = pia).
A. A, D, P
B. D, P, A
C. P, A, D
D. D, A, P
E. A, P, D

69. A vaccine mostly results in
A. passive immunity.
B. active immunity.
C. production of antibodies.
D. both **B** and **C**.
E. both **A** and **C**.

70. An organism makes and gives off useful chemical compounds. It is carrying on the life process of
A. secretion.
B. photosynthesis.
C. catalysis.
D. cellular respiration.
E. hormonal control.

71. Calcitonin
A. decreases serum calcium.
B. has no effect on serum calcium.
C. is made in the parathyroid gland.
D. is a steroid.
E. increases serum calcium.

72. All of the following are families in Suborder Eubacteriineae, except
A. rhizobiaceae.
B. chlamydobacteriales.
C. achromobacteriaceae.
D. parvobacteriaceae.
E. polyangium lichenicolum.

73. Select the *incorrect* statement concerning the parasympathetic system.
A. Ganglia are located near the end-organ
B. Increases the heart rate
C. Maintains homeostasis
D. Increases digestive actions
E. None of the above

74. All of the following are *infections* except
A. typhoid.
B. botulism.
C. common flu.
D. strep throat.
E. mononucleosis.

5.1.3 Explanatory Solutions for Biology Sample Test

Question 1: [D] Topic: diversity of life. Choice **1** refers to heterotrophic organisms, and the other choices to some, not all, autotrophs.

Question 2: [A] Topic: cell and molecular biology. ATP is the main short term energy storage molecule and is not an electron carrier.

Question 3: [B] Topic: cell and molecular biology. Translation is the conversion of a nucleotide sequence to an amino acid sequence. Responses **A**, **D**, and **E** have no connection at all to the question.

Question 4: [C] Topic: cell and molecular biology. The cell membrane is composed of phospholipids and proteins.

Question 5: [D] Topic: cell and molecular biology. Mitosis is a nucleocytoplasmic division. There is only one division of the cell into two identical diploid (2n) daughter cells. Meiosis has two phases, (i) is a reduction division in which daughter cells contain the haploid number of chromosomes and (ii) is similar to mitosis except that the cell has the haploid number of chromosomes.

Question 6: [C] Topic: cell and molecular biology. Some ions, lipid soluble substances, and very small molecules (such as ethanol, glycerol, and urea) can diffuse through membranes. Polar molecules, ions (especially cations), and larger molecules such as sugars and amino acids must cross the membrane by other means.

Question 7: [D] Topic: cell and molecular biology. Oxidation is the removal of hydrogen, or more generally a loss of electrons. Water is formed as a by-product of oxidation; it is not the primary function of oxidation.

Question 8: [A] Topic: vertebrate anatomy and physiology. This question specifically requires knowledge of the hormones secreted by the posterior pituitary gland. All of the other hormones are secreted by the anterior pituitary gland.

Question 9: [D] Topic: developmental biology. This question tests your knowledge of embryology, specifically those factors that cause cells to differentiate.

Question 10: [D] Topic: vertebrate anatomy and physiology. This question tests your knowledge of the brain and its role in respiration. The key in selecting the correct answer is to know the function of the other parts of the brain as well as the diaphragm.

Question 11: [C] Topic: vertebrate anatomy and physiology. None of the other hormones are associated with the stomach.

Question 12: [A] Topic: cellular and molecular biology, origin of life. This question tests your general knowledge of the theories relating to the origin of living things.

Question 13: [C] Topic: evolution, ecology, and behavior. This question tests your understanding of the ecosystem and its composition at various levels.

Question 14: [A] Topic: cellular and molecular biology. A reduced compound has all (or mostly) hydrogens and not oxygens. The fatty acid has many more hydrogens and fewer oxygens so it is more reduced. The more reduced a compound, the higher the energy that can be released when it is oxidized to CO_2 and H_2O.

Question 15: [C] Topic: genetics. This question tests your understanding of alleles carried on the X or Y chromosomes and the probability of this trait being expressed based on which chromosome it is attached to.

Question 16: [B] Topic: enzymology. This question discusses conditions under which enzymes function. The function of a cellular enzyme should be maximal at those conditions found in the internal milieu of a cell or a particular compartment of a cell. This would generally be conditions similar to the whole organism. The temperature of 37^oC is the normal human body temperature and the normal pH of blood is 7.40. The other conditions are extreme, but there are enzymes that can function at or near most of these--some in the human, some not.

Question 17: [B] Topic: organelle structure and function. This question tests your understanding of characteristics of fungi.

Question 18: [C] Topic: organelle structure and function. This question discusses cell geometry. The reasoning is as follows: the nutritional and energy requirements and waste production are proportional to the volume of the cell. The volume of a cell is proportional to a linear dimension (l = length) cubed, i.e., l^3. The flux (i.e., the exchange rates) of materials in (nutrients) and out (wastes) is proportional to the surface area of a cell. The surface area is proportional to a linear dimension squared, i.e., l^2. As the cell increases in size (as volume increases), the requirements, given by l^3, increase much more rapidly than supply and waste removal, give by l^2. Hence, a balance between surface area and volume is required such that supply (and waste removal) can keep in balance with cell requirements.

Question 19: [A] Topic: structure and function of muscular system. This question tests your understanding of various types of muscles.

Question 20: [C] Topic: structure and function of the immunological system. The structure and functions of lymph nodes are tested in this question.

Question 21: [A] Topic: structure and function of the digestive system. This question tests your understanding of bile composition and production.

Question 22: [C] Topic: structure and function of the respiratory system. This question tests your understanding of physiology of the respiratory system.

Question 23: [E] Topic: structure and function of the urinary system. This question tests your understanding of anatomy of the kidney.

Question 24: [A] Topic: structure and function of the nervous system. This question tests your understanding of anatomy of a neuron.

Question 25: [C] Topic: structure and function of the endocrine system. This question is designed to check if you remember the major glands and hormones secreted by them.

Question 26: [B] Topic: origin of life. This question checks your understanding of work done on spontaneous generation.

Question 27: [A] Topic: biological organization and relationship of major taxa. This question checks your fundamental knowledge of major taxonomic groups.

Question 28: [D] Topic: structure and function of the immunological system. This question relates causes of various diseases to the type of microorganism.

Question 29: [C] Topic: cell metabolism. True catalysis occurs when the activation energy is lowered and this lowering is accomplished by the enzyme's active site environment. Coenzymes serve the accessory function of transferring chemical groups.

Question 30: [C] Topic: structure and function of the nervous system. Impulse transmission in neurons is tested in this question. Draw a clear sketch showing one-way impulse conduction to understand neuronal pathways for impulses.

Question 31: [A] Topic: structure and function of the endocrine system. This question checks to see if you remember hormonal secretion glands and hormones secreted by each gland.

Question 32: [B] Topic: structure and function of the immunological system. This question tests your understanding of the lymphatic system, in particular the flow pattern of lymphatic fluid.

Question 33: [D] Topic: structure and function of the digestive system. The absorption of chemical elements or compounds occurs in various parts of the digestive system. You should memorize with reasons what chemicals are absorbed in which specific parts of the digestive system.

Question 34: [D] Topic: structure and function of the nervous system. This question tests your understanding of anatomy of the autonomic nervous system.

Question 35: [D] Topic: structure and function of the endocrine system. This question tests your understanding of the endocrine glands.

Question 36: [D] Topic: structure and function of the urinary system. Understanding the functions of different parts of the kidney, e.g., nephron, glomerulus, calyx, etc. is being tested in this question.

Question 37: [B] Topic: structure and function of the immunological system. This question tests your understanding of heterotrophs and autotrophs.

Question 38: [C] Topic: relationship of major taxonomic groups. This question tests your understanding of classification characteristics of taxonomic groups.

Question 39: [C] Topic: structure and function of immunological systems. This question tests your understanding of viral diseases, infections, and microbiological characteristics.

Question 40: [D] Topic: major differences between eukaryotic and prokaryotic cells. This question tests your understanding of reproductive characteristics of fungi.

Question 41: [C] Topic: structure and function of muscular system. This question tests your understanding of striated muscle anatomy. Technically, the band is visible as such because of the myosin, but within the limits of the band, actin is also present.

Question 42: [E] Topic: structure and function of immunological system. This question tests your understanding of characteristics of lymph nodes and factors which cause swelling of the node.

Question 43: [B] Topic: structure and function of the digestive system. This question tests your understanding of digestive enzymes.

Question 44: [A] Topic: structure and function of respiratory system. This question tests your understanding of the anatomic structures in the respiratory system.

Question 45: [B] Topic: structure and function of the endocrine system. This question tests your understanding of secretion of ADH and its functions.

Question 46: [C] Topic: structure and function of the urinary system. This question tests your understanding of Reabsorption sites in the renal system.

Question 47: [D] Topic: structure and function of the nervous system. This question tests your understanding of myelin sheaths encasing the neuron.

Question 48: [C] Topic: structure and function of the endocrine system. This question tests your understanding of endocrine glands, hormones, and their effects and functions.

Question 49: [E] Topic: cell metabolism (including photosynthesis). This question tests your understanding of biochemical reactions and conversions.

Question 50: [A] Topic: biological organization of chordates. This question is designed to see if you remember characteristics of vertebrates.

Question 51: [D] Topic: immunology and basic pathology. This question tests your knowledge about fungal diseases.

Question 52: [D] Topic: structure and function of the renal system. The question discusses the flow of filtered blood through the kidney. A flow diagram of the renal system would be helpful to develop visual skills.

Question 53: [A] Topic: reproduction in eukaryotic cells. This question tests your understanding of sexual and asexual reproduction.

Question 54: [A] Topic: Characteristics of prokaryotic and eukaryotic cells. Pseudopods are cytoplasmic extensions that aid in motion as found in amoeba. Microvilli are evaginations (out pouches) of the cell membrane which increase its surface area. Its function is to permit more area for flux of materials in and out of cells, as in the gut.

Question 55: [D] Topic: structure and function of the digestive system. This question tests your understanding of enzymology of the digestive system.

Question 56: [C] Topic: structure and function of the respiratory system. This question tests your understanding of respiratory rate and how it is changed by ionic tension.

Question 57: [D] Topic: structure and function of the circulatory system. This question tests your understanding of components of blood and their chemical characteristics.

Question 58: [D] Topic: structure and function of the nervous system. This question tests your understanding of nerve cells and chemistry of ionic transmission.

Question 59: [C] Topic: biological classification. This question tests your knowledge of arthropods.

Question 60: [B] Topic: infectious diseases. This question tests your understanding of microorganisms and diseases caused by these organisms.

Question 61: [A] Topic: structure and function of the renal system. Your knowledge of the function of the glomerulus is tested in this question.

Question 62: [A] Topic: structure and function of endocrine glands. This question tests your understanding of pancreatic enzymes.

Question 63: [A] Topic: structure and function of the nervous system. Your understanding of neurophysiology is tested through this question.

Question 64: [C] Topic: structure and function of the nervous and endocrine system. In the long feedback loop, the specific hormone (cortisol) of the gland (adrenal) feeds back past the pituitary to the hypothalamus.

Question 65: [A] Topic: structure and function of the urinary system. This question tests your understanding of chemical structure of urea.

Question 66: [A] Topic: modes of cellular transport. This question tests your understanding of ionic equilibrium between extracellular and intracellular fluids.

Question 67: [D] Topic: bacteria types and their origins. This question tests your memory on various types of bacteria.

Question 68: [D] Topic: structure and function of the nervous system. This question is best answered if you have a sequential diagram of the meninges from outside inward.

Question 69: [D] Topic: structure and function of the immune system. This question tests your understanding of the immune system (antibodies and antigens).

Question 70: [A] Topic: cellular metabolism. This question tests your understanding of the biochemical reactions of various organisms.

Question 71: [A] Topic: structure and function of the endocrine system. This question tests your understanding of hormonal effects.

Question 72: [B] Topic: bacterial classification. this question tests your understanding of bacterial classes and subclasses.

Question 73: [B] Topic: structure and function of the parasympathetic system. This question tests your understanding of neuroanatomy related to the parasympathetic system.

Question 74: [B] Topic: infectious diseases. This question tests your understanding of infectious diseases.

5.2 GENERAL CHEMISTRY

This section outlines, with brief introductions, the topics in general chemistry required for the OAT. The material is divided into content groups with a short listing of the topics that should be mastered. Several sample problems are included with explained solutions. Use these questions to gauge your understanding of the general chemistry required on the OAT and identify specific topics requiring more independent study and review. It is important to note that a periodic table will be included on the OAT for your reference. As mentioned in Section 5.1, consult the *The Betz Guide: A Complete Preparation for the MCAT* and the GRE subject test books, as and when needed.

5.2.1 General Chemistry Outline

A. Stoichiometry
- **1.** Review of Chemical Compounds
  - **a.** Mole (Definition, Equation, Application)
  - **b.** Equivalent and Gram Equivalent Weight
  - **c.** Percentage Composition
    - **(i)** Structural Formula
    - **(ii)** Molecular Formula
    - **(iii)** Empirical Formula
    - **(iv)** Application to Determine Structural Formula, Molecular Formula, and Empirical Formula
  - **d.** Applications of Mole in Stoichiometry
  - **e.** Use of Mole in Balancing Equations
- **2.** Stoichiometry Problems
  - **a.** Weight/Weight Problems
  - **b.** Weight/Volume Problems
  - **c.** Density Problems

B. Atomic Arrangements in Molecules
- **1.** Definition
  - **a.** Ionic Bond
  - **b.** Covalent Bond
  - **c.** Coordinate Bond
- **2.** Shapes of Molecules
  - **a.** Switching Shapes
  - **b.** Covalent Molecules
    - **(i)** Polar
    - **(ii)** Non-Polar
- **3.** Valence Shell Electron Pair Repulsion Theory
- **4.** Bohr's Atomic Structure
  - **a.** Electron Energy States
  - **b.** Quantum Theory
    - **(i)** Quantum Numbers
    - **(ii)** Pauli Exclusion Principle
    - **(iii)** Electron Configuration in Orbitals
    - **(iv)** Hund's Rule
- **5.** Condensed Phases and Bonds
  - **a.** Intermolecular Forces
  - **b.** Van der Waals Forces
  - **c.** Hydrogen Bonding Forces
  - **d.** Hydrophobic Bonding Forces

C. Periodic Properties of Elements
- **1.** The Periodic Table
  - **a.** Periods
  - **b.** Groups
  - **c.** Metals
  - **d.** Atomic Radius
  - **e.** Transition Metals
  - **f.** Non-Transition Metals
  - **g.** Metalloids
- **2.** Periodic Trends of Elements
  - **a.** Ionization Energy
  - **b.** Electron Affinity
  - **c.** Electronegativity
  - **d.** Atomic Radius

    e. Oxidation State
    f. Diamagnetism
    g. Ferromagnetism
    h. Paramagnetism

D. Gases
  1. Kinetic Molecular Theory of Matter
  2. Laws for Gases
    a. Boyle's Law
    b. Charles' Law
    c. Gay-Lussac's Law
    d. Dalton's Law of Partial Pressures
    e. Avogadro's Law
    f. Graham's Law of Gas Diffusion
    g. Universal Gas Equation for Ideal Gases
      (i) Van der Waal's Real Gas Law
      (ii) Molar Volume of a Gas

E. Review of Colligative Properties
  1. Phase Equilibrium
    a. Phase Changes
      (i) Boiling Point Elevation
      (ii) Freezing Point Depression
      (iii) Effects of solutes on BP and FP
    b. Definitions
      (i) Suspension
      (ii) Colloid
      (iii) Emulsion
      (iv) Foam
      (v) Gel
    c. Molality

F. Acids, Bases, and Buffers
  1. Three Common Definitions of Acids and Bases
    a. Arrhenius
    b. Bronsted-Lowry
    c. Lewis
  2. Strength
    a. Strong and weak acids
    b. Weak and Strong Bases
    c. Conjugate Acid and Base
    d. pH as a Strength Indicator
    e. Molarity
    f. Normality
  3. Solubility Rules for Acids and Bases
    a. Ionization Constant, Percent of Ionization
    b. Common Ion Effect
      (i) Le Chatelier's Principle
      (ii) Buffers (equilibrium constants and pH)

G. Chemical Equilibrium
  1. Reversible Reactions
  2. Le Chatelier's Principle and Reactants
    a. Effect of Concentration
    b. Effect of Pressure
    c. Effect of Temperature
  3. Equilibrium Constant Calculations

H. Thermodynamics and Thermochemistry
  1. Energy Changes in Reactions
    a. Law of Constant Heat Summation
    b. Heat of Formation, Hess's Law
    c. Gibbs Law
      (i) Free Energy
      (ii) Entropy
      (iii) Enthalpy
      (iv) Spontaneous Reactions
    d. Exothermic and Endothermic Reactions

I. Rate Processes in Chemical Reactions/Kinetics
   1. Activation Energy Diagram
      a. Reversibility of Reaction
      b. Reaction Rate
         (i) Forward
         (ii) Backward
      c. Equilibrium Constant
J. Electrochemical Concepts and Calculations
   1. Oxidation and Reduction Reactions
      a. Oxidation
      b. Reduction
      c. Anode
      d. Cathode
   2. Types of Cells
      a. Electrolytic
      b. Galvanic
      c. Concentration
   3. Faraday's Laws of Electrolysis
      a. Steps to Balance Redox Reactions
      b. Problems in Electrolysis
K. Nuclear Structure and Reactions
   1. Binding Energy of an Atom
      a. Nuclear Binding Energy
      b. Fission
      c. Fusion
   2. Stability of Atoms
   3. Nuclear Reactions
      a. Radioactive Decay
      b. Half life
   4. Atomic and Quantum Physics
      a. Absorption and Emission Spectra
      b. Fluorescent Emission

5.2.2 Basic Concepts and Stoichiometry, With Sample Questions

This section covers concepts related to density, the classification of matter, the law of definite proportions, nomenclature of common polyatomic ions, formula weight of a substance, percent composition, moles, empirical formulas, molecular formulas, the law of conservation of mass, how to balance a chemical equation, the use of a balanced chemical equation, and other information to calculate the quantities of reactants consumed or products produced in a chemical reaction, and how to determine a limiting reactant with percent yield.

1. The chemical compound with the formula of PCl_3 has the name
   A. phosphorus trichlorite.
   B. phosphorus trichloride.
   C. phosphorus trichlorate.
   D. phosphorus trichorine.
   E. phosphorus pentachlorite.

2. The chemical compound with the name of barium oxide has the formula of
   A. BaO.
   B. BaO_2.
   C. Ba_2O.
   D. Ba_2O_3.
   E. Ba_2O_2.

3. Of the following compounds, which contains the *lowest* % carbon by mass?
   A. CH_4
   B. CH_3CO_2H
   C. $Na_2C_2O_2$
   D. $C_6H_{12}O_6$
   E. C_2H_4

4. A compound has the empirical formula CH_2Cl and molecular mass of 198 g mole^{-1}. The molecular formula is
   A. CH_2Cl.
   B. $C_2H_4Cl_2$.
   C. $C_3H_6Cl_3$.
   D. $C_4H_8Cl_4$.
   E. $C_2H_{10}Cl_2$.

5. Balance the following hypothetical equation using the minimum integral coefficients.

$$CrPO_4 + Bi_2(SiO_4)_3 \rightarrow BiPO_4 + Cr_2(SiO_4)_3$$

   The correct coefficient for $BiPO_4$ is
   A. 1.
   B. 2.
   C. 3.
   D. 4.
   E. 5.

6. A chemist, trying to identify the main component in a commercial record cleaner, finds that 25 mL of the substance has a mass of 20 g. Which of these compounds is the most likely choice?
   A. Chloroform, density = 1.5 g/cm^3
   B. Diethyl ether, density = 0.7 g/cm^3
   C. Isopropyl alcohol, density = 0.8 g/cm^3
   D. Toluene, density = 0.9 g/cm^3
   E. Benzyl bromide, density = 1.4g/cm^3

7. How many grams of HCl are required to react completely with 1 mole of Zn?

$$HCl_{(aq)} + Zn_{(s)} \rightarrow ZnCl_2(aq) + H_{2(g)}$$

   A. 18 g
   B. 36 g
   C. 54 g
   D. 72 g
   E. 90g

5.2.3 Gases, With Sample Questions

Material to be reviewed in this section includes Boyles's Law, Charles's Law, Gay-Lussac's Law, Avogadro's Law, the ideal gas law, and Dalton's Law of Partial Pressures. Other useful topics are gas stoichiometry, STP, kinetic molecular theory, and diffusion.

8. The total pressure of a mixture of gases is
   A. obtained by multiplying the individual pressures by the number of moles and averaging.
   B. the sum of the partial pressures of the components.
   C. dependent only on the pressure of the gas that is present to the greatest extent.
   D. the product of the partial pressures of the components.
   E. dependent on the diffusion rates of each component.

9. What volume is occupied by 2.00 moles of methane (CH_4) at 273 K and 2.00 atm?
   A. 22.4 liters
   B. 11.2 liters
   C. 10.00 liters
   D. 44.8 liters
   E. 60.0 liters

10. Four identical 1.0 L flasks contain the following gases each at 0° C and 1 atm of pressure. Which gas has the lowest density?
A. He
B. Cl_2
C. CH_4
D. C_3H_6
E. All gases above have the same density.

11. One liter of nitrogen and one liter of carbon dioxide initially at one atmosphere pressure are forced into a single 500 mL vessel. What is the new nitrogen pressure if the temperature remains unchanged?
A. 1 atm
B. 2 atm
C. 3 atm
D. 4 atm
E. 5 atm

12. Given the following reaction (not balanced), $N_{2(g)} + Br_{2(g)} \rightarrow NBr_{3(g)}$, how many liters of gaseous bromine are needed to react with 2 liters of nitrogen?
A. 1 liter
B. 3 liters
C. 4 liters
D. 6 liters
E. 8 liters

5.2.4 Liquids and Solids, With Sample Questions

This section covers phase changes, intermolecular forces, solutions, colligative properties (freezing point depression, boiling point elevation, and osmotic pressure), hydrogen bonding and hydrophobic bonding forces.

13. You are given the following boiling point data: ethylene glycol bp = 198°, water bp = 100°, formamide = 111°, ethanol bp = 79°, methanol bp = 65°.
Which of the compounds has the highest vapor pressure at room temperature?
A. ethylene glycol
B. water
C. ethanol
D. methanol
E. formamide

Questions 14 and 15 refer to the following phase diagram.

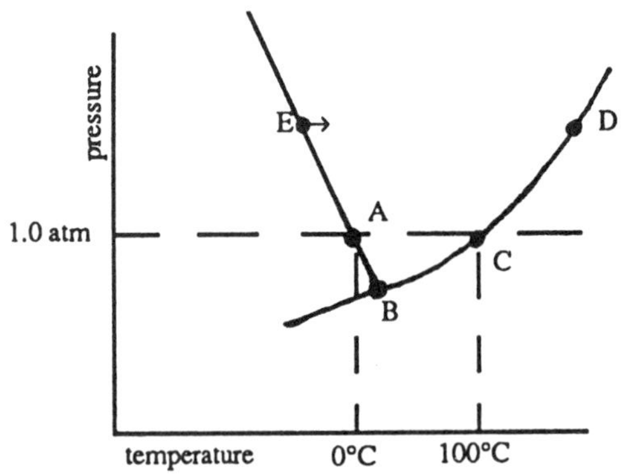

14. The triple point of water is located at the temperature and pressure represented by
A. A.
B. B.
C. C.
D. D.
E. E.

15. The arrow labeled "E" represents the physical change called
  A. sublimation.
  B. condensation.
  C. melting.
  D. deposition.
  E. boiling.

16. The addition of a nonvolatile solute into a solvent
  A. lowers the freezing point and raises the boiling point.
  B. raises the freezing point and lowers the boiling point.
  C. raises both the freezing and boiling points.
  D. lowers both the freezing and boiling points.
  E. lowers the boiling point only.

17. In any cubic lattice, an atom lying at the corner of a unit cell is shared equally by how many unit cells?
  A. 1
  B. 2
  C. 8
  D. 16
  E. 20

5.2.5 Solutions, With Sample Questions

Solution chemistry involves the ideas of concentration, intermolecular forces, and the properties of the solute and solvent.

18. Electrolytes are
  A. solutions that contain solvated electrons.
  B. solutions that conduct an electric current.
  C. solutions that contain soluble salts, strong acids, or strong bases.
  D. both **B** and **C**.
  E. both **A** and **D**.

19. What volume of 2.0 M HCl must be used to prepare 10.0 liters of a 0.50 M HCl solution?
  A. 25 L
  B. 2.5 L
  C. 0.25 L
  D. 250 L
  E. 12 L

20. A student has 500 L of a 4×10^{-3} M solution of NaOH. How many atoms of sodium are contained in this sample?
  A. 6.02×10^{23}
  B. 3.01×10^{23}
  C. 1.2×10^{24}
  D. 4.50×10^{22}
  E. 2.4×10^{21}

21. Which of the following pairs of liquids would be infinitely miscible?
  A. Ethanol and water
  B. Benzene and water
  C. Ether and water
  D. Chloroform and water
  E. Hexane and water

22. Which of the following compounds is nonpolar?
  A. Ammonia, NH_3
  B. Boron trichloride, BCl_3
  C. Water, H_2O
  D. Carbon monoxide, CO
  E. Sulfur dioxide, SO_2

5.2.6 Acids and Bases, With Sample Questions

Topics reviewed in this section are definitions of acids, conjugate acid/base pairs, neutralization reactions, titrations, buffers, and hydrolysis reactions of salts.

23. What is the conjugate acid of NH_3?

A. OH^-

B. NH_2^-

C. H_3O^+

D. NH_4^+

E. Cl^-

24. When sodium acetate, $NaC_2H_3O_2$, is dissolved in water, the resulting solution is
A. acidic.
B. basic.
C. neutral.
D. colligative.
E. not enough information was given.

25. Which of the following systems is a buffer?
A. 10 mL of 0.1 M NH_4Cl and 10 mL of 0.1 M HCl
B. 10 mL of 0.1 M NH_4Cl and 10 mL of 0.1 M NaCl
C. 10 mL of 0.1 M NH_4Cl and 10 mL of 0.1 M NH_3
D. 10 mL of 0.1 M NH_4Cl and 10 mL of 0.1 M NaOH
E. 10 mL of 0.1 M NH_4Cl and 10 mL of 0.1 M KOH

26. Given the following reaction, $HCl + Ba(OH)_2 \rightarrow BaCl_2 + H_2O$, what volume of 1 N of HCl is required to react completely with 10 mL of 1 N $Ba(OH)_2$?
A. 5 mL
B. 10 mL
C. 15 mL
D. 20 mL
E. 25 mL

27. Given the following reaction, $B_2H_6 + 2\ N(CH_2CH_3)_3 \rightarrow 2\ H_3B\text{-}N(CH_2CH_3)_3$, the best description of the role of $N(CH_2CH_3)_3$ in this reaction is as
A. Lewis acid.
B. Lewis base.
C. Bronsted-Lowry acid.
D. Bronsted-Lowry base.
E. conjugate base.

5.2.7 Chemical Equilibrium, With Sample Questions

This section reviews how chemical equilibrium can be treated in a quantitative manner. First review the basic principles of chemical equilibrium in the gas phase. Other important equilibria are acid/base and solubility.

28. Consider the equilibrium, $4\ NH_{3(g)} + 3\ O_{2(g)} \rightleftharpoons 2\ N_{2(g)} + 6\ H_2O_{(l)}$, $\Delta H = -303$ kcal, which of the following will cause the equilibrium to shift to the right?
A. An increase in temperature
B. Selectively absorb the water
C. Add a catalyst
D. Selectively absorb the O_2
E. Selectively absorb the ammonia

29. Given the reaction, $2\,XY_{(g)} \rightleftharpoons X_{2(g)} + Y_{2(g)}$, K = 0.9 at 243 K, 1 mole of XY was injected into a 1 liter container at 243 K. What is the correct equilibrium expression?

A. $0.9 = \frac{(1-2x)^2}{x^2}$

B. $0.9 = \frac{x^2}{(1-2x)^2}$

C. $0.9 = \frac{x^2}{(1-2x)}$

D. $0.9 = \frac{(1-2x)}{x^2}$

E. $0.9 = \frac{(1-2x)^2}{2x}$

30. Which of the following compounds is the most soluble in water?

A. $CaSO_4$, Ksp = 10^{-5}
B. CuI, Ksp = 10^{-12}
C. AgI, Ksp = 10^{-16}
D. CuS, Ksp = 10^{-45}
E. $BaSO_4$, Ksp = 10^{-10}

31. What would be the concentration of silver in a saturated silver iodide solution?

A. 10^{-16} M
B. 10^{-32} M
C. 10^{-4} M
D. 10^{-8} M
E. 10^{-6} M

32. The K_{sp} of $Fe(OH)_2$ is 10^{-15}. You are given a system at equilibrium that is a brown solution, $Fe(OH)_{2(aq)}$, and a brown solid, $Fe(OH)_{2(s)}$. If you add 50 mL of NaOH, what will you observe?

A. Additional solid forms, solution color pales
B. Some solid dissolves, solution color deepens
C. A gas is evolved, solution color changes to green
D. No change would be observed
E. No precipitate forms, solution color deepens

5.2.8 Thermodynamics, With Sample Questions

Spontaneity of a reaction, the enthalpy change (ΔH), the entropy change (ΔS), and the free energy change (ΔG) are presented with regards to the Second Law of Thermodynamics.

33. The heat of formation of an element in its standard state is

A. the ΔH of its reaction with hydrogen.
B. the ΔH of its reaction with oxygen.
C. zero.
D. determined by use of the molecular mass.
E. none of the above.

34. When a sample was burned in a bomb calorimeter containing 1.00 kg of water, the temperature of the water increased 1° C. If the heat capacity of the system was 0kJ/K and the specific heat of water is 4.18 J/K g, how much heat was evolved?

A. 2.09 kJ
B. 8.36 kJ
C. 1.00 kJ
D. 4.18 kJ
E. 6.43 kJ

35. Calculate the heat of formation of ethanol, C_2H_5OH, using the following information:

$$C_2H_5OH_{(l)} + 3\,O_{2(g)} \rightarrow 2\,CO_{2(g)} + 3\,H_2O_{(l)}, \quad \Delta H = -1300\text{kJ}$$
$$C_{(s)} + O_{2(g)} \rightarrow CO_{2(g)}, \quad \Delta H = -400\text{ kJ}$$
$$H_{2(g)} + 0.5\,O_{2(g)} \rightarrow H_2O_{(l)}, \quad \Delta H = -300\text{ kJ}$$

A. –2000 kJ
B. +2000 kJ
C. –400 kJ
D. +400 kJ
E. +1000 kJ

36. In which case *must* a reaction be spontaneous, independent of T?
A. $\Delta H = 0, \Delta S > 0$
B. $\Delta H = 0, \Delta S < 0$
C. $\Delta S = 0, \Delta H > 0$
D. $\Delta H < 0, \Delta S > 0$
E. $\Delta H > 0, \Delta S < 0$

5.2.9 Kinetics, With Sample Questions

To control the rates of reactions, you must understand the factors that influence the rate. For this section, review the effect of concentration of the reactants, the temperature, the presence of a catalyst, and activation energy.

37. Which of the following is the rate of a unimolecular reaction?
A. $k[A]$
B. $k[A]^2$
C. $k[A][B]$
D. $k[A][B]^2$
E. $k[B]^3$

38. The rate constant for a certain first order reaction is 0.40 min^{-1}. What is the initial rate in mol L^{-1} min^{-1}, if the initial concentration of the compound is 0.50 M?
A. 0.90
B. 0.10
C. 0.20
D. 0.40
E. 0.60

39. Which of the following is necessary for a reaction to occur between two molecules?
A. A particular collision between two molecules has an energy greater than the E_a.
B. A particular collision between two molecules has an energy less than the ΔH of the reaction.
C. The activated complex has sufficient vibrational energy to begin bond breaking.
D. The activated complex has less potential energy than the reaction products.
E. None of the above.

Questions 40 and 41 refer to the following diagram.

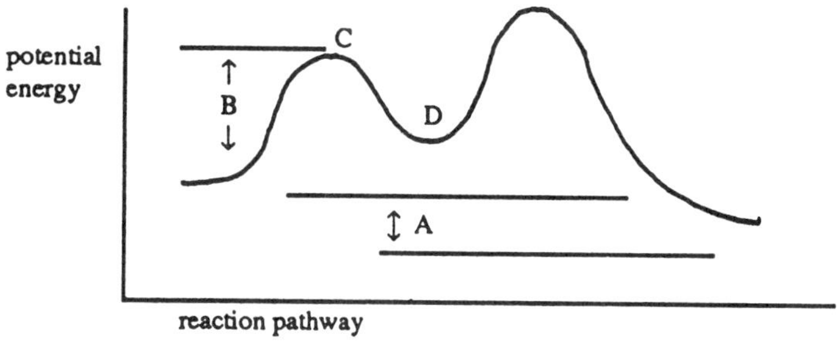

40. What point on the reaction diagram represents a reaction intermediate?
A. A
B. B
C. C
D. D
E. None of the above

41. What point on the reaction diagram represents a transition state?
A. A
B. B
C. C
D. D
E. None of the above

5.2.10 Redox Reactions, With Sample Questions

This section considers the use of electrical energy to carry out chemical reactions. Important topics include oxidation numbers, the Nernst Equation, and redox chemistry.

Questions 42 and 43 refer to the following information and cell diagram.

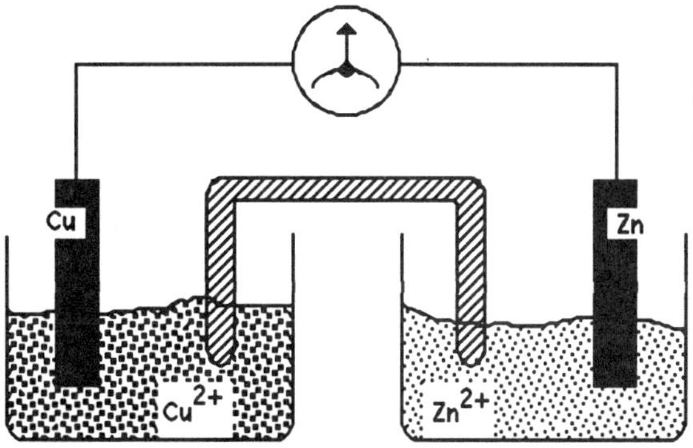

$Zn^{2+} + 2e^- \rightarrow Zn \quad E° = -0.76$ V

$Cu^{2+} + 2e^- \rightarrow Cu \quad E° = +0.34$ V

42. Which of the following reactions will give a spontaneous reaction ($\Delta G < 0$) for the above cell?
A. $Cu^{2+} + Zn \rightarrow Cu + Zn^{2+}$
B. $Cu + Zn^{2+} \rightarrow Cu^{2+} + Zn$
C. $Cu^{2+} + Zn^{2+} \rightarrow Cu + Zn + 4e^-$
D. $Cu + Zn + 4e^- \rightarrow Cu^{2+} + Zn^{2+}$
E. $Cu + Zn + 2e^- \rightarrow Cu^+ + Zn^+$

43. If the above cell contains 1.0 M $CuSO_4$ and 1.0 M $ZnSO_4$, what is the potential, E, of this cell?
A. –1.10 V
B. +1.10 V
C. +2.20 V
D. –2.20 V
E. +3.30 V

44. What is the oxidation state of nitrogen in NO_3^-?
A. –3
B. 0
C. +3
D. +5
E. –5

45. Based on the following information, which metal is the strongest reducing agent?

(i) $Zn^{2+} + Fe \rightarrow$ no reaction
(ii) $Fe^{2+} + Zn \rightarrow Zn^{2+} + Fe$
(iii) $Mg^{2+} + Zn \rightarrow$ no reaction
(iv) $Zn^{2+} + Mg \rightarrow Mg^{2+} + Zn$
(v) $Cu^{2+} + Zn \rightarrow Cu + Zn^{2+}$

A. Cu
B. Fe
C. Mg
D. Zn
E. All metals are oxidizing agents

5.2.11 Atomic and Molecular Structure, With Sample Questions

Important topics to review in this section include electron configuration, Hund's Rule, the Pauli Exclusion Principle, the Aufbau Principle, quantum numbers, Lewis dot structures, and the octet rule.

46. Oxygen has 6 valence electrons. Consider the following electron arrangements. Which represents the ground state for oxygen (O)?

A.
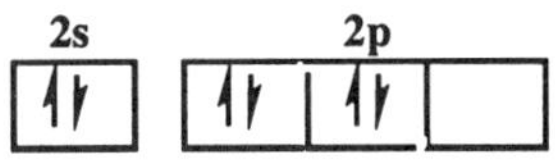

B.
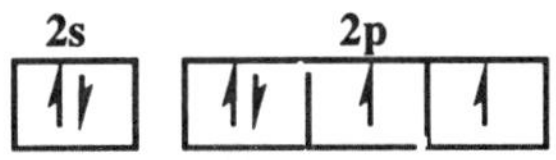

C.
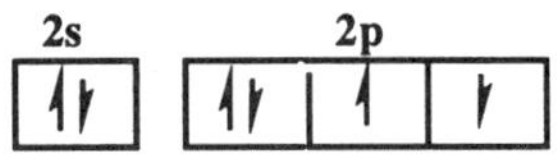

D.
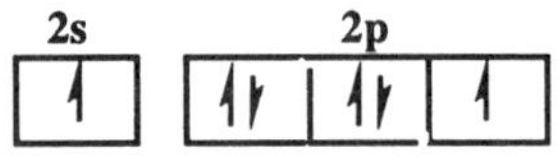

E.
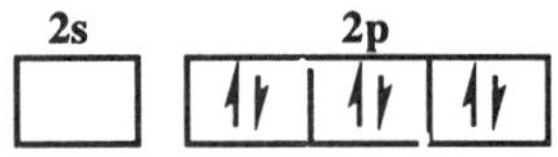

47. Which of the following ions is isoelectronic with Ar?
A. Ca^+
B. S^-
C. K^+
D. P^{2-}
E. Cu^+

48. Which of the following best describes the bonding in HCN?
A. ionic only
B. 2 sigma bonds and 2 π-bonds
C. 3 sigma bonds and 1 π-bond
D. 4 sigma bonds
E. 1 sigma bond and 3 π-bonds

49. How many electrons can occupy a shell with n = 3?
   A. 2
   B. 8
   C. 18
   D. 42
   E. 24

50. How many electrons can occupy a subshell with $l = 2$?
   A. 2
   B. 6
   C. 10
   D. 14
   E. 8

51. Which of the following elements does not have to obey the octet rule?
   A. C
   B. Ne
   C. P
   D. H
   E. O

52. What element has this electron configuration, [Kr] $4d^5 5s^2$?
   A. Mn
   B. Tc
   C. Re
   D. Uns (#107)
   E. Fe

5.2.12 Periodic Properties, With Sample Questions

Areas to be reviewed include named groups (halogens, alkali metals, alkaline earth, noble gases, semi-metals, transition metals), and periodic trends (size, ionization potential, electronegativity).

53. Which of the following elements is classified as a semi-metal or metalloid?
   A. Carbon
   B. Sulfur
   C. Arsenic
   D. Lead
   E. Oxygen

54. Which of the following elements is a liquid at room temperature?
   A. F_2
   B. Cl_2
   C. Br_2
   D. I_2
   E. H_2

55. Which of the following lists of elements are known collectively as the noble gases?
   A. He, Ne, Ar, Kr, Xe
   B. F, Cl, Br, I, At
   C. Be, Mg, Ca, Sr, Ba, Ra
   D. Li, Na, K, Rb, Cs, Fr
   E. N, P, As, Sb, Bi

56. Which of the following elements is the most electronegative?
   A. B
   B. C
   C. N
   D. O
   E. F

57. Which of the following orderings of atoms are listed in *increasing* size?

I Al, Si, P, S
II S, P, Si, Al
III I, Br, Cl, F
IV F, Cl, Br, I

A. I and III
B. II and IV
C. I and IV
D. II and III
E. III and IV

58. What is the value of 1 for a 3d orbital?
A. 0
B. 1
C. 2
D. 3
E. 4

59. Which of the following atoms require the *most* energy to remove a valence electron?
A. Li
B. Na
C. K
D. Rb
E. Cs

60. Which of the following metals yields an oxide with the formula MO when reacted with oxygen?
A. Sodium
B. Potassium
C. Aluminum
D. Magnesium
E. Lithium

61. Which of the following compounds is caustic soda?
A. NaOH
B. Na_2CO_3
C. NaCl
D. Na_2SO_4
E. KOH

5.2.13 Nuclear Reactions, With Sample Questions

Several topics should be reviewed, including balancing nuclear equations, decay processes, and particles.

62. Which of the following radioactive decay processes does not involve a change in atomic number?
A. Electron capture
B. Gamma emission
C. Positron emission
D. Beta emission
E. Neutrino capture

63. The half-life of iodine-131 is 8.0 days. How many grams of iodine-131 remain after 16.0 days in a sample that initially contained 1.00 gram of iodine-131?
A. 0.50 g
B. 0.25 g
C. 0.13 g
D. 0.05 g
E. 0.01 g

64. What is the missing product of the following reaction? ${}^{43}_{19}\text{K} \rightarrow {}^{43}_{20}\text{Ca} + ?$

A. ${}^{4}_{2}\text{He}$
B. ${}^{0}_{-1}\text{e}$
C. ${}^{0}_{1}\text{e}$
D. γ
E. none of the above

65. What is the missing product of the reaction shown? ${}^{80}_{28}\text{Ni}^* \rightarrow {}^{80}_{28}\text{Ni} + ?$

A. ${}^{4}_{2}\text{He}$
B. ${}^{0}_{-1}\text{e}$
C. ${}^{0}_{1}\text{e}$
D. γ
E. none of the above

5.2.14 Answers and Explanations for General Chemistry

Question 1: [B] Topic: nomenclature. When naming small inorganic compounds, always list the more electropositive element first. The other element is named as an anion. Anion endings are -ide for elemental and -ite and -ate for oxygen-containing polyatomic anions (the ending -ine is the ending used for elements).

Question 2: [A] Topic: nomenclature. Barium is a +2 cation and oxide is a –2 anion. The correct formula would contain 1 barium and 1 oxide.

Question 3: [C] Topic: percent composition. Determine the molecular weight of each species. A = 16 g/mole; B = 61 g/mole; C = 102 g/mole; D = 192 g/mole; E = 28 g/mole. Next divide the mass of carbon by the molecular weight. A = 12/16 = 0.75; B = 24/61 = 0.40; C = 24/102 = 0.24; D = 72/196 = 0.37; E = 24/28 = 0.86.

Question 4: [D] Topic: empirical/molecular formula. Determine the mass of empirical formula unit (49 g). Divide into molecular mass (= 4). This means the molecule contains four empirical units.

Question 5: [B] Topic: balancing equations. Start with the most complicated molecule, $Bi_2(SiO_4)_3$. Balance Bi with 2 on product side and $CrPO_4$ with 2.

Question 6: [C] Topic: Density is the ratio of mass to volume. Divide mass of sample by volume.

Question 7: [D] Topic: stoichiometry. First balance the equation by placing 2 with HCl. Mole ratio calculation gives 2 moles of HCl per 1 mole of Zn. Molecular weight of HCl is 36 g/mole.

Question 8: [B] Topic: Dalton's Law of partial pressure. This is the definition of this gas law.

Question 9: [A] Topic: ideal gas law and Avogadro's Gas Law. Remember that at STP one mole of an ideal gas occupies 22.4 L. Avogradro's Gas Law states that the amount of gas present (moles) is directly proportional to the pressure. If the number of moles doubles and the pressure doubles, the volume and temperature are constant.

Question 10: [B] Topic: ideal gas law. Substitute mass/MW for n in the ideal gas law. Solve for density using mass/V. Density is proportional to molecular weight.

Question 11: [B] Topic: Boyle's Law. Boyle's Law states that the pressure of a gas is inversely proportional to its volume. To halve the volume, double the pressure.

Question 12: [D] Topic: law of combining volumes. The law of combining volumes allows us to substitute volumes of gas for moles in stoichiometric calculations in gas-phase reactions.

Question 13: [D] Topic: vapor pressure. The definition of boiling point is when the vapor pressure of the liquid equals the atmospheric pressure. The lower the boiling temperature, the closer the vapor pressure is to the atmospheric pressure.

Question 14: [B] Topic: phase diagrams. **A** = normal freezing point. **C** = normal boiling point. **D**= critical point.

Question 15: [C] Topic: phase changes. The change occurring is from solid to liquid.

Question 16: [A] Topic: colligative properties. The addition of an impurity to a material increases the boiling point according to $\Delta T_b = k_b m$ (ΔT_b is the change in boiling point, k_b is a constant, and m is the molality of the solution). The addition of an impurity lowers the freezing point (why we use salt to melt ice in the winter) according to $\Delta T_f = k_f m$.

Question 17: [C] Topic: cubes. Any atom on the corner of a cube is 1/8 in that cube, so any corner atom is shared by eight atoms. Get 8 shoe boxes and try it.

Question 18: [D] Topic: solutions. Electrolytes are solutions that conduct electrons and are either soluble salts or acids/bases. Any compound that ionizes in solution is an electrolyte.

Question 19: [B] Topic: concentration units. Using the formula $C_1V_1 = C_2V_2$ for this dilution problem, solve for V_1.

Question 20: [C] Topic: concentration units. The definition of molarity is mole per liter. Multiply the concentration by the volume to get moles. Avogradro's number tells us there are 6.02×10^{23} molecules per mole. So there are 2 moles of NaOH and in solution it ionizes to 2 moles of Na^+ atoms.

Question 21: [A] Topic: polarity. "Like dissolves like." Water is polar, only another polar compound will be totally miscible.

Question 22: [B] Topic: polarity. You need to draw the molecule in a three-dimensional view and look for a permanent dipole moment.

Question 23: [D] Topic: conjugates. When ammonia ionizes in aqueous solution the reaction is $NH_3 + H_2O \leftrightarrow NH_4^+ + OH^-$. The definition of a base is a proton acceptor, which makes NH_4^+ the correct response.

Question 24: [B] Topic: salt hydrolysis. Acetate, $C_2H_3O_2^-$, is the conjugate base of a weak acid, acetic acid. The resulting conjugate base of a weak acid is a strong conjugate base that reacts with water.

Question 25: [C] Topic: buffers. The definition of a buffer includes a weak base (acid) and the salt of its conjugate acid (base). See question 23. **A** has a strong acid, **B** has two salts, and **D** has a strong base.

Question 26: [B] Topic: neutralization reaction. Notice the unit of concentration, N (normality). Normality is defined as gram-equivalent weight of a particular substance dissolved in 1 liter of solution. HCl has one reactive H per molecule, giving a gram-equivalent weight equal to the molecular weight. $Ba(OH)_2$ has two reactive hydroxyl ions (each being equivalent to a proton). Therefore, the gram-equivalent weight is one-half the molecular weight. So equal volumes of equal normality solutions are needed for complete reaction.

Question 27: [B] Topic: acid definition. The definition of a Lewis Acid is an electron pair acceptor. A Lewis Base is an electron pair donor. Bronsted-Lowry Acid is a proton donor. Bronsted-Lowry Base is a proton acceptor. In the course of the reaction no proton is exchanged, ruling out choices **C** and **D**. By knowing the Lewis Dot Structures of the reactants, N possesses a lone pair of electrons [$:N(CH_2CH_3)_3$], making it an electron donor.

Question 28: [B] Topic: equilibrium. The removal of a product will cause a shift to the right, whereas the addition of a product will cause a shift to the left. **C** has no effect because catalysts do not cause the equilibrium to shift. Selective absorption of H_2O will cause the equilibrium to remain on the right side or shift to the right as shown in **B**.

Question 29: [B] Topic: equilibrium calculations. To solve any similar problem (gas phase, acid/base, or solubility equilibriums) think of the problem in 3 phases.

	$2\,XY_{(g)} \leftrightarrow$	$X_{2(g)}$ +	$Y_{2(g)}$	(phase I)
t_o	1M	0	0	
Δ	$-2x$	$+x$	$+x$	(phase II)
t_{eq}	$1-2x$	x	x	(phase III)

(1) t_o, concentration at the start. (2) Δ, concentration change, and (3) t_{eq}, equilibrium concentration. Place the information into the equilibrium expression for the reaction in question. The general form of an equilibrium expression is [for x A + y B $\leftrightarrow$ aX + bY]

$$K = \frac{\text{concentration of products}}{\text{concentration of reactants}} = \frac{[X]^a\,[Y]^b}{[A]^x\,[B]^y}$$

where a, b, x, and y are the coefficients from the balanced chemical equation.

Question 30: [A] Topic: equilibrium. Since all of the salts in question form the same number of ions in solution, we can compare the K_{sp} values. If the salts formed different numbers of ions in solutions, you would have to calculate the *molar solubility.*

Question 31: [D] Topic: solubility equilibrium. The expression for Ksp for this equilibrium is K_{sp} = $[Ag^+][I^-]$; substitute x for the concentration and solve for x. The K_{sp} value was given in the previous question.

$$AgI_{(s)} \leftrightarrow Ag^+_{(aq)} + I^-_{(aq)}$$

$$\qquad\qquad x \qquad\quad x$$

Question 32: [A] Topic: common ion effect (Le Chatelier's Principle). The chemical equation describing the equilibrium is $Fe(OH)_{2(s)} \leftrightarrow Fe^{2+}_{(aq)} + 2\,OH^-_{(aq)}$. The problem states you have added NaOH, a strong base. Strong bases ionize completely in water, $NaOH_{(aq)} \rightarrow Na^+_{(aq)} + OH^-_{(aq)}$. Notice both equations have hydroxide as a product. The addition of product of the equilibrium will cause reactants to form.

Question 33: [C] Topic: heat of formation. The heat of formation is the heat needed to form a compound from its component elements. Elements do not need to be formed.

Question 34: [D] Topic: calorimetry. Heat q, evolved in a calorimeter, is q = CΔT (C is heat capacity = specific heat × mass and ΔT is the change in room temperature). C = (4.18 J/Kg)(1.00 kg) = 4.18 kJ/K. q then is equal to (4.18 kJ/K)(1K) = 4.18 kJ.

Question 35: [C] Topic: Hess's Law. Hess's law states that the energy of a chemical reaction is the same regardless of how you get there. We can use the three given reactions and add them up to the desired reaction. Heat of formation is the formation of the compound from the component elements, in this case $2\,C + 3\,H_2 + 1/2\,O_2 \rightarrow C_2H_5OH$. The first given reaction contains information on ethanol, but as a reactant. To reverse the reaction is equivalent to multiplying by –1. This changes the sign of the heat, ΔH. To remove unwanted species we will use the other reaction to cancel. We need to remove 2 carbon dioxides as reactants. To cancel out you need two carbon dioxides as products. Similar reasoning will remove the water. The problem solved is shown below:

$$-1[C_2H_5OH + 3\,O_2 \rightarrow 2\,CO_2 + 3\,H_2O\ \Delta H = -1300\text{ kJ}] = \cancel{2\,CO_2} + \cancel{3\,H_2O} \rightarrow C_2H_5OH + \cancel{6/2\,O_2} \quad \Delta H = +1300\text{ kJ}$$

$$2[C_{(s)} = O_{2(g)} \rightarrow CO_{2(g)}\ \Delta H = -400\text{ kJ}] = 2C_{(s)} + \cancel{4/2\,O_{2(g)}} \rightarrow \cancel{2\,CO_{2(g)}} \quad \Delta H = -800\text{ kJ}$$

$$3[H_{2(g)} = 1/2\,O_{2(g)} \rightarrow H_2O_{(l)}\ \Delta H = -300\text{ kJ}] = 3H_{2(g)} + (1/2)\cancel{3/2}\,O_{2(g)} \rightarrow \cancel{3\,H_2O_{(l)}} \quad \Delta H = -900\text{ kJ}$$

$$2\,C + 3\,H_2 = 1/2\,O_2 \rightarrow C_2H_5OH,\ \Delta H = -400\text{ kJ}$$

Question 36: [D] Topic: spontaneity/Gibbs free energy. Free energy is the relationship between enthalpy (ΔH, heat that seeks a minimum value) and entropy (ΔS, which seeks a maximum value). The relationship is $\Delta G = \Delta H - T\Delta S$, resulting in

ΔH	ΔS	ΔG	
>0	>0	>0 <0	at low temp (nonspontaneous) at high temp (spontaneous)
>0	<0	>0	at all temperatures (never spontaneous)
<0	>0	<0	at all temperatures (always spontaneous)
<0	<0	>0 <0	at high temp (nonspontaneous) at low temp (spontaneous)

Figure 5.1 — Gibbs Free Energy Related to Entropy, Enthalpy

Question 37: [A] Topic: rate laws. Unimolecule refers to one molecule. Bimolecular would refer to two and relates to either **B** or **C** (it doesn't distinguish between two different molecules or two of the same molecules). **D** is trimolecular. The "order" of the reaction is the sum of the coefficients in the rate law and refers to the number of molecules participating in the rate determining step.

Question 38: [C] Topic: reaction rates. See solution for question 37 above and substitute 0.4 for k and 0.5 for the concentration and multiply. A unimolecular reaction is first-order.

Question 39: [A] Topic: activation energies. The criteria for a successful reaction are for the molecules to collide in the correct orientation and with sufficient energy to overcome the activation energy barrier.

Question 40: [D] Topic: reaction diagrams. In a reaction diagram, several concepts are presented. A is the change in enthalpy, ΔH is the energy difference between the reactants and the products, B is the energy of activation, E_a is the energy required for the reactants to react, C is the transition state (an energy maximum), and D is an intermediate (an energy minimum located between the reactants and products).

Question 41: [C] Topic: reaction diagram.

Question 42: [A] Topic: spontaneity. For the reaction to occur spontaneously, the potential (E°) for the cell must be greater than 0. In thermodynamics, $\Delta G°$ is less than 0 for a spontaneous reaction and $\Delta G° = -nFE°$(n = number of electrons transferred and F is Faraday's constant).

Question 43: [B] Topic: Nernst Equation. Since the concentrations of the ions are equal, $\log Q = 0$, so $E = E°$.

Question 44: [D] Topic: oxidation states. Since O is –2 and three Os give –6, what positive charge is needed to give a –1? Nitrogen has a charge of +5.

Question 45: [C] Topic: redox reactions. A reducing agent in a redox reaction is the species that is oxidized. Simply stated for metals, it prefers to be a cation, not the neutral element. By comparing the given reactions, Mg always reacts and Mg^{2+} never does.

Question 46: [B] Topic: electron configurations. The Aufbau principle states that the orbitals of lowest energy must fill first, so this rules out choices **D** and **E** (s orbitals are of lower energy than p orbitals). Hund's rule states that the lowest electron configuration has the maximum number of unpaired spins. This means the unpaired spins need to be in the same direction (rules out choices **A** [not enough spin, all electrons are paired], and **C** [unpaired electrons but spins in opposite direction]).

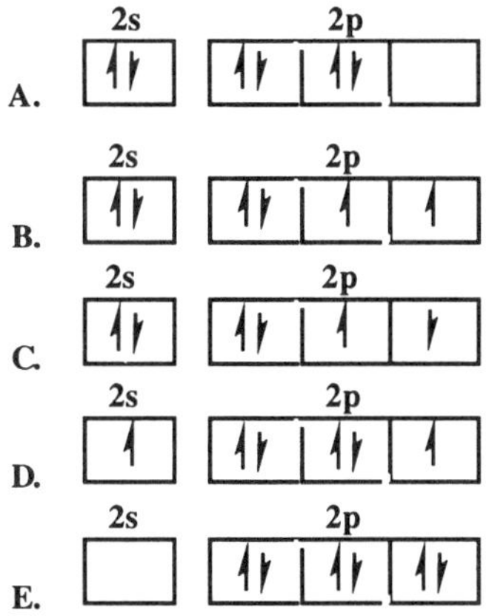

Question 47: [C] Topic: electron configurations. The electron configuration of argon is [Ne]$3s^2 3p^6$. The electron configurations of the choices are

A. [Ar]$3s^1$
B. [Ne]$3s^2 3p^5$
C. [Ar] or [Ne]$3s^2 3p^6$
D. [Ne]$3s^2 3p^5$
E. [Ar]$3d^{10}$

Question 48: [B] Topic: bonding. Since ionic bonding usually occurs in compounds consisting of metals and nonmetals and HCN contains only nonmetals, choice **1** is ruled out. To answer this question you need to draw the Lewis Dot structure of HCN. Remember this general rule—H forms 1 bond, N forms 3 and C forms 4, (O will form 2), you will get this result: H–C≡N. The first bond between atoms will be a sigma bond and if multiple bonds are present, all bonds after the first will be π-bonds. The total number of sigma bonds will be 2, and 2 π-bonds are present.

Question 49: [C] Topic: quantum numbers. For principle quantum number 3, s, p, and d orbitals are allowed. The 3s orbital can contain 2 electrons, the 3 p orbital can contain 6 electrons, and the 3 d orbital can contain 10 electrons, for a total of 18 allowed electrons.

Question 50: [C] Topic: quantum numbers. The azimuthal quantum number refers to the shape of an orbital. $l = 0$ means s, $l = 1$ means p, $l = 2$ means d, and $l = 3$ means f. Since choice **A** was 2, the question refers to a d orbital that can hold 10 electrons.

Question 51: [C] Topic: octet rule. The elements C, N, O, F, Ne, and H must always obey the octet rule. To violate the octet rule most elements use d orbitals, which for these elements are not allowed by quantum mechanics. Their principle quantum number is 2 (or less), which gives for l (allowed values of O → n–1, 0 and l) only s and p orbitals. These orbitals can hold a maximum of 8 electrons.

Question 52: [B] Topic: electron configurations.

Question 53: [C] Topic: metalloids. Most periodic tables have a "red" zig-zag line snaking through the p-block. Elements along this line are metalloids.

Question 54: [C] Topic: halogens. Flourine and chlorine are gases, bromine is one of two liquid elements (mercury is the other), iodine is a solid. As a general rule, the greater the molecular weight for a series of related compounds, the higher the melting and boiling points.

Question 55: [A] Topic: group names. The name groups are (A) noble gases, (B) halogens, (C) alkaline earths, (D) alkali metals, and (E) group V elements.

Question 56: [E] Topic: electronegativity. F is the most electronegative element, O is the second most. Electronegativity decreases as you move away from F in the periodic chart.

Question 57: [B] Topic: periodic trends. Size increases as you go down the periodic chart and size increases as you go to the *left* across the periodic chart.

Question 58: [C] Topic: quantum numbers. The values of 1 refer to: 0→s, 1→p, 2→d, and 3→f.

Question 59: [A] Topic: ionization energy trends. Ionization energies decrease as you go down the periodic chart. Ionization energies increase as you go *right* across the chart.

Question 60: [D] Topic: ionic compounds. O is a –2 anion and needs a +2 cation to form a 1:1 ionic compound.

Question 61: [A] Topic: descriptive chemistry. Sodium hydroxide is known generically as caustic soda, while NaCl is called "salt."

Question 62: [B] Topic: decay process. Gamma radiation is only release of energy. Electron capture and positron emission decrease the atomic number by 1, and beta emission increases the atomic number by 1.

Question 63: [B] Topic: half life. Sixteen days represents two half-life periods, in the first 50% of the sample decayed [1 g→ 0.5 g], in the second 50% of the sample decayed [0.5 g → 0.25g].

Question 64: [B] Topic: nuclear reactions. The atomic mass is unchanged but the atomic number has increased by one (beta emission).

Question 65: [D] Topic: nuclear reactions. The atomic mass and atomic number are unchanged, only energy has been released (gamma emission).

5.3 ORGANIC CHEMISTRY

This section outlines with brief introductions the subject of organic chemistry required for the OAT. The material is divided into area groups with a short listing of the topics that should be mastered. Specific concepts are covered briefly. Several sample problems are included with explained solutions. Use these questions to gauge your understanding of the organic chemistry required on the OAT and to identify specific topics requiring further independent study and review. As mentioned in Section 5.1, consult the *The Betz Guide: A Complete Preparation for the MCAT* and the GRE special subject test books, as and when needed.

5.3.1 Organic Chemistry Outline

A. Chemical Bonding
- **1.** Atomic Orbitals
  - **a.** Aufbau Principle
  - **b.** Pauli's Exclusion Principle
  - **c.** Hund's Rule
- **2.** Molecular Orbitals
  - **a.** Energy and Intermolecular Distance Diagram
  - **b.** Types of Orbitals
    - **(i)** Overlapping Bonding Orbital
    - **(ii)** Overlapping Antibonding Orbital
- **3.** Hybridization
  - **a.** sp^3 hybrids
  - **b.** sp^2 hybrids
  - **c.** sp hybrids
- **4.** Lewis Structures
  - **a.** Lewis Acids
  - **b.** Lewis Bases
  - **c.** Atomic Bonds
    - **(i)** π bonds (pi)
    - **(ii)** σ bonds (sigma)
- **5.** Resonance and Bond Characteristics
  - **a.** Bond Length
    - **(i)** Single Bonds
    - **(ii)** Double Bonds
    - **(iii)** Polar Covalent Bonds
    - **(iv)** Dipole Moment
  - **b.** Bond Angles
    - **(i)** VSEPR Theory
    - **(ii)** Molecule Shapes

B. Mechanism of Reactions
- **1.** Energetics
- **2.** Structure and Stability of Intermediates
  - **a.** S_N1 Reactions
  - **b.** S_N2 Reactions
  - **c.** Elimination Reactions
  - **d.** Addition
- **3.** Free Radical Mechanisms
- **4.** Substitution Mechanisms

C. Properties of Molecules
- **1.** Stability
- **2.** Solubility
- **3.** Polarity
  - **a.** Polar
  - **b.** Non-Polar
- **4.** Inter/Intra Molecular Forces
  - **a.** Separation of Molecules
  - **b.** Purification of Molecules

D. Organic Analysis of Compounds
- **1.** Introduction to Infrared Spectroscopy
- **2.** H-NMR Spectroscopy
- **3.** Simple Chemical Tests

E. Stereochemistry
  1. Conformational Analysis
  2. Optical Activity
  3. Chirality
    a. Chiral Centers
    b. Places of Symmetry
    c. Enantiomers
    d. Diastereomers
    e. Meso Compounds
F. IUPAC Nomenclature
  1. Identification of Functional Groups
  2. Naming conventions for Various Functional Groups
  3. Reactions of Major Functional Groups
    a. Prediction of Reaction Products
    b. Important Mechanistic Generalities
G. Acid-Base Chemistry
  1. Resonance Effects
  2. Inductive Effects
  3. Prediction of Products
  4. Equilibria
H. Chemistry of Aromatic Compounds
  1. Concept of Aromaticity
  2. Electrophilic Aromatic Substitution
  3. Synthesis (Simple Sequence of Reactions)
    a. Identification of the Product
    b. Identification of Reagents

5.3.2 Structure and Stereochemistry, With Sample Questions

Covalent bonds are formed by two atoms sharing a pair of electrons. Covalent bonds generally form between atoms of similar electronegativity (as a rule, the nearer they are to each other in the periodic table the farther apart atoms are located, and the greater the difference in electronegativity the greater likelihood of ionic bonding; for example, NaCl). There are two types of bonds: sigma bonds (orbital overlap in one area in space) and π-bonds (orbital overlap in two areas of space). Topics to be reviewed for this section should include the octet rule, resonance structures, dipoles, optical activity, and assignment of configurations.

1. What is the best description of the bonding in CO_2?
  A. One sigma bond and three pi bonds
  B. Three sigma bonds and one pi bond
  C. No sigma bonds and four pi bonds
  D. Two sigma bonds and two pi bonds
  E. Four sigma bonds and no pi bonds

2. Which of the following molecules violates the octet rule?
  A. BH_3
  B. CH_4
  C. NH_3
  D. H_2O
  E. C_6H_6

3. Which of the following molecules represents "molecule 1" in a Fisher projection?

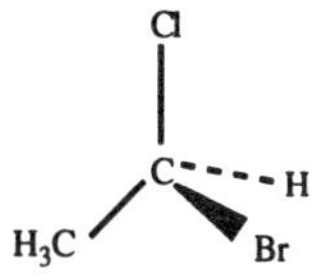

molecule 1

A. 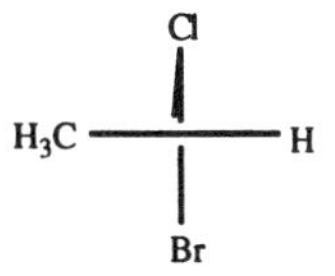

B. 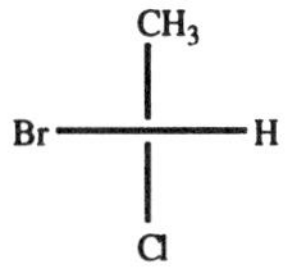

C. 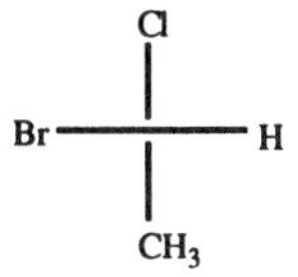

D. 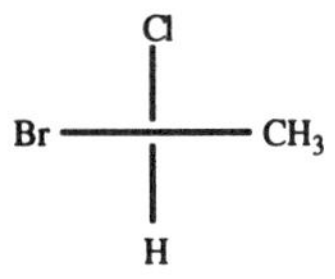

E. 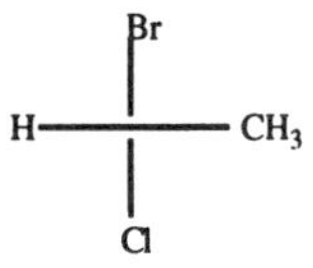

4. Which of the following molecules is in the "S" configuration?

A. 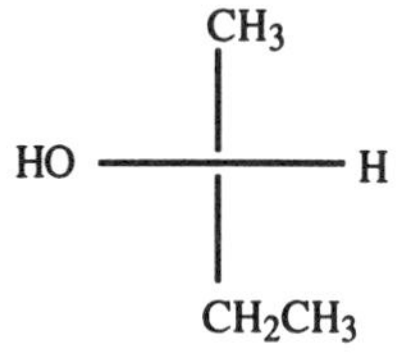

B. 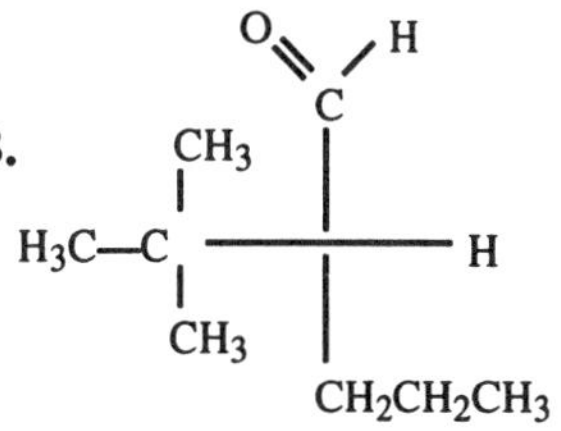

C. 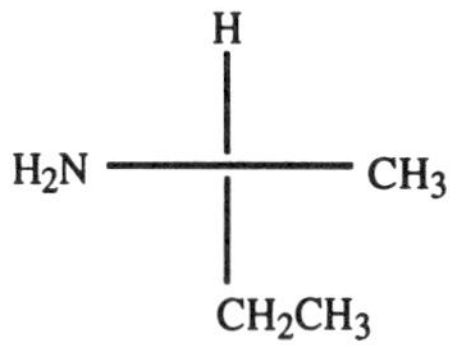

D. 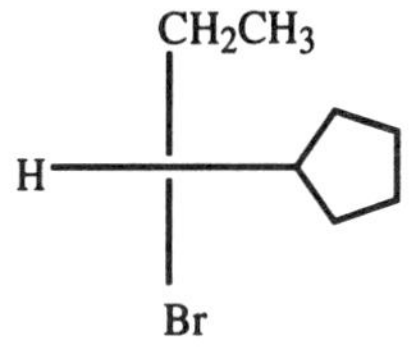

E. 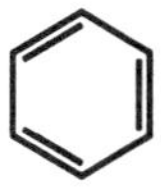

5. Which of the following molecules is an enantiomer of "molecule 2"?

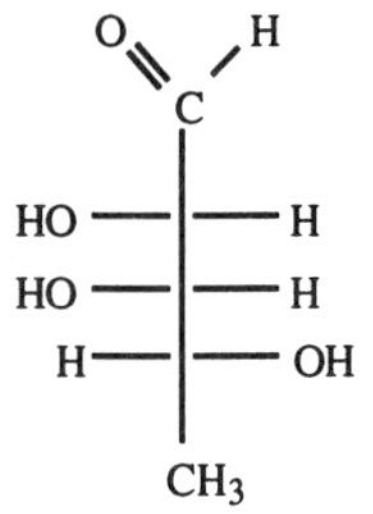

molecule 2

A.

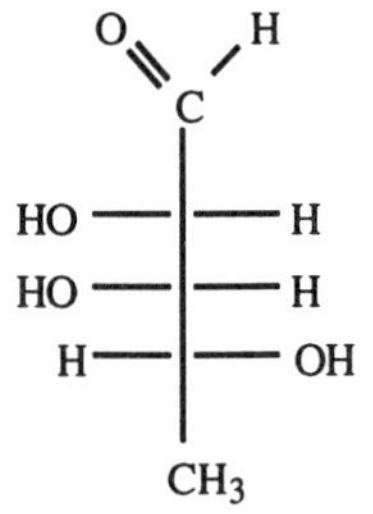

B.

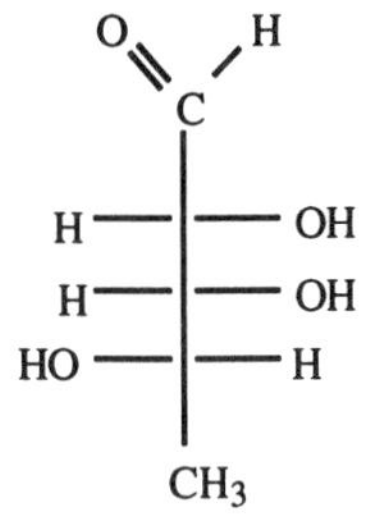

C.

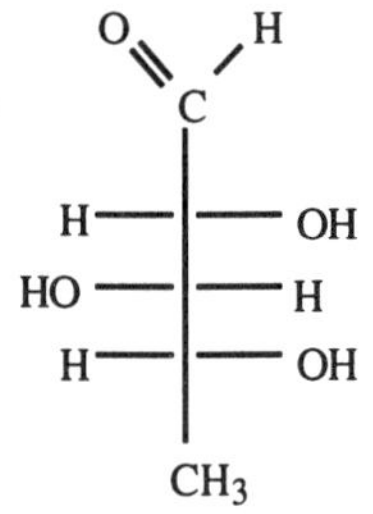

D.

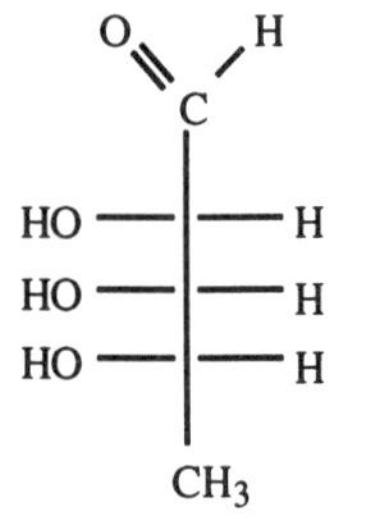

E.

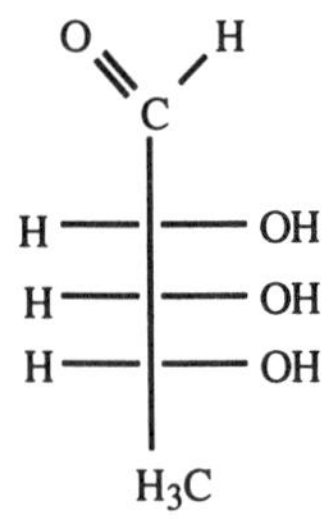

6. How many stereoisomers of "molecule 3" exist?

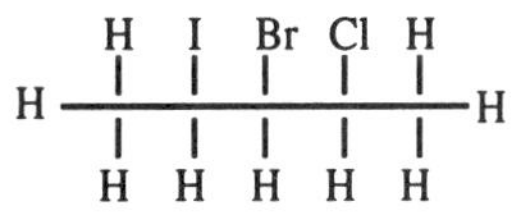

molecule 3

A. 4
B. 8
C. 16
D. 32
E. 0

Note: For all of the following sections you should review the IUPAC rules for nomenclature of organic compounds relating to the topic. For all sections you should review nomenclature, physical properties, preparation, and reactions.

5.3.3 Alkanes, Alkenes, and Aromatics, With Sample Questions

A few concepts to remember for this section are as follows: Alkanes: the general formula is C_xH_{2x+2}, all names end in -ane, and fragments end in -yl.

Physical properties: (1) the higher the molecule mass the higher the boiling point, (2) branched compounds have lower boiling points than related straight chain compounds, (3) cyclic compounds have higher boiling points than open chains, (4) low densities, and (5) nonpolar.

Unsaturated: the general formula is C_xH_{2x} for one double bond and C_xH_{2x-2} for one triple bond. Alkenes use the ending -ene and alkynes use the ending -yne. Geometric isomers are possible for alkenes, cis, and trans or Z and E.

Aromatics: aromaticity requires (1) cyclic, (2) planar, (3) sp^2 or sp hybrids, and (4) obey Huckel's Rule (number of π-electrons = 4n + 2).

7. Of the labelled carbons in "molecule 4," which represents a tertiary carbon?

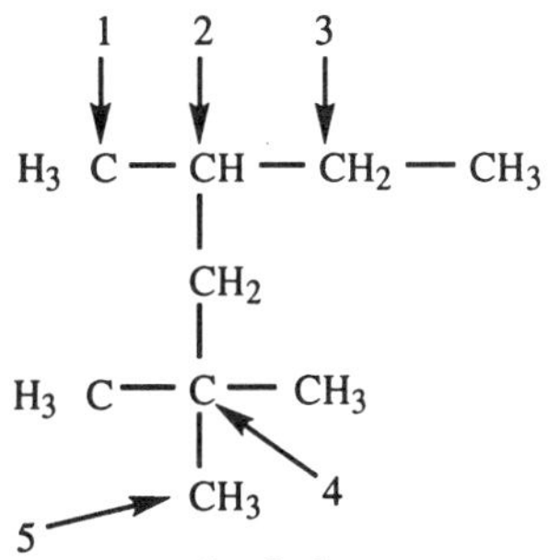

molecule 4

A. 1
B. 2
C. 3
D. 4
E. 5

8. Which of the following compounds has the highest boiling point?
A. n-hexane
B. 2-methylpentane
C. 2,3-dimethylbutane
D. Cyclohexane
E. Methane

9. Which of the following Newman projects represents the highest energy configuration?

A. 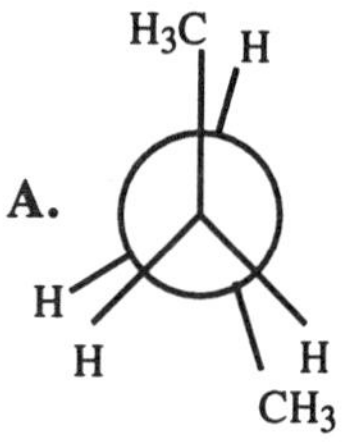

B. 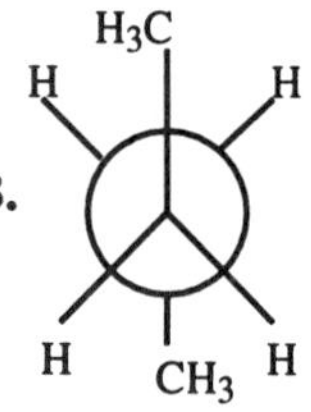

C. 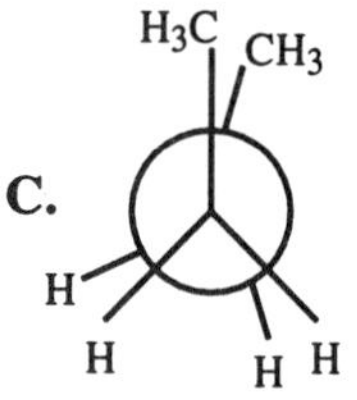

D. 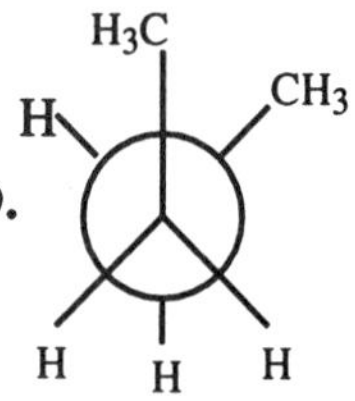

E. 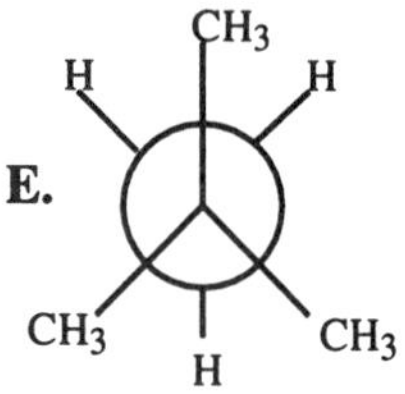

10. What would be the product of the following reaction?

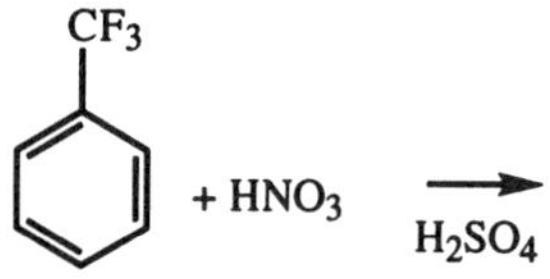

A. 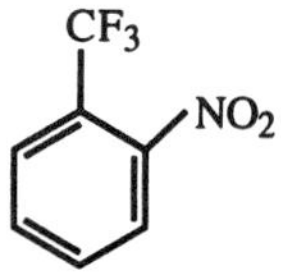

B. 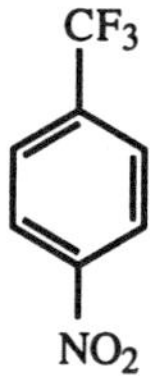

C. 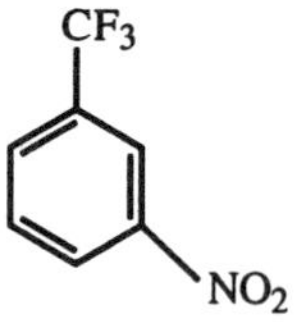

D. 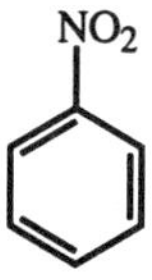

E. 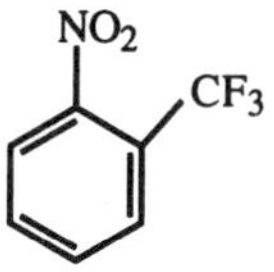

11. Which of the following compounds is not aromatic?

A. 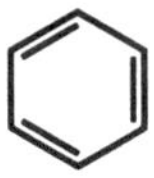

B. 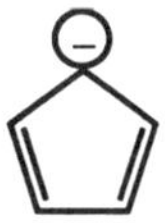

C. 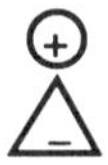

D. 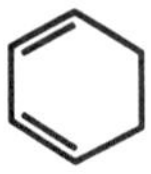

E. 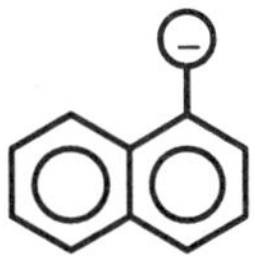

12. What is the product of the following reaction?

$H_3CCH{=}CH_2 + HBr \longrightarrow\ ?$

A. $H_3C\underset{|}{\overset{}{C}}H{-}\underset{|}{C}H_2$ (Br on CH, H on CH_2)

Br H

B. $H_3C\underset{|}{C}H{-}\underset{|}{C}H_2$ (H on CH, Br on CH_2)

H Br

C. $H_3CCH{=}C\begin{smallmatrix}H \\ Br\end{smallmatrix}$

D. $H_3CC(Br){=}CH_2$

E. CH3 = Br = CH2

5.3.4 Alcohols, Aldehydes and Ketones, Ethers, and Phenols, With Sample Questions

Oxygen-containing groups are as follows:

–OH **Alcohols:** unusually high boiling points, more soluble in water, polar, name using longest carbon chain plus -ol ending.

Ph-OH **Phenols**

O
||
R-C-H **Aldehydes:** name using longest carbon chain with group and ending -al. Carbons are numbered beginning at aldehyde end.

O
||
R-C-R **Ketones:** use the longest chain, numbered to give carbonyl lowest possible number, and use the ending -one.

R-O-R **Ethers:** somewhat polar, name using two allyr ñames plus ether.

13. The reaction of a primary alcohol with CrO_3 yields

A. an aldehyde.
B. a carboxylic acid.
C. a ketone.
D. an ether.
E. no reaction occurs.

14. The Williamson Ether Synthesis is the reaction of

A. ROH and R'X
B. RCOOH and R'X
C. RONa and R'X
D. ROH and R'Na
E. ROR and ROH

15. Which of the following is the correct name for

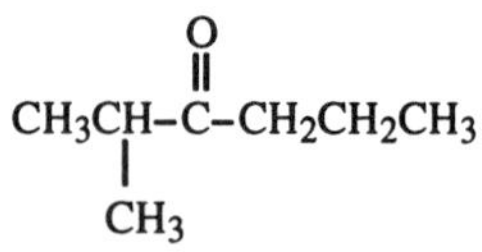

A. 2-methyl-3-hexanal
B. 1-methyl-3-hexanal
C. 2-methyl-3-hexanone
D. 1-methyl-3-hexanone
E. 1 methyl-2-hexanal

16. Which of the following species represents a ketal?

A. 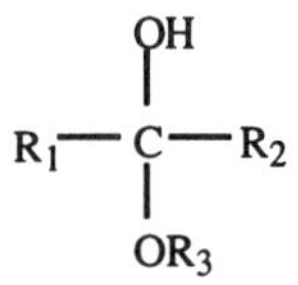

B. 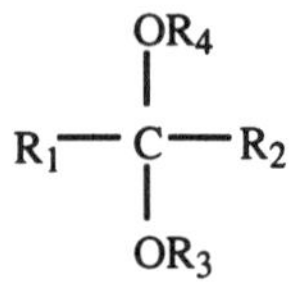

C. 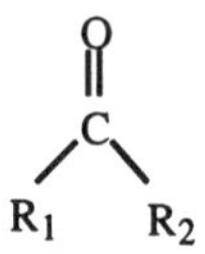

D. 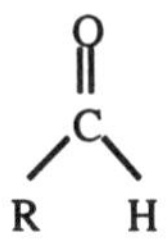

E. 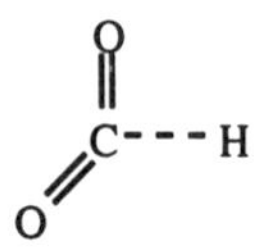

17. Which of the following would be the major product in this reaction?

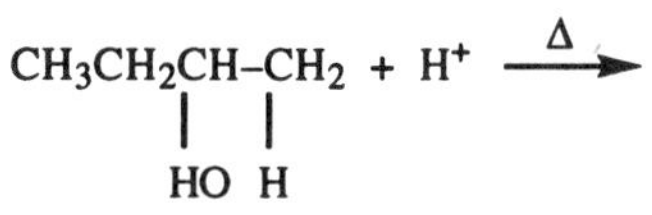

A. $CH_3CH_2CH{=}CH_2$

B. $CH_3CH{=}CH{-}CH_3$

C. 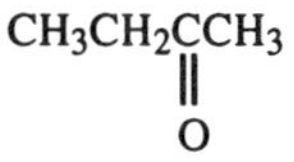

D. $CH_3CH_2CH_2CH_3$

E. $CH_3CH_2CHCH_2CH_3$

18. Alcohols have higher boiling points than the corresponding alkanes (for example, methane boils at –164°C while methanol boils at 65°C). Which of the following accounts for this fact?

A. Higher molecular mass
B. Hydrogen bonding
C. London Dispersion Forces
D. Higher density
E. Low freezing point

5.3.5 Carboxylic Acids and Their Derivatives, With Sample Questions

Carboxylic acids are named using the longest carbon chain and the ending -oic acid.

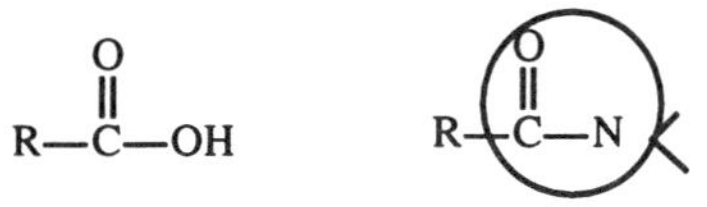

is the amide group.

Anhydrides are formed by the removal of water from two-COOH groups. Anhydrides are more reactive than the corresponding acids. Esters are named by changing -oic to -ate.

19. Which of the following carboxylic acids is the strongest acid?

A. 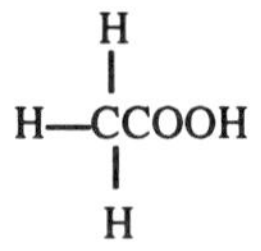

B. 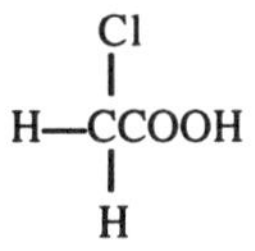

C. 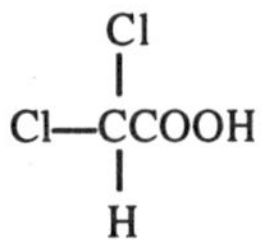

D. 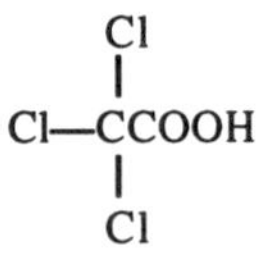

E. 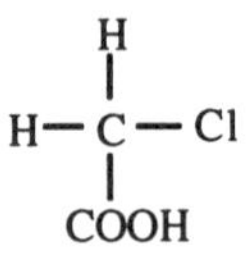

20. The reaction of a carboxylic acid and an alcohol will produce
- **A.** an anhydride.
- **B.** an ether.
- **C.** an ester.
- **D.** an acid with a longer carbon chain.
- **E.** an amide.

21. Which of the following is the correct name for the compound shown?

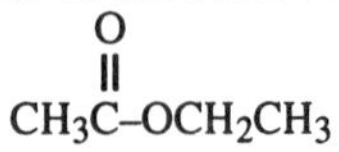

- **A.** Ethanoic acid
- **B.** Ethanoic anhydride
- **C.** Ethyl ethanoate
- **D.** Ethanamide
- **E.** Ethyl Methyl Ketone

22. A general reagent for the conversion of an acyl chloride to an ester is
- **A.** excess ammonia.
- **B.** an alcohol in the presence of pyridine.
- **C.** a dialkyl cadmium compound.
- **D.** hydrogen in the presence of Pd.
- **E.** an ester in the presence of benzene.

23. Which of the following compounds has the lowest melting point?
- **A.** Ethanamide
- **B.** N-ethylethanamide
- **C.** N, N-diethylethanamide
- **D.** N, N-diethylethanamidiumchloride
- **E.** Not enough information given

5.3.6 Amines, With Sample Questions

Amines are weak bases, named either as (organic group) amine or using the longest carbon chain numbered to give the amine-N the lowest possible number.

24. Which of the following compounds is the strongest base in the gas phase?

A. Trimethylamine
B. Dimethylamine
C. Methylamine
D. Ammonia
E. Hydrogen Chloride

25. What is the product of the following reaction?

$$RC(=O)NH_2 + LiAlH_4 \longrightarrow$$

A. $R\text{–}C \equiv N$

B. RCH_2NH_2

C. $RC(=O)H$

D. $RC(=O)NH_3^+$

E. $R\text{—}C(=O)\text{—}R$

26. What is the product of the following reaction?

$$CH_2 = CHC \equiv N + H_2/Pt \rightarrow ?$$

A. $CH_3CH_2C \equiv N$
B. $CH_2{=}CHNH_2$
C. $CH_3CH_2CH_2NH_2$
D. $CH_3CH_2CH{=}NH$
E. $CH_3CH_2CH_2CH_3$

27. Which of the following compounds is aniline?

A. 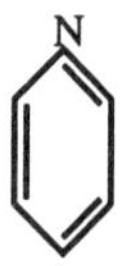

B. 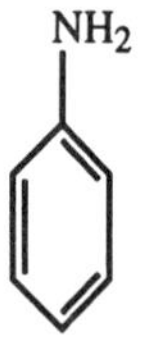

C. 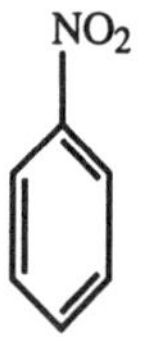

D. 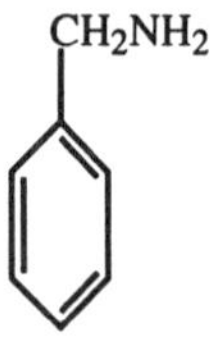

E. 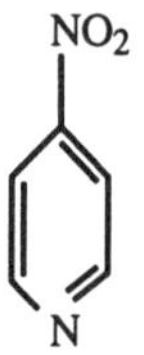

5.3.7 Amino Acids and Proteins, With Sample Questions

Amino acids can act as zwitterions, ions that have both a cation site and anion site in a single molecule, have high melting points, and are soluble in water.

Proteins are divided into two broad classes, fibrous and globular. These classifications are related to function. The structure of proteins is divided into primary, 1°, secondary, 2°, tertiary, 3°, and quaternary, 4°. The primary structure relates the way the atoms of the protein molecule are linked by covalent bonds. The secondary structure yields information on the way the chains are arranged in space (for example: coils or sheets). The tertiary structure involves more details on the intramolecular interactions (hydrogen bonding, van der Waals interactions). The quaternary structure deals with the intermolecular interactions between protein chains.

28. A peptide linkage between two amino acids is best described by
- **A.** the condensation of two carboxylic acids groups on amino acids.
- **B.** interaction between amine and carboxyl groups of amino acids.
- **C.** a hydrogen bond formed between the –COOH group and $-NH_2$ groups of amino acids.
- **D.** a new carbon-carbon interaction between amino acids.
- **E.** none of the above.

29. The isoelectric point of amino acids is defined as
- **A.** occurring when all –COOH sites are protonated.
- **B.** occurring when all $-NH_2$ sites are deprotonated.
- **C.** occurring when the amino acid present as a zwitterion is at a minimum.
- **D.** occurring when the amino acid present as a zwitterion is at a maximum.
- **E.** all of the above.

30. One useful method for determining the N-terminal amino acid residue is the "Sanger Method." In this reaction, using 2,4-dinitrofluorobenzene, the terminal amino acid contains
   A. a nitro group.
   B. a fluorophenyl group.
   C. a 2,4-dinitrophenyl group.
   D. a fluoro group.
   E. none of the above.

31. Which of the following functional groups are not commonly found in amino acids?
   A. thiol, –SH
   B. nitrosyl, –NO
   C. hydroxyl, –OH
   D. amino, $-NH_2$
   E. methyl, $-CH_3$

32. How many amino acids occur naturally in proteins?
   A. 10
   B. 12
   C. 18
   D. 20
   E. 16

33. What is the product of the reaction of glycine with benzoyl chloride and $NaOH_{(aq)}$?

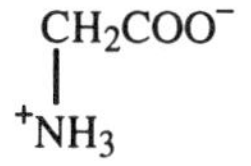

glycine

   A. $PhC(=O)NHCH_2COOH$
   B. $(Cl^-)(^+H_3NCH_2COOH)$
   C. H_2NCH_2COOCl
   D. $H_2NCH_2COOCH_2C_6H_5$
   E. $CH_3CH_2CH_2CH_2OH$

34. Which of the following is not characteristic of globular proteins?
   A. Insoluble in water
   B. Intramolecular hydrogen bonding
   C. Folded into compact units
   D. Functions usually related to regulation of life processes
   E. All of the above

35. Stereochemical studies of naturally occurring amino acids have shown they all have the same configurations about the carbon bonded to the alpha-amino group as
   A. D-gylceraldehyde.
   B. L-glyceraldehyde.
   C. D-Tartaric acid.
   D. L-Tartaric acid.
   E. D-Ethanediol.

5.3.8 Carbohydrates, With Sample Questions

Carbohydrates are polyhydroxy aldehydes, ketones, or related compounds. Monosaccharides cannot be hydrolyzed to simpler compounds, disaccharides can be hydrolyzed to two, and polysaccharides hydrolyzed to many monosaccharides. If it contains an aldehyde group it is an aldose, if it contains a ketone group it is a ketose. For example, a five-carbon monosaccharide containing an aldehyde is classified as an aldepentose.

36. Which of the following labeled carbons is the anomeric carbon?

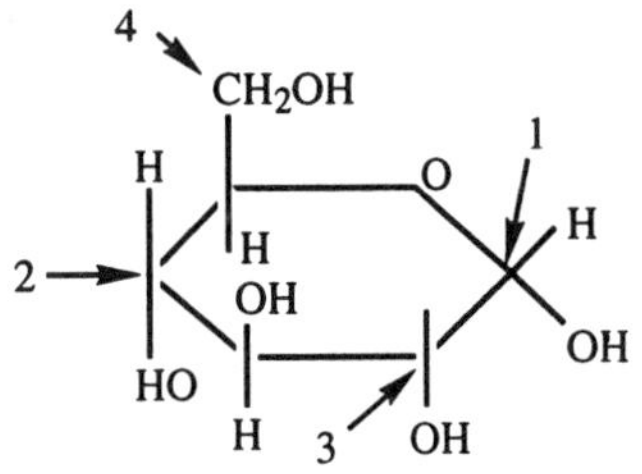

A. 1
B. 2
C. 3
D. 4
E. 5

37. Which of the following straight chain aldoses gives the following cyclic structure?

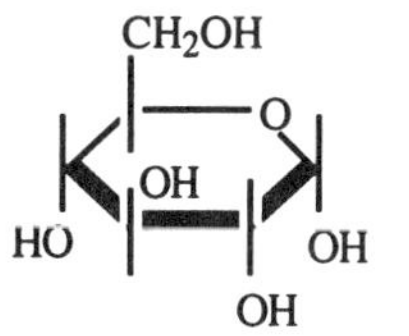

A.

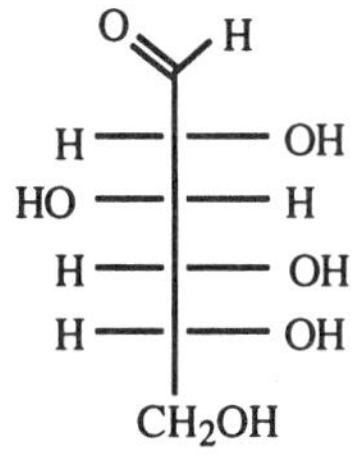

B.

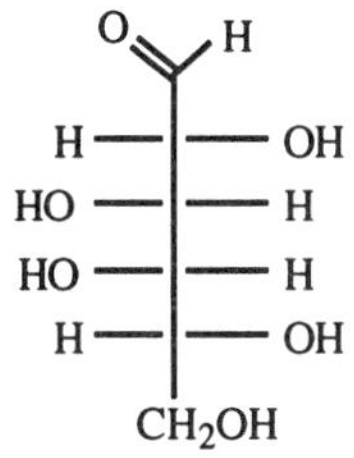

C.

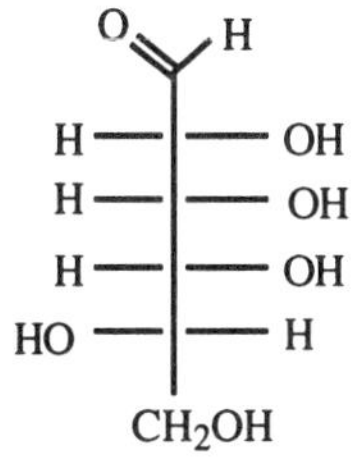

D.

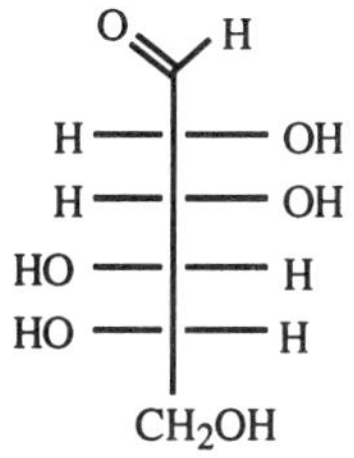

E.

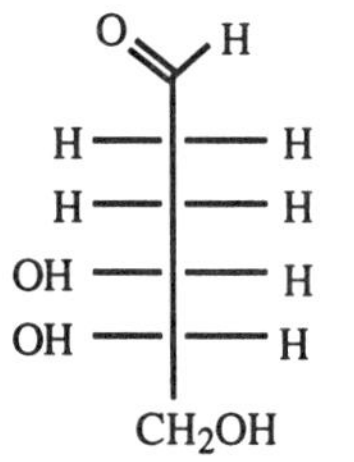

38. Which of the following procedures is used in the Kiliani-Fischer synthesis to lengthen the carbon chain of aldoses?

A. Reaction with H_2CO_3 followed by hydrolysis
B. Reaction with $H_2C{=}O$ followed by hydrolysis
C. Reaction with H_3COH followed by hydrolysis
D. Reaction with HCN followed by hydrolysis
E. Reaction with HCHO followed by hydrolysis

39. What is the product of a Ruff Degradation starting with

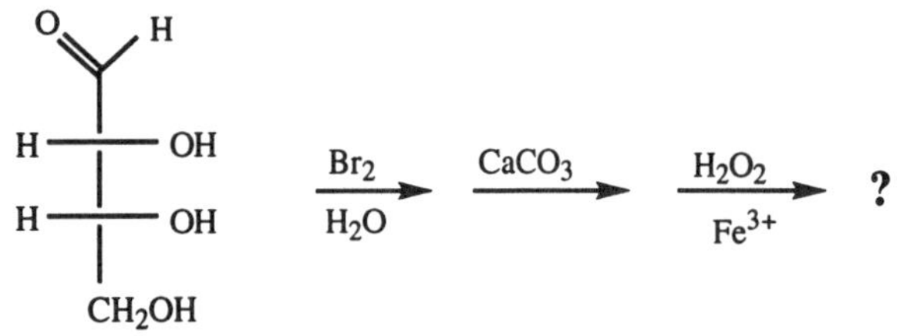

A. 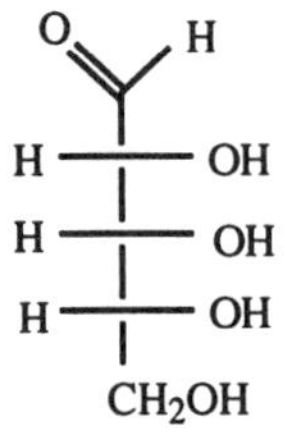

B. 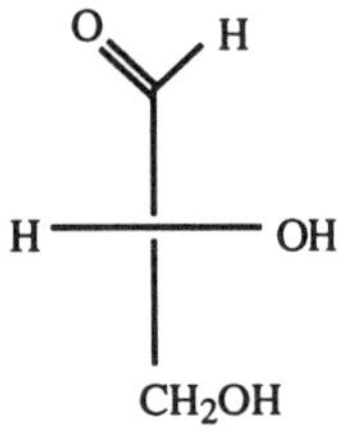

C. 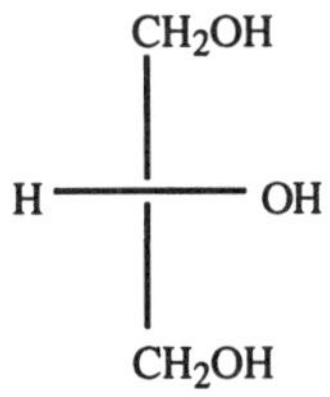

D. 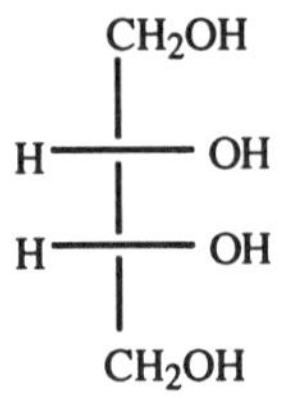

E. 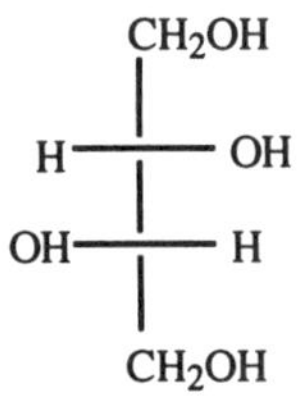

40. Which of the following reagent tests can be used to differentiate aldoses and ketoses?
A. Fehling's Reagent
B. Tollen's Reagent
C. Bromine water
D. Benedict's Solution
E. Mevalonic acid

5.3.9 Spectroscopy, With Sample Questions

This section reviews identification of organic compounds using IR and ^1H NMR data. A few important correlations are as follows (ranges given are approximate values):

IR

Functional group	cm^{-1}	Notes
-OH	3640–3610	usually broad peaks
amines	3500–3300	1° amines = doublet, 2° amines = singlet
≡ C-H	3315–3270	
-C-H	3100–3000	aromatics
$=CH_2$	3080	
$-CH_3$, $-CH_2-$	2990–2890	methyl groups have weak intensity, other alkyls are strong
C ≡ N	2300–2200	
C=O	1750–1740	ester
	1740–1720	aldehyde
	1720–1700	ketone

^{1}H NMR

Group	Chemical shift (∂ in ppm)	Notes
Methyl	0.9	
methylene	1.3	
Benzylic	2.3–3	Ar-**CH**
Vinyl	4.5–6.0	C = C -**H**
Amino	2.0–2.8	R**CH**$_2$NH$_2$
	1–5	R**NH**$_2$
Ketones	2.0–2.7	R**CH**$_2$C(= O)R
Alcohols	3.4–4.0	R**CH**$_2$COH
	1–5	RCH$_2$CO**H**
Ethers	3.3–5.0	R**CH**$_2$COR
Esters	3.7–4.1	RC(= O)O**CH**$_2$R
	2.0–2.2	R**CH**$_2$C(= O)OR
Aromatic	6.0–8.5	Ar-**H**
Aldehydic	9–10	
Carboxylic acids	10–12	

41. High-resolution mass-spectrometric analysis of compound A gave a molecular formula of $C_9H_{10}O_2$. The infrared spectrum showed strong absorption at 1715 cm^{-1} as well as many other medium-intensity bands. The NMR spectrum consisted of three sharp peaks at S = 7.22 ppm (area 5), δ = 5.00 ppm (area 2), and δ = 1.96 ppm (area 3). What is the structure of compound A?

A. 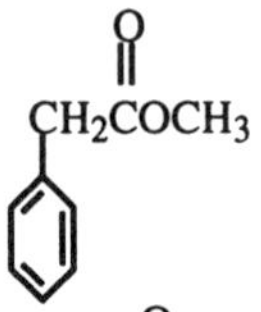

B. 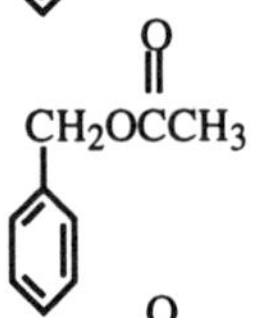

C. 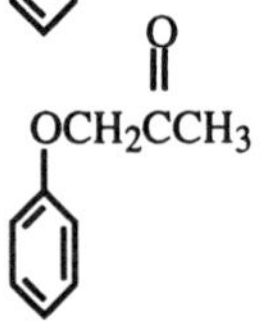

D. 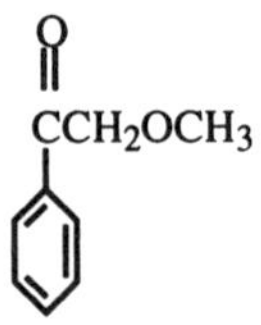

E. 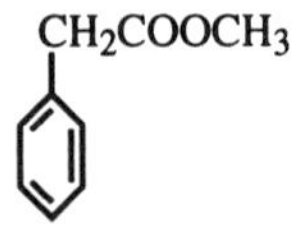

42. From a high-resolution mass spectrum of compound B, a molecular formula of $C_6H_{14}O$ could be assigned. In the infrared, the strongest absorption above 1400 cm^{-1} occurred at 2900 cm^{-1}. In the NMR, compound B showed a septet at ∂ = 3.62 ppm (area 1), J = 7 Hz, and a doublet at ∂ = 1.10 (area 6), J = 7 Hz. What is the structure of compound B?

A. 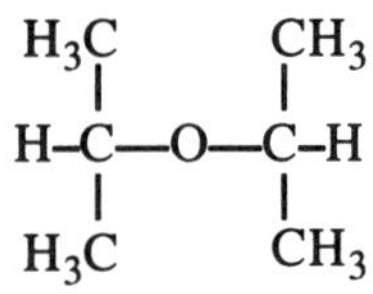

B. 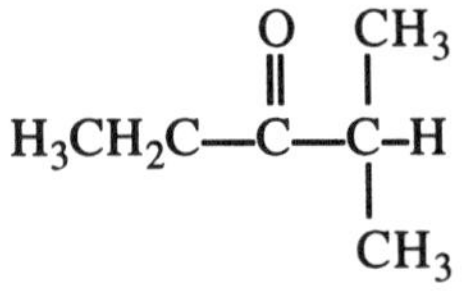

C. $H_3CH_2CH_2C–O–CH_2CH_2CH_3$

D. 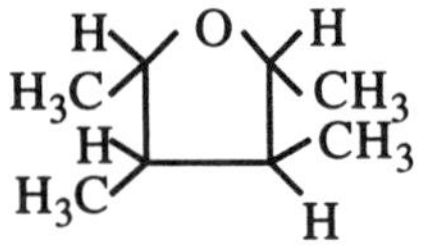

E. $C_6H_5CH_2CH_2OH$

5.3.10 Solutions and Explanations for Organic Chemistry

Question 1: [D] Topic: covalent bonding. The first step to solve this problem is to draw a Lewis Dot structure: O=C=O. In forming covalent bonds, the first bond between atom pairs is a sigma bond and further, multiple bonds are π-bonds.

Question 2: [A] Topic: octet rule. Choices **B-D** have 8 valence electrons. [CH_4 has 4 pairs of bonding electrons, NH_3 has 3 bonding pairs and 1 lone pair, and H_2O has 2 bonding pairs and 2 lone pairs]. BH_3 has 3 bonding pairs but no lone pairs for a total of 6 valence electrons.

Question 3: [C] Topic: stereoview. In a Fisher projection, the horizontal bonds represent bonds pointing out of the page and vertical bonds represent bonds behind (or into the page). Rotating the molecule to the right by about 60° gives the proper orientation.

Question 4: [C] Topic: Cahn-Ingold-Prelog rules. To assign an absolute configuration, (1) assign a rank to the four atoms/groups attached to the chiral carbon by mass. The largest mass is the highest range, #1, and (2) "draw" an arrow from 1 to 2 to 3 to 4. If it is clockwise, assign R for rectus. If it is counterclockwise, assign S for sinister, *unless* the #4 group is in a horizontal position, then reverse the arrow.

Question 5: [B] Topic: enantiomers. An enantiomer is a nonsuperimposable mirror image. Enantiomers have similar chemical and physical properties, except for rotation of light and reactions with chiral reagents. Diastereomers are stereoisomers that are not mirror images. They possess similar chemical properties but different physical properties.

Question 6: [B] Topic: stereoisomers. The number of stereoisomers is 2^n, where N is the number of chiral carbons present.

Question 7: [B] Topic: carbon types. Carbon atoms are typed by the number of carbon-carbon bonds formed. A primary 1° carbon has formed 1 C-C bond, a secondary 2° carbon has formed 2 C-C bonds, a tertiary 3° carbon has formed 3 C-C bonds, and a quaternary 4° carbon has formed 4 C-C bonds.

Question 8: [D] Topic: physical properties of alkanes. Cyclic hydrocarbons have a higher boiling point than straight chain analogs. This is due to London Dispersion Forces.

Question 9: [C] Topic: conformations of alkanes. The highest energy form will have the highest amount of steric interactions. In choice **C** the methyl groups are located in the closest possible arrangement.

Question 10: [C] Topic: directors in aromatic electrophilic substitution reactions. The group $-CF_3$ is a meta director. Some other groups and their influences are:

Activators: ortho & para directors	$-NH_2$, $-O\overset{\overset{O}{\|}}{C}R$, $-R$, $-OH$, $-NH\overset{\overset{O}{\|}}{C}R$, $-Ph$
Deactivators: meta directors	$-NO_2$, $-\overset{\overset{O}{\|}}{C}-R$, $-NH_3^+$, $-\overset{\overset{O}{\|}}{C}-OR$
Deactivators: ortho & para directors	Halogens

Question 11: [D] Topic: aromaticity. This compound is not planar and all of the carbons in the ring are not sp^2 or sp hybrids.

Question 12: [A] Topic: addition reactions. This is an addition across a C-C double bond. This class of reaction follows Markovnikov's Rule, which is that the carbon with the most hydrogens gets the H added. If this were a radical reaction, the reverse would be true.

Question 13: [A] Topic: oxidation reactions of alcohols. CrO_3 is an average oxidizing agent and will oxidize 1° alcohols to aldehydes. To produce a carboxylic acid you need to use a stronger oxidizing agent, like $KMnO_4$. Oxidizing agents will react with 2° alcohols to form ketones and will not react with 3° alcohols. For a reaction to occur, the alcohol carbon must possess an H.

Question 14: [C] Topic: name reactions. The Williamson Ether Synthesis is the reaction of an alkoxide and alkyl halide.

Question 15: [C] Topic: nomenclature. The compound is a ketone so the ending is -one. The longest carbon chain is 6 (hexane). Finally, use the lowest number combination from an end.

Question 16: [B] Topic: reaction products. A ketal is produced in the reaction of a ketone with two alcohols under acidic conditions. Choice **A** is the hemi-ketal, which is produced by reaction with one alcohol. Further reaction will produce the ketal. If your starting material is an aldehyde, you will produce an acetal.

Question 17: [B] Topic: reaction products. The reaction in question is a dehydration, which results in a C=C. The major product is the most substituted double bond, due to a rearrangement. Choice **A** would be a minor product.

Question 18: [B] Topic: physical properties. Alcohols meet the criteria for hydrogen bonding (electronegative element, N, O, or F, with an H attached and a lone pair of electrons). This is the strongest intermolecular force and gives the higher boiling points.

Question 19: [D] Topic: acid strength. Cl is an electron withdrawing group. The inductive effect results in a withdrawing of electrons from the O-H bond, weakening the bond, and resulting in a stronger acid. The higher the degree of substitution, the larger the effect.

Question 20: [C] Topic: reaction products. Anhydrides are formed by the removal of water from two carboxylic groups and ethers would form from alcohols in the Williamson Ether Synthesis.

Question 21: [C] Topic: nomenclature. The compound in question is an ester, named by changing the acid ending with -ioc to -ate, and naming the organic group attached to the oxygen. The others would be

A. CH_3COOH (common name = acetic acid) **B.** $CH_3\overset{\overset{O}{\|}}{C}O\overset{\overset{O}{\|}}{C}CH_3$ **D.** $CH_3\overset{\overset{O}{\|}}{C}NH_2$ **E.** $CH_3\overset{\overset{O}{\|}}{C}CH_2CH_3$

Question 22: [B] Topic: reaction reagents. Acyl chlorides, PhC(=O)Cl show these general reactions (to name a few):

1. with excess ammonia to form amides
2. with an alcohol to form esters
3. with a dialkyl cadium compound, R_2Cd, to form ketones
4. with H_2/Pd to form aldehydes

Question 23: [C] Topic: Physical properties. The trisubstituted N does not possess a bond for use in hydrogen bonding. This would result in a lower melting point. Both choices **A** and **B** can form strong hydrogen bonds resulting in higher melting and boiling points. Choice 4 is a salt.

Question 24: [A] Topic: physical properties. In the gas phase, the inductive effect of the donor group, Me, results in increasing the electron density on the central N. The higher the degree of substitution, the larger the effect. This is similar to question 19.

Question 25: [B] Topic: reaction products. $LiAlH_4$ is a reducing agent. The product will generally contain more Hs along a unit of unsaturation. This example reduces a C=O group to a CH_2 group. This is a typical reaction result with $LiAlH_4$.

Question 26: [C] Topic: reaction products. H_2/M is also a reducing agent. The product will generally contain hydrogens along a unit of unsaturation. In this example there are two units of unsaturation, C=C and C≡N. Both units are reduced by this strong reducing agent.

Question 27: [B] Topic: nomenclature. The correct names are

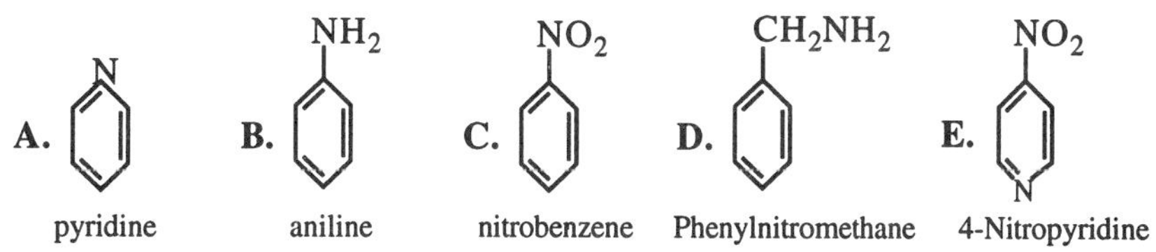

Question 28: [B] Topic: peptides. A peptide linkage is formed by loss of water from the –COOH and –NH_2 groups on amino acids. The formation is shown and the correct way to draw the peptide. For example:

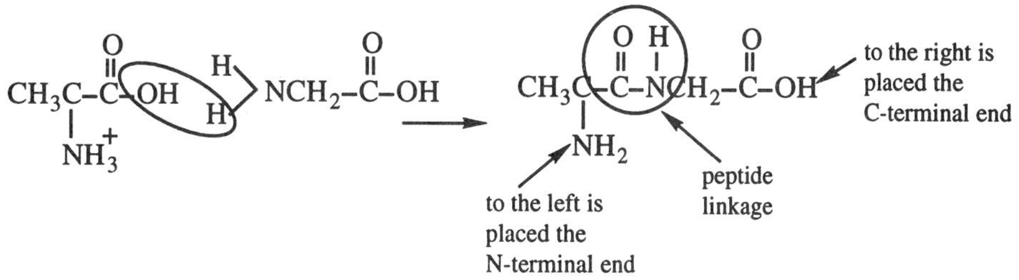

Question 29: [D] Topic: properties. The isoelectric point is when the rate of reaction 1 is equal to the rate of reaction 2, and the concentration of the zwitterion is maximized.

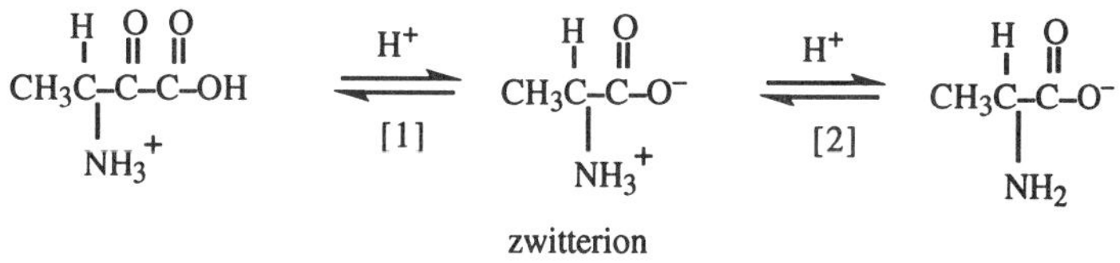

Question 30: [C] Topic: reaction types. The Sanger method labels the N-terminal end with 2,4-dinitrophenyl group. The DNFB will react with any free amino group, but only an α-amino group is at the N-terminal end.

Question 31: [B] Topic: amino acids. Nitrosyl groups are normally found bonded to transition metals.

Question 32: [D] Topic: amino acids. There are 20 naturally occurring amino acids.

Question 33: [A] Topic: reactions. Amino acids exhibit the reactions the functional groups possess. Amines react with acid chlorides, and -Cl is replaced by the -NHR group yielding the observed product.

Question 34: [A] Topic: globular proteins. Hemoglobin and lysozyme are globular proteins that are soluble in water. Globular proteins have low molecular weights, e.g., lysozyme is an enzyme with a molecular weight of 14,600.

Question 35: [B] Topic: configuration of amino acids. All naturally occurring amino acids have the same configuration as L-glyceraldehyde.

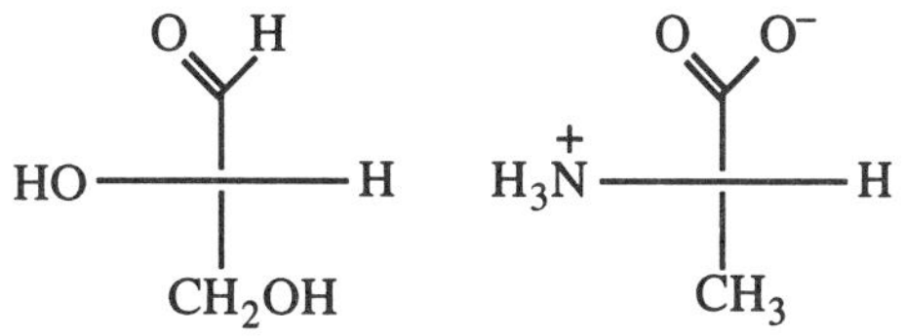

L-Glyceraldehyde   L-Alanine

Question 36: [A] Topic: diastereomeric forms. The "1" carbon in a cyclic representation of the structure is called the anomeric carbon. The forms are designated as the α-anomer or the β-anomer, depending on the orientation of the OH group. The α-anomer refers to the -OH in the down orientation and β-anomer has the -OH in the up orientation. Which is this one?

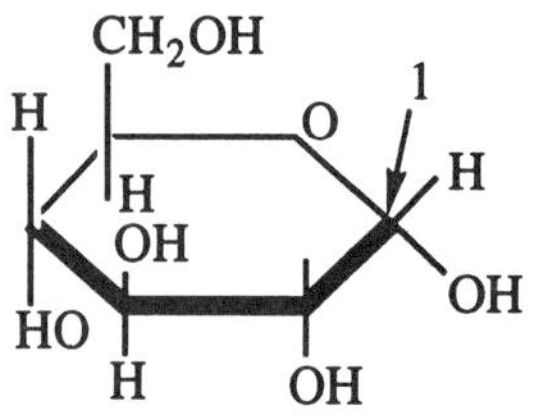

Question 37: [A] Topic: sugar structures. To relate a linear structure to a cyclic structure, follow this procedure:

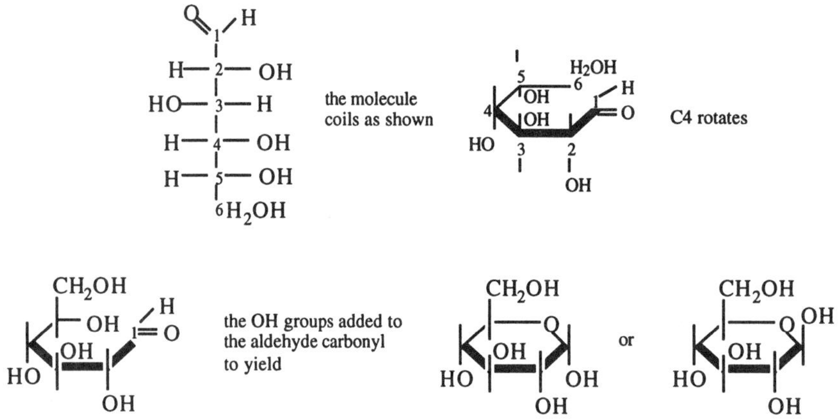

Question 38: [D] Topic: name reactions. The Kiliani-Fischer synthesis uses HCN followed by hydrolysis to lengthen the carbon chain by one unit.

Question 39: [B] Topic: name reactions. The Ruff degradation shortens the carbon chain by one H-C-OH unit. It is the reverse reaction of the Kiliani-Fischer synthesis.

Question 40: [C] Topic: chemical tests. Fehling's Reagent, Tollen's Reagent, and Benedict's Solution are all tests for sugars. They do not differentiate between aldoses and ketoses. Bromine water will only react with aldoses. It converts aldoses to an aldonic acid.

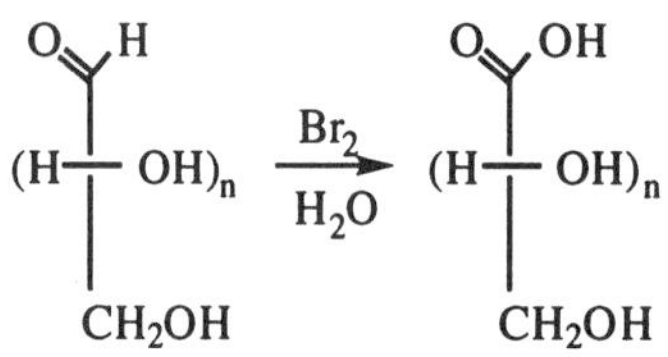

Question 41: [C] Topic: spectroscopy. The IR signal at 1715 cm^{-1} indicates a ketone (this rules out choices **A** and **B**). The NMR signal at 7.22 indicates C_6H_5, the other signals are not coupled. A peak of area 2 suggests CH_2 and a peak of area 3 suggests CH_3. A group neighboring an O is in the range of 3–5 and this suggests choice **C**.

Question 42: [A] Topic: spectroscopy. The IR information suggests there is no carbonyl, C=O, in this molecule (rules out choice **B**). The formula tells you that there are only 6 carbons (rules out choice **D**). The NMR data of a doublet at 1.10 ppm suggests a group next to a carbon with one hydrogen, and the septet suggests a group next to carbon(s) with six hydrogens. This is choice **A**.

5.4 REFERENCES

1. Jacob, Stanley W., M.D., and Clarice A. Francone, *Structure and Function of Man*, 3rd Edition. W. B. Saunders Company, 1974.
2. Masterton, W., and C. Hurley Pub., *Test Bank for Chemistry*. Saunders College Pub., 1989.
3. Burkett, A., and J. Sedenair, *Test Bank for Chemistry*, 2nd Edition. Allen and Baker, 1989.

PART 3

Sample OAT Test

6.0 INTRODUCTION TO TEST-TAKING SKILLS

The OAT requires a little over half a day for administration (approximately five hours). The OAT is given every year in February and October. Examinees should report to the testing center by 8:00 a.m. The exam will usually begin at 8:20 a.m. and end at 1:40 p.m. **There is a fifteen-minute break, but no lunch break.** Any other breaks are decided by the proctor and vary from test center to test center.

There are 240 test items on the exam, but the time allowed for each section may vary slightly depending on the length and difficulty of the questions in that section. Writing on the test booklet is allowed, including marking with highlighter pens. Calculators and electronic watches are not allowed. When the OAT is given, the order of the sections may be randomized. For example, in California, Reading Comprehension might come first, whereas Quantitative Reasoning Test might come first in Alabama. This information is based on previous data and it may or may not happen at your test center. Special test-taking skills are outlined in this chapter.

6.1 SELF-ASSESSMENT

This chapter trains you to be test-wise. By now you are familiar with the OAT test item format. You have developed your skills for accuracy, even if you are not yet working at OAT speed; you have reviewed the natural science sections, concentrating to master weak areas while maintaining your mastery of strong areas. You have also practiced Reading Comprehension, Quantitative Reasoning, and Problem Solving skills through test-item practice. Can you concentrate for two and a half hour segments, including short, structured breaks?

Now is the moment for honesty. If you have procrastinated, you may consider postponing your test date until the next application. Doing poorly on the test is personally demoralizing and does not enhance your standing with application committees. On the other hand, you may have spent the disciplined time required for OAT preparation, and you may now be ready to develop your test-taking strategies.

6.2 OAT TEST-TAKING SPEED

If your accuracy level (without time considerations) is high on all sections of the OAT, now you add speed as a variable. The actual OAT takes four hours. The following chart provides information on the timing requirements of each subtest.

TEST DAY SCHEDULE

Subtest	No. of Test Items	Time Allotted	Average Time/ Test Item	Comments
• Survey of the Nat Sciences		90 min.	54 secs/item	Total No. of Items = 100
Biology	40			
General Chemistry	30			
Organic Chemistry	30			
• Physics Test	40	50 min.	75 secs/item	—
Break	—	15 min.	—	—
• Pretest (not scored)	—	25 min.	—	Content/no. of items are variable
• Reading Comprehension Test	50	50 min.	60 secs/item	3 passages (1,300 words each)
• Quantitative Reasoning Test	50	45 min.	54 secs/item	30 math problems and 20 word problems

*The early morning session lasts for about 140 minutes followed by a late morning session for 120 minutes. Thus the total OAT time is approximately 240 minutes (4 hours). The remaining time is divided into a 15-minute rest break followed by a 25-minute pretest (not scored) used for field testing of new items. The student should note the pacing of various parts of the examination; for example, the response time (the time it takes to answer one test item in a subtest) varies from about 54 seconds/item test-taking to 75 seconds/item. The student should prepare for the OAT keeping the "variable pace" or speed in mind.

Figure 6.1 — OAT Timing Requirements by Subtest

Managing your time well on the OAT is a major ingredient of test-wiseness. First, you have to keep in mind that there are no extra points for finishing a subtest. You need to develop your speed, but speed is always a trade-off with accuracy, so you will need to gauge for yourself what is the best speed/accuracy ratio for the highest score. On the real test, you are interested only in getting the highest score you possibly can. Second, it is clear from the chart that your speed will have to vary from section to section. On average, you have approximately 25% more time for the physics items than for the reading comprehension items. But in addition, within each subtest, some questions are designed to take longer than others. This means that the test-wise student will not spend an equal amount of time on each item within a given subtest, but rather will take less time on those that are "easy," thereby saving time for the more difficult items.

A good test-taking strategy is to work the relatively easy questions quickly, thereby earning the more certain points and saving time for the harder questions. Keep in mind that there are no extra points for answering the single hardest question. If you take the same time you spent on that single hardest question to answer three easier questions, that would be a better strategy.

Separate subscores are given for each topic. The Survey of the Natural Sciences part of the test is undifferentiated. It is natural to spend more time on the science topics you like, avoiding those areas you don't like. If you have studied in accord with the suggestions in this manual, you should be fairly disciplined in your approach, knowing better than to dawdle in biology, simply because you are in no hurry to get to organic chemistry. On the other hand, the pressure of real testing situations has a tendency to make everyone revert to past behaviors. Don't let the test take you!

6.2.1 How to Work on Speed

Serious work on increasing your speed should begin approximately six weeks before the exam.

Work with a clock in front of you. Take approximately ten items at a time, work first for accuracy and note how much time it takes you to get the accuracy level you need. On the next set of practice items, push yourself to work just a little faster. If your accuracy level stays the same, work just a little bit faster on the next practice set. At the point where your accuracy level begins to suffer, work at that speed to bring the accuracy level back up. Increase your speed only when the accuracy level is high. Work in this way on all the subtests.

As you work on building your test-taking speed, look for "short-cuts." Would a quick estimate have allowed you to eliminate several answer possibilities quickly? Were there other ways to answer a question that would have been quicker? Did you become stubborn about answering a question that simply ate up too much time? (Note: this might be a virtue when you are a practicing optometrist, but not when you are taking the OAT!)

6.3 THREE WEEKS BEFORE THE TEST

1. Plan to take **a full simulated or mock OAT** about three or four Saturdays before the actual test. The AOA-provided OAT practice test could be used for this purpose. From the results you should be able to determine both whether you are ready to take the OAT and how you might spend your last few weeks of study most profitably. The practice test provided in this manual will also help you understand your weaknesses.

   If you can get others to participate in the simulation with you, so much the better. But remember, even if you do it on your own, the closer you simulate the real thing, the more benefit you can derive from the experience. For example, if you take the test at home, do not play the radio or take phone calls while you take the test. Carefully follow the time limits in the AOA test booklet.

2. Part of the benefit, of course, will be **a careful analysis** of the results. Score one point for each correct answer. There is no penalty for incorrect or unanswered items. Now make a percentage to discover your raw score. For example, if there are fifty questions and you answered thirty-five correctly, your raw score is 70 percent. You will now be able to tabulate your converted or scaled score exactly the way the AOA does. It varies from test to test, depending on test hardness, item analysis, and other variables. Simplified charts are presented in figures 6.2 and 6.3 to illustrate the scoring process.

1990 - 1993 Test Preparation Materials
Optometry Admission Testing Program Standard Score-Raw Score Conversions

STD SCORE	QRT	RCT	BIO	GEN CHEM	ORG CHEM	PHY	Total SCI
400	42–50	48–50	36–40	30	27–30	37–40	122–140
390	40–41	47	35	29	26	36	120–121
380	38–39	46	33–34	28	25	33–35	114–119
370	36–37	44–45	—	27	24	—	110–113
360	34–35	42–43	31–32	26	23	31–32	105–109
350	32–33	40–41	30	25	21–22	30	99–104
340	29–31	38–39	28–29	23–24	20	29	96–98
330	27–28	35–37	27	22	18–19	27–28	90–95
320	26	34	25–26	20–21	16–17	25–26	86–89
310	24–25	31–33	23–24	18–19	15	24	81–85
300	22–23	29–30	22	16–17	13–14	22–23	76–80
290	21	27–28	20–21	15	12	21	71–75
280	19–20	25–26	19	13–14	11	20	67–70
270	17–18	23–24	17–18	12	10	18–19	62–66
260	16	21–22	14–16	10–11	9	17	57–61
250	15	19–20	13	9	8	16	53–56
240	14	17–18	12	8	7	15	50–52
230	11–13	15–16	11	7	6	14	47–49
220	10	14	10	6	5	13	43–46
210	9	12–13	8–9	5	4	12	40–42
200	0–8	0–11	0–7	0–4	0–3	0–11	0–39

Figure 6.2 — OAT Standard/Raw Score Conversion Chart

Note: On the actual OAT, the scores for the four most recent tests are released on the official scorecard. The total number of times the OAT was taken is also recorded on the official scorecard.

Standard Deviation	Coded Score		Percentile Band Equivalents
+2 1/2	400–	.9%	99.3–100
+2 1/4	390–	.8%	98.5–99.2
+2	380–	1.4%	97.1–96.4
+1 3/4	370–	2.2%	96–97
+1 1/2	360–	3.2%	93–95
+1 1/4	350–	4.5%	88–92
+1	340–	6.0%	82–87
+3/4	330–	7.5%	75–81
+1/2	320–	8.8%	66–74
+1/4	310–	9.6%	56–65
MEAN	300–	10.3%	46–55
–1/4	290–	9.6%	36–45
–1/2	280–	8.8%	27–35
–3/4	270–	7.5%	20–28
–1	260–	6.0%	14–19
–1 1/4	250–	4.5%	9–13
–1 1/2	240–	3.2%	6–8
–1 3/4	230–	2.2%	3.2–5
–2	220–	1.4%	1.8–3.1
–2 1/4	210–	.8%	1–1.7
–2 1/2	200–	.9%	0.0–0.9

Figure 6.3 — OAT Scores Interpretation Guide

There is no advantage in taking the test just to learn that you were not yet ready. You can take the OAT as many times as you want, but all your scores will be forwarded to the schools where you apply.

3. Insofar as is possible, **maintain an OAT daily schedule.** This includes the time you get up, what you do when you get up, diet (do not forget to eat a reasonable breakfast), and what time you go to sleep. You cannot be at your best on a morning test if you have maintained a night-study schedule up until the test day.

6.4 THE LAST WEEK BEFORE THE TEST

1. If possible, on the Saturday before the actual OAT, drive to the **testing location** at the same time as you will on the day the OAT is given. Pay attention to route, traffic, parking, etc. Locate the testing room, bathroom, snack bar. Over-preparation is a good antidote to anxiety.

2. Schedule review sessions that emphasize **short-term memory tasks.** The rest of your OAT study time should be spent working item sets from each section under timed conditions. During these final sessions, **simulate real test situations** as closely as possible. For example, do not allow yourself to spend too much time solving one problem. In a good simulation, the adrenaline should be flowing just enough so you feel the stress, but not enough to make you anxious.

3. In these final practice sessions, **stick to the strategies** you have developed and practiced. Be deliberate. Consider carefully and mark the answer clues in the question. Cross out wrong answers. Work with the

watch that you intend to bring to the real OAT. It should have a large, clear face and a minute hand. Remember, **no** calculators are allowed. Remember, accuracy and speed are a trade-off. You should know beforehand what speed on each subtest gives you the highest level of accuracy.

4. Put yourself **on the OAT schedule,** doing each morning what you intend to do on the test day itself. Working with your plan of things to do today should now be a **habit.**

6.5 THE TEST DAY ITSELF

1. **Prepare in advance what you will take with you.** This may include your watch, three or four well-sharpened pencils with erasers, small boxes of raisins (raisins are a better source of quick energy than a candy bar. They metabolize fast and you do not risk the same sugar "low" that you can get from candy, and as an added bonus, opening the little box makes no noise!), and juice or water.
2. The night before the test eat a **high-carbohydrate dinner.** Called "carbohydrate packing," athletes do this the night before a game because the carbohydrates convert to energy by morning.
3. The morning before the test, eat **a high-protein breakfast.** Research at Johns Hopkins shows that protein at breakfast is particularly important for problem-solving activities. Get up in time to have your breakfast calmly.
4. **Get to the testing room in plenty of time to settle in.**
5. Once the test starts, you may want to note down certain short-term memory items.
6. Remember to **stick to your strategies throughout the test.** Do not be distracted by what others are doing around you. **Periodically make sure your mark on the answer sheet corresponds to the number of the question you are answering.**
7. If you go blank reading the first item, go on to the next. Continue until you **find one you can answer.** Then go back. Once started, **keeping to the pace** that you know from the practice sessions gives you the highest level of accuracy.
8. Do not omit any items. For those you don't know, simply fill in your **predetermined "guess answer."** There is no penalty for wrong answers.
9. During breaks, do not talk to other test takers. **Keep your energies focused on the test.**
10. **Stay in control** of your time and energy. Remember, you are taking the test. Do not let the test take you.

6.6 AFTER THE TEST

1. If you feel sick during the exam or you realize that you are not adequately prepared, you *cannot* void your test. If you must leave the test center before taking all the sections, you will receive a zero for the missed sections. Candidates are permitted to apply and retake the OAT as many times as they want.
2. After the test is over, do not compare what you remember answering with what someone else remembers answering. It is unreliable at best and often depressing. Be good to yourself!
3. Both preparation and luck have a part in any event that is going to occur at a specific time. If you have not performed as well as you needed to, you can take the test again. Do not waste too much time in depression; rather, analyze your weaknesses and figure out the best ways to correct them.

6.7 REFERENCES

1. *Optometry Admission Testing Program*, application and preparation materials (1993); Association of Schools and Colleges of Optometry, Optometry Admission Testing Program, 1992.
2. *Optometry Admission Test Preparation Materials*, Optometry Admission Testing Program, 1990.
3. Coury, V. M., J. E. Wells, and M. W. Reed, *Pretest Preparation for the Dental Admission Test.* McGraw-Hill Book Company (out of print).

Optometry Admission Test: Model Examination

7.0 INTRODUCTION

The model test consists of four separate examinations, one each in Reading Comprehension, Quantitative Reasoning, Survey of the Natural Sciences, and Physics. The model test is designed in accordance with the AOA Optometry Admission Test and proper course outlines. We emphasize that this examination is not a copy of the actual exam, which is guarded closely and may not be duplicated. The exam you'll take may have more difficult questions in some areas than you will encounter on this sample test, or some questions may be easier.

The time allotted for each subtest in the sample model test is based on a careful analysis of all the information currently available. The time we allot for each test, therefore, merely suggests in a general way approximately how much time you should spend on each subject when you take the actual exam. We have not, in every case, provided precisely the number of questions you will actually get on the examination. It's just not possible to know what the examiners will finally design for the actual test. It might be a good idea to jot down your "running" time for each test and make comparisons later on. If you find that you're working faster, you may assume you are making progress. Remember, we have timed each test uniformly. If you follow all our directions, your scores will be comparable.

The actual OAT is given with a different schedule from the one in this book. The chart below shows the schedule for the actual OAT:

Actual Test Schedule	Time Allowed
Survey of Natural Sciences	90 minutes
Physics Test	50 minutes
Rest	15 minutes
Pretest (Not Scored)	25 minutes
Reading Comprehension Test	50 minutes
Quantitative Reading Test	45 minutes

7.1 READING COMPREHENSION

Read each passage to get the general idea. Then reread the passage more carefully to answer the questions based on the passage. For each question read all choices carefully. Then select the answer you consider correct or most nearly correct. Blacken the answer space corresponding to your best choice, just as you would do on the actual examination.

Time limit: 50 minutes

Passage #1
Growth and Formation of Bones

The "cartilage" skeleton is completely formed at the end of three months of pregnancy. During subsequent months of gestation, ossification and growth occur.

Longitudinal growth of bones continues in a definite sequence until approximately fifteen years of age in the female and sixteen in the male. Longitudinal growth should not be confused with bone maturation and remodeling, which are processes continuing until the age of twenty-one in both the male and female. This pattern of maturation is so regular that an individual's age can be determined with amazing accuracy from radiologic examination of his or her bones.

It is sometimes stated that bone is preformed in the cartilage, since the majority of embryonic bones do resemble the future skeleton in shape and composition; however, it is incorrect to state that cartilage actually turns into bone. Cartilage merely represents the environment in which the bone develops.

Formation

Chemical Composition

The strong protein matrix of bone is responsible for its resilience when tension is applied, whereas the salts deposited in this matrix prevent crushing when pressure is applied. A substance known as hydroxyapatite $[Ca_3(PO_4)_2]_3 \cdot Ca(OH)_2$ makes up the major portion of salts present in bone. Small amounts of calcium carbonate ($CaCO_3$) are also present.

Deposition of Bone

Bone develops from spindle-shaped cells called **osteoblasts**, which are found beneath the periosteum (the fibrovascular membrane covering the bone) and in the endosteum, which lines the marrow cavity. The first function of the osteoblasts is that of secreting a protein substance that polymerizes to form the tough, leather-like matrix. Calcium salts are then precipitated within the matrix, giving the bone its characteristic quality of hardness. For these salts to be deposited it is necessary that calcium first combine with phosphate, producing calciumphosphate ($CaHPO_4$); this substance is slowly converted over a period of several weeks into hydroxyapatite.

Regulation of Deposition

Deposition of bone is regulated partially by the amount of strain on the bone—the more strain the greater the deposition. Bones in casts, therefore, will waste away, whereas continued and excessive strain will cause the bone to grow thick and strong. In addition, a break in the bone will stimulate injured osteocytes to proliferate, secreting large quantities of matrix for the deposition of new bone.

Reabsorption of Bone

Large cells called **osteoclasts** are present in almost all cavities of bone, and function to cause reabsorption of bone. It is thought that this is brought about by the secretion of enzymes that digest the protein portion of bone and split the salts. These phosphate and calcium salts are then absorbed into the surrounding extracellular fluid.

The strength and, in some instances, the size of the skeletal bone will depend on the comparative activity of the bone. For example, it is obvious that during the growth period deposition is more active than reabsorption. The role of the osteoclast has not been definitely established, but it is known to be associated with the removal of dead bone from the inner side during remodeling. As a result, the medullary cavity enlarges, and the bone itself is prevented from becoming overly thick and heavy. Osteoblastic deposition continues to counteract the never ending process of reabsorption, even when the bones are no longer capable of growth.

It is possible for crooked bones to become straight due to this continual process. A broken bone that has healed crooked in a child will straighten in a matter of a few years.

During the four-day flight of Gemini IV in 1965, one of the astronauts lost between 1 and 12 percent of his bone mass, as measured by x-ray of his hands and feet. The flight of Gemini V, which lasted eight days, caused losses of more than 20 percent. As a result of these findings, exercises in flight were prescribed that were found to reduce this loss.

Intramembranous Ossification

There are two types of ossification. The first of these is intramembranous ossification, a process in which dense connective membranes are replaced by deposits of inorganic calcium salts, thus forming bone. The membrane itself becomes the **periosteum** (around bone), while immediately within the periosteum can be found compact bone with an inner core of **spongy** or **cancellous bone.**

Endochondral Ossification

Most bones form by the process of **endochondral ossification,** the replacement of cartilaginous structures with bone. Growth in length of a bone occurs at the growth plate, which consists of a number of layers of cartilage cells lying between the epiphysis (knoblike extremity of a bone) and the diaphysis (the shaft or central portion of a bone). The basal layer of cells is abundantly supplied with blood, and this layer proliferates, producing more cartilage cells and adding to the length of the bone. The upper layers of cells are thus lifted away from the source of blood and nutrients and are subsequently ossified.

As a long bone increases in length, there is a proportional increase in its diameter owing to periosteal deposition of layers of compact tissue. These layers are thickest in the middle of the shaft and taper toward the epiphysis, which remains essentially cancellous. Simultaneously, the cancellous interior of the diaphysis is destroyed, leading to the formation of the marrow canal. The spongy bone of the epiphysis is left intact.

Ossification of the epiphysis follows a generally predictable pattern. The age of the skeleton can be determined by the presence and size of various mes-ossification centers. For instance, the physician can determine if a baby is at term by ascertaining whether or not the distal femoral epiphysis is ossified.

Longitudinal growth is dependent, then, on the growth plate at the junction of the diaphysis and epiphysis. Growth in the diameter of bone occurs primarily by the deposit of bony tissue beneath the periosteum. In a short time, only two thin strips of tissue, the growth plates, remain between the epiphysis and the diaphysis. When these two final sites have filled with osseous tissue, longitudinal growth is complete and growth is no longer possible. The initial shape assumed by a bone during its formation is genetically determined. Extrinsic factors such as muscle strength, mechanical stress, and biochemical environment assume a function in determining the shape of a bone. Wolff's law reflects the role of mechanical forces acting on bone and, briefly stated, suggests that the structure of a bone is dependent on its function.

1. Which of the following is NOT a function of the skeletal system?
   A. Support tissues
   B. Protect vital organs and other tissues
   C. Hematopoiesis
   D. Filtration of blood
   E. Storage of minerals and salts

2. The skeletal system is composed of ________ bones?
   A. 1,206
   B. 601
   C. 2,010
   D. 206
   E. 156

3. Which of the following is NOT a part of the appendicular skeletal system?
   A. Shoulders
   B. Vertebrae
   C. Pelvic girdle
   D. Arms
   E. Legs

4. Ossification of the skeletal system begins
   A. at birth.
   B. during puberty.
   C. during first three months of pregnancy.
   D. after the first three months of pregnancy.
   E. immediately after implantation.

5. The major portion of salts found in bone is represented by
   A. hydroxyapatite.
   B. calcium carbonate.
   C. calcium chloride.
   D. sodium chloride.
   E. calcium phosphate.

6. Bone develops from cells responsible for secreting a protein matrix, in which salts are precipitated. These cells are called
   A. osteoclast.
   B. fibroblast.
   C. ameloblast.
   D. osteocytes.
   E. osteoblast.

7. Bone deposition is regulated *primarily* by
   A. genetic coding.
   B. stress.
   C. age.
   D. cartilage.
   E. calcium.

8. Before hydroxyapatite can be formed, calcium must first combine with
   A. phosphate.
   B. protein.
   C. oxygen.
   D. carbon.
   E. chloride ions.

9. Phosphate and calcium salts freed as a result of bone reabsorption are absorbed into the
   A. small intestine.
   B. lymphatic system.
   C. extracellular fluids.
   D. bone matrix.
   E. bone marrow.

10. Bones of the face and skull are formed by the process of
    A. endochondral ossification.
    B. osteoclastic activity.
    C. intramembranous ossification.
    D. Wolff's Law.
    E. cartilage deposition.

11. Longitudinal growth of bones continues until age
    A. 25 in males and 24 in females.
    B. 16 in males and 15 in females.
    C. 19 in males and 18 in females.
    D. puberty in males and females.
    E. menopause in males and females.

12. The bone found immediately beneath the periosteum is called
    A. spongy bone.
    B. compact bone.
    C. cancellous bone.
    D. long bone.
    E. intramembranous bone.

13. Growth in bone length occurs
    A. in the shaft.
    B. at the sutures.
    C. at the epiphysis.
    D. in the growth plate.
    E. in the diaphysis.

14. Which statement is incorrect?
    A. Longitudinal growth of bone is complete when the growth plates are completely ossified.
    B. Cartilage skeletal will turn to bony skeletal.
    C. Strain and injury will cause bone to grow thick and strong.
    D. Osteoclast is known to be associated with bone reabsorption.
    E. Only bones of the skull form completely by intramembranous ossification.

15. The fibrovascular membrane covering bone is called the
    A. peritoneum.
    B. osseous membrane.
    C. endosteum.
    D. periosteum.
    E. none of the above.

16. All of the following statements are correct EXCEPT
   A. Reabsorption is less active than deposition in the growth period of the bone.
   B. Some bones form by the process of mitrochondrial ossification.
   C. In a long bone, the periosteal deposition of layers makes the bone taper toward the cancellous epiphysis.
   D. The age of the skeleton can be determined by the location and size of mesossification centers.
   E. In a child, crooked bones become straight due to the process of reabsorption and osteoblastic deposition.

Passage #2
Mitosis and Meiosis

All organisms that reproduce sexually develop from a single cell, the **zygote**, produced by the union of two cells, the **germ cells** or **gametes** (a **spermatozoon** from the male and an **ovum** from the female). The union of an egg and a spermatozoon is called **fertilization**. The zygote produced by fertilization develops into a new individual of the same species as the parents. Every cell of the individual with the exception of gametes contains the same number of chromosomes. In the somatic cells of a plant or an animal, chromosomes are paired, one member of each pair originally derived from one parent, the other member from the other parent. The member of a pair of chromosomes is called a **homologue**, and commonly we speak of pairs of chromosomes (or of homologues) when we refer to the chromosome number of a species. Man has forty-six chromosomes or twenty-three pairs, the onion has eight pairs, a toad has eleven pairs, a mosquito has three pairs, and so on. Homologues of each pair are alike, but the pairs are generally different. The original chromosome number of each cell (diploid number) is preserved during successive nuclear divisions involved in the growth and development of a multicellular organism.

Mitosis

The continuity of the chromosomal set is maintained by **cell division**, which is called **mitosis.** At the time of cell division the nucleus becomes completely reorganized. Mitosis takes place in a series of consecutive stages known as prophase, anaphase, and telophase. In a somatic cell the nucleus divides by mitosis in such a fashion that each of the two daughter cells receives exactly the same number and kind of chromosomes as the parent cell.

Each chromosome duplicates some time during **interphase** before the visible mitotic process begins. At this stage and at early **prophase** chromosomes appear as extended and slender threads. At late prophase chromosomes become short, compact rods by a process of spiral packing. A spindle arises between the two centrioles and the chromosomes line up across the equatorial plane of the spindle at the **metaphase** plate. At **anaphase** each chromosome separates, forming two daughter chromosomes, which go to opposite poles of the cell. Finally, at **telophase** the daughter chromosomes at each pole resolve themselves into a reticulum and two daughter nuclei are formed.

In mitosis the original chromosome number is preserved during the successive nuclear division. Since the somatic cells are derived from the zygote by mitosis, they all contain the normal double set, or diploid number (2n), of chromosomes.

Meiosis

If the gametes (ovum and spermatozoon) were diploid, the resulting zygote would have twice the diploid chromosome number. To avoid this, each gamete undergoes a special type of cell division called **meiosis**, which reduces the normal diploid set of chromosomes to a single (**haploid**) set (**n**). Thus when the ovum and spermatozoon unite in fertilization, the resulting **zygote** is diploid. The meiotic process is characteristic of all plants and animals that reproduce sexually and it takes place in the course of gametogenesis.

Meiosis is the reduction of the chromosome number by means of two nuclear divisions, the **first** and **second meiotic divisions**, that involve only a single division of the chromosomes.

The essentials of the process are simple. The homologous chromosomes, distinguished by their identical morphologic characteristics, pair longitudinally; they lie in close contact, forming a bivalent. Each chromosome is composed of two spiral filaments called the **chromatids**. The bivalent thus contains four chromatids and is also called a **tetrad**. In the tetrad each chromatid of the homologue has a single pairing partner. Portions of these paired chromatids may be exchanged from one homologue to the other, giving rise to cross-shaped figures, which are called **chiasmata**. Chiasma is a cytologic manifestation of an underlying genetic phenomenon called **crossing over**.

At metaphase I the bivalents arrange themselves on the spindle, and at anaphase I the homologous chromosomes and their two associated chromatids migrate to opposite poles. Thus in the first meiotic division the monologous pairs of chromosomes are segregated. After a short interphase, the two chromatids of each homologue separate in the second meiotic division, so that the original four chromatids are distributed into each of the four gametes. The result is four nuclei with only a single set of chromosomes.

In the male, all four cells develop into spermatozoa. In the female, one cell develops into an ovum, and the other three become small **polar bodies**. The formation of germ cells in plants is complicated because before fertilization the haploid products of meiosis undergo two or more mitotic divisions. However, the essential features of the meiotic process are similar in all sexually reproducing plants and animals.

17. All organisms that reproduce sexually develop from the
- **A.** gamete.
- **B.** zygote.
- **C.** ovum.
- **D.** homologue.
- **E.** tetrad.

18. The chromosomes duplicate during
- **A.** anaphase.
- **B.** telophase.
- **C.** interphase.
- **D.** prophase.
- **E.** metaphase.

19. The zygote contains the _____ number of chromosomes
- **A.** haploid.
- **B.** tetraploid.
- **C.** quadroploid.
- **D.** diploid.
- **E.** triploid.

20. Which statement is NOT true of mitosis?
- **A.** It is a process of cell division.
- **B.** In mitosis the original chromosome number is preserved.
- **C.** The daughter cells will have the haploid number of chromosomes.
- **D.** The nucleus is completely reorganized.
- **E.** Mitosis and Meiosis results are the same but the method is different.

21. The process of gametogenesis occurs during
- **A.** mitosis.
- **B.** fertilization.
- **C.** implantation.
- **D.** meiosis.
- **E.** ovulation.

22. Meiosis is the process by which
- **A.** nuclear division occurs with the original number of chromosomes.
- **B.** the zygote is formed.
- **C.** the diploid number of chromosomes is preserved.
- **D.** continuity of chromosomal set is maintained.
- **E.** nuclear division occurs with a reduction in the chromosomes to the haploid number.

23. The bivalent contains four chromatids, it is also called
- **A.** tetrad.
- **B.** polar bodies.
- **C.** homologues.
- **D.** gametes.
- **E.** chiasma.

24. During meiosis the homologous chromosomes and their chromatids migrate to opposite poles during
- **A.** second meiotic division.
- **B.** metaphase I.
- **C.** first meiotic division.
- **D.** anaphase II.
- **E.** formation of the polar bodies.

25. In mitosis the chromosomes line up across the equatorial plate during
- **A.** anaphase.
- **B.** metaphase.
- **C.** prophase.
- **D.** interphase.
- **E.** telophase.

26. During the first meiotic division the major accomplishment is when
- **A.** tetrads are formed.
- **B.** gametes are formed.
- **C.** chromosomes comes together to form the bivalent.
- **D.** the homologous chromosomes are segregated.
- **E.** daughters are formed.

27. A member of a pair of chromosomes is called a
- **A.** polar body.
- **B.** ovum.
- **C.** sperm cell.
- **D.** homologue.
- **E.** centriole.

28. The chromosomes become coiled and visible and the nuclear membrane disintegrates. This is what phase of mitosis?
- **A.** Interphase
- **B.** Prophase
- **C.** Metaphase
- **D.** Telophase
- **E.** Intraphase

29. The correct sequence of steps in mitosis is
- **A.** Prophase, metaphase, interphase, Anaphase, Telophase.
- **B.** Interphase, anaphase, metaphase, prophase, telophase.
- **C.** Interphase, prophase, metaphase, anaphase, telophase.
- **D.** Anaphase, prophase, interphase, metaphase, telophase.
- **E.** Interphase, prophase, anaphase, telophase, metaphase.

30. The number of mature gametes resulting from meiosis in the male is
- **A.** 1
- **B.** 2
- **C.** 3
- **D.** 4
- **E.** 5

31. The key difference(s) in Anaphase I of meiosis and anaphase of mitosis is
   - **A.** crossing over occurs in Anaphase I of meiosis.
   - **B.** centromeres divide in Anaphase I of meiosis.
   - **C.** homologous chromosomes move to opposite poles in Anaphase I of meiosis.
   - **D.** anaphase in mitosis creates polar bodies.
   - **E.** all of the above.

32. A key difference in the mechanism of mitosis and meiosis is
   - **A.** mitosis has crossing over of homologous chromosomes during prophase.
   - **B.** meiosis has a second duplication of DNA during interphase I.
   - **C.** meiosis has alignment of homologous chromosomes in metaphase I and separation of homologous chromosomes in anaphase I.
   - **D.** mitosis has a reductional division.
   - **E.** mitosis leads to meiosis.

33. The main difference in the outcome of mitosis versus meiosis is
   - **A.** meiosis produces identical daughter cells and mitosis produces different daughter cells.
   - **B.** mitosis occurs only in vertebrates.
   - **C.** meiosis produces somatic cells.
   - **D.** meiosis results in haploid cells and mitosis results in diploid cells when the parent cells are diploid.
   - **E.** mitosis occurs only in birds.

Passage #3
Viruses and Bacteria (Procaryotes)

Procaryotes (bacteria and blue-green algae) differ from eucaryotes by the latter having (1) genetic material in a nucleus and DNA conjugated with proteins, (2) organelles bound within membranes, (3) subcellular structural units to carry out specific functions (e.g., ATP production, photosynthesis), and (4) presence of cell walls made of cellulose or chitin versus murein (amino sugars and amino acids) as in procaryotes. The DNA of procaryotes is found in a nonmembrane region called the nucleoid; enzymes for metabolism and energy production are either free in the cytoplasm or bound to the cell membrane, and the ribosomes are smaller than in eucaryotes. Viruses are not procaryotes or eucaryotes but constitute their own group.

Viruses

Viruses are usually called "nonliving" and differ from bacteria and other "living" organisms because they (1) don't contain both DNA and RNA, (2) have no metabolic machinery for energy production or protein synthesis, (3) do not arise directly from other viruses but depend on the host's metabolic machinery to synthesize them, and (4) have no membranes to regulate exit and entry. Structurally, most viruses consist of a protein coat surrounding a core (center) of either DNA or RNA.

There are many variations of the basic life cycle of a virus given below. A cell may have a special receptor or region that is recognized by the virus. The virus attaches and may enter via a process similar to phagocytosis. In the cell, the central core of DNA or RNA and occasionally special enzymes or proteins take over the host's metabolic machinery to produce new coat proteins and new viral DNA or RNA. This may occur in the nucleus or the cytoplasm or both. The viral coat and viral core (DNA or RNA) then combine to form complete viral particles. At a certain point, the host cell lyses (bursts) and releases the new viral particles as well as uncombined viral coats and viral cores. Sometimes the viral particles exit by a process similar to reverse phagocytosis and incorporate part of the host's cell membrane onto their protein coat in doing so. The above is typical of a virus that attacks an animal or plant cell.

Viruses that attack bacteria are called bacteriophages. Bacteriophages in general consist of a head made of a protein coat and a core as before, and they also contain a tail made of protein that is specialized for attaching to bacteria. A bacteriophage attaches to the surface of a bacterium and the core of RNA or DNA is injected into the bacteria and the protein coat remains on the surface. Then the cycle may proceed as described above for viruses and is called lytic or virulent. However, the bacteriophage nucleic acid may become combined with the bacterial nucleic acid and remain as such for long periods before new bacteriophages are produced and cell rupture occurs. In this case, the bacteriophage is called lysogenic or temperate. The nucleic acid from the bacteriophage is called a prophage. Newly-released bacteriophages may contain some of the bacterias' nucleic acid that may be passed onto other bacteria when they are attacked by these bacteriophages. This is the mechanism of transduction.

Bacteria

The general characteristics of bacterial structure are discussed above under procaryotes. More specifically, from inside out, a bacteria may have a capsule that is usually made of a polysaccharide mucoid-like material and protects the bacteria from phagocytosis. Inside the capsule is the cell wall, and this prevents the hyperosmotic bacteria from bursting. Inside the cell wall is the cell membrane that may contain invaginations called mesosomes where localization of enzymes concerned with similar functions may be found. The cytoplasm and nucleoid are as described above. The DNA is circular and is haploid. Some bacterias contain flagella or cilia for locomotion—these are structurally different than their eucaryotic counterparts.

Bacteria have three common shapes: cocci (spherical or ovoid), bacilli (cylindrical or rod-like), and spirillia (helically coiled). The cocci are often found in clusters: diplococci (two bacteria together), streptococci (linear chains of cocci), or staphylococci (grape-like clusters of cocci). All of these are made up of individual bacteria with distinct cell walls.

Metabolically, bacteria may be aerobic or anaerobic. Anaerobic bacteria may use fermentation (where an organic molecule such as pyruvate lactate is the final electron acceptor) or inorganic substances as final electron receptors (such as S — H_2S). An obligate anaerobe is one that is killed if exposed to oxygen. This is usually because they cannot handle the peroxides (very toxic) produced in oxidative metabolism. A facultative anaerobe can metabolize in the presence or absence of oxygen. Bacteria may use a great variety of molecules as nutrients. Some are photosynthetic, others heterotrophic (using organic molecules made by other organisms) and others are chemosynthetic (making organic molecules and energy from inorganic precursors). The last group are important in fixation of nitrogen for use by all organisms. The variety of metabolic nutrients required and products produced are extremely important in studying basic questions of genetics as well as biochemistry, and also in differentiating between the different types of bacteria.

Most bacteria reproduce asexually by the process of binary fission that produces two identical haploid daughter cells by the simple process of mitosis. Genetic recombination (e.g., transfer and rearrangement of genetic information) may occur by three distinct means: transformation, transduction, and conjugation. Transformation involves a bacterium picking up free DNA from a medium, the free DNA being from a different bacterium. Transduction is the transfer of parts of DNA between bacteria by bacteriophages. In conjugation there is pairing of "male" and "female" forms. DNA is passed sequentially between them via structures called pili. All or a fraction of the DNA may be passed in this way. The above three genetic mechanisms allow extraordinary adaptability and variability of bacterium. Since bacteria can reproduce in a span as short as twenty minutes, a new trait such as drug resistance can spread rapidly in a given population.

34. Bacteriophages
   A. cause disease in humans.
   B. are viruses.
   C. are bacteria.
   D. can reproduce by binary fission.
   E. all of the above.

35. Select the substance(s) not ordinarily found in viruses.
   A. Carbohydrates
   B. Proteins
   C. RNA
   D. DNA
   E. All of the above

36. Viruses
   A. are considered to be living organisms.
   B. consist of protein, lipids, and carbohydrates only.
   C. do not arise from other viruses directly.
   D. have an incomplete metabolic machinery for energy production.
   E. may be either procaryotes or eucaryotes.

37. Eucaryotes are characterized by all except
   A. genetic material in a nucleus.
   B. organelles bound within membranes.
   C. presence of cell walls made of murein.
   D. subcellular structural units to carry out specific functions.
   E. **A** and **B** only.

38. "Contains DNA or RNA, no means of energy production, cannot reproduce self directly" would be a description of a
   A. animal cell.
   B. plant cell.
   C. bacteria.
   D. virus.
   E. fungi.

39. In the replication of a virus in a host cell
   A. the virus directs the metabolic machinery of the host.
   B. the host directs synthesis of new viral particles.
   C. viral particles are made as a single unit (i.e., coat and core).
   D. coat and core structures are released from the host and then combined.
   E. viruses attack only gametes capable of reproduction.

40. Structurally, bacteriophages differ from the usual virus by
   A. having a protein coat.
   B. having a core of DNA or RNA.
   C. being able to replicate independent of a host cell.
   D. having a tail region made of protein for attaching to cells.
   E. their ability for energy production.

41. The part of the cycle of a bacteriophage that may be different from that of a typical virus is
   A. taking over of host cells metabolic machinery.
   B. incorporation of its nucleic acid into the host cell's.
   C. lysis of host cell.
   D. synthesis by host cell of coat and core separately and then combining to form complete particle.
   E. uses special enzymes or proteins to take over host cells.

42. Which structure may protect a bacteria from phagocytosis by white blood cells?
   A. Mesosome
   B. Capsule
   C. Nucleoid
   D. Cell wall
   E. Specialized tail

43. Select the incorrect association.
   A. Cocci–spherical
   B. Bacilli–rod-like
   C. Diplococci–two cocci
   D. Staphylococci–linear combinations of cocci
   E. Spirillia–helically coiled

44. The process whereby a bacterium picks up DNA from a medium and incorporates it into its own DNA is called
   A. binary fission.
   B. conjugation.
   C. transformation.
   D. transduction.
   E. transmutation.

45. Bacteria transfer (exchange) genetic information between themselves by all except
   A. transformation.
   B. transduction.
   C. budding.
   D. conjugation.
   E. none of these.

46. Methods used to distinguish between bacteria may include all of the following except
   A. shape.
   B. nutrient requirements.
   C. products of metabolism.
   D. all are possible methods.
   E. **A** and **C** only.

47. A form of hepatitis (inflammation of the liver) is caused by a virus. The serum of patients with hepatitis may contain antigens from the virus, HB_SAg (hepatitis B surface antigen) and HB_CAg (hepatitis B core antigen). (An antigen is a substance foreign to the body capable of eliciting an immune response.) Select the correct statement.

A. This information is inconsistent with what is known about modes of viral replication.
B. The HB_CAg is probably a lipid.
C. The HB_SAg is probably a protein.
D. Enzymes found in liver cells probably do not increase in the serum during the acute disease.
E. The HB_SAg is probably a bacteriophage.

48. Which of the following would interfere most with the replication of a virus? Assume all agents can only affect the host cell and its contents.

A. An agent that blocks synthesis of lipids.
B. An agent that blocks synthesis of carbohydrates.
C. An agent that blocks synthesis of proteins.
D. An agent that blocks synthesis of lysogenic enzymes.
E. All of the above.

49. In the treatment of viral infections, a drug is discovered that directly blocks the synthesis of the viral protein coat. This drug

A. probably adversely affects protein synthesis by the host cell and hence may cause side affects in the host.
B. probably does not affect host protein synthesis.
C. probably destroys final electron receptors.
D. probably makes the viral protein coat thicker to penetrate.
E. probably unblocks the viral infection site.

50. Given a bacterial population without resistance to a certain drug, all of the following may cause introduction of bacterial resistance except

A. transformation.
B. binary fission.
C. transduction.
D. conjugation.
E. **A, C,** and **E.**

7.2 QUANTITATIVE REASONING

Each test item is a question or incomplete statement followed by suggested answers or completions. Read the item, decide which choice is the best, and circle only one answer per item.

Time Limit: 45 minutes

1. Find the largest of four consecutive even integers, which is two less than twice the smallest. Which of the following is the largest?
   A. 8
   B. 10
   C. 6
   D. 14
   E. 18

2. Which line is perpendicular to the Y-axis?
   A. $y = 3$
   B. $x = 3$
   C. $x = y$
   D. $y = 1 - x$
   E. $x = 1 - y$

3. $\left(\frac{1}{x}\right)^6 + \left(\frac{2}{x^2}\right)^3 =$
   A. $\frac{3}{x^2}$
   B. $\frac{9}{x^6}$
   C. $\frac{12}{x^6}$
   D. $2x^6$
   E. $6x^6$

4. What is the probability of obtaining heads in five tosses of a fair coin?
   A. $\frac{1}{2}$
   B. $\frac{3}{5}$
   C. $\frac{2}{5}$
   D. $\frac{5}{8}$
   E. $\frac{5}{32}$

5. What is the slope of a line containing the points (–2, 4) and (1, 3)?
   A. 3
   B. $\frac{1}{3}$
   C. –3
   D. $-\frac{1}{3}$
   E. 2

6. The value of $\frac{2}{3} + \frac{1}{4} - \frac{1}{2}$ is
   A. $\frac{2}{3}$
   B. $\frac{-1}{2}$
   C. $\frac{1}{12}$
   D. $\frac{1}{6}$
   E. $\frac{5}{12}$

7. The value of $\frac{2}{3} \times \frac{3}{4} \times \frac{4}{5}$ is
   A. $\frac{9}{12}$
   B. $\frac{2}{5}$
   C. $\frac{1}{4}$
   D. $\frac{3}{8}$
   E. 4

8. If $ax^2 = 2y$, then $\frac{a}{y} =$
   A. 2
   B. $2x^2$
   C. $\frac{2}{x^2}$
   D. $\frac{x^2}{2}$
   E. x^2

9. $\frac{\sqrt{15}\sqrt{3}}{\sqrt{10}} =$
   A. $\frac{3}{2}$
   B. $2\sqrt{5}$
   C. $9\sqrt{5}$
   D. $\frac{3\sqrt{2}}{2}$
   E. $\frac{\sqrt{2}}{2}$

10. If $2^{x/3} = 16$, then $x =$
    A. –2
    B. 4
    C. 6
    D. 12
    E. –3

11. If the perimeter of a square is 5.2, what is the area?
A. 1.3
B. 1.69
C. 52
D. 13
E. 16

12. If an ordinary coin is tossed four times, what is the probability that all four tosses will be tails?
A. $\frac{1}{16}$
B. $\frac{1}{4}$
C. $\frac{1}{2}$
D. $\frac{1}{8}$
E. $\frac{1}{3}$

13. Which of the following is equal to $(\tan \theta)(\csc \theta)$?
A. $\sin \theta$
B. $\cos \theta$
C. $\sec \theta$
D. $\csc \theta$
E. $\cot \theta$

14. Find the perimeter of the composite figure. Use 3.14 for π.

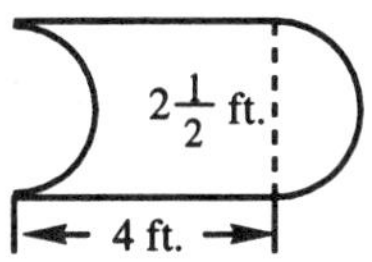

A. 15.85 ft.
B. 13.25 ft.
C. 10.5 ft.
D. 13 ft.
E. 7.87 ft.

15. The angles of a triangle are in the ratio of 2:3:5. What is the measure of the smallest angle?
A. 48°
B. 36°
C. 90°
D. 45°
E. 60°

16. If the area of the triangle BCE is 32, what is the area of the square ABCD?

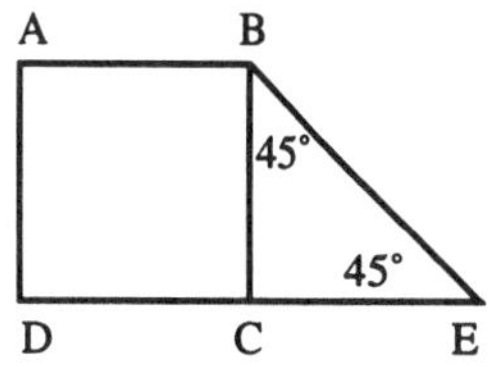

A. 64
B. 32
C. 16
D. 8
E. 4

17. A child withdraws from his piggy bank 20% of the original sum in the bank. If he must add 80 cents to bring the amount in the bank back up to the original sum, what was the original sum in the bank?
A. $1.00
B. $1.80
C. $2.60
D. $4.00
E. $5.60

18. $-4 - 3\{2 + 1[3 - (2 + 3) + 2] + 2\} + 4 =$
A. −12
B. 0
C. 2
D. 8
E. −4

19. 0.01% of 10 =
A. 1
B. 0.1
C. 0.01
D. 0.001
E. 0.0001

20. If $2x - y = 7$ and $x + y = 2$, then $x - y =$
A. 6
B. 4
C. $\frac{3}{2}$
D. 0
E. −5

21. The distance between Jimmy's house and the zoo is 12 miles. Jimmy rode his bicycle from his house to the zoo at an average speed of 12 miles per hour. He walked home from the zoo at an average speed of 6 miles per hour. Since he took the same route in both directions, what was his average speed?
A. 8 miles per hour
B. 12 miles per hour
C. 16 miles per hour
D. 20 miles per hour
E. 24 miles per hour

22. Ned is three years older than Mike, who is twice as old as Linda. If the ages of the three total 28 years, how old is Mike?
    A. 5 years old
    B. 8 years old
    C. 9 years old
    D. 10 years old
    E. 12 years old

23. Paul drove his car until the gas tank was 1/6 full. He stopped to refill the tank to capacity by putting in 20 gallons. What is the capacity of the gas tank?
    A. 20
    B. 21
    C. 24
    D. 28
    E. 25

24. In dentistry a mixture of gold and platinum is sometimes used to fabricate crowns (caps) for teeth, usually in the ratio 3:2 by weight. If the crowns made of these metals weigh 0.4 ounces, how many ounces of gold does the crown contain?
    A. 0.20
    B. 0.24
    C. 0.32
    D. 0.36
    E. 0.48

25. Simplify $\sqrt{\frac{3x^2}{9}+\frac{4x^2}{36}}$
    A. $\frac{3x}{4}$
    B. $\frac{2x}{3}$
    C. 4x
    D. $\frac{2x^2}{3}$
    E. $\frac{3x^2}{4}$

26. Three times the first of three consecutive odd integers is five more than twice the third. Find the third integer.
    A. 11
    B. 13
    C. 15
    D. 17
    E. 19

27. Barbara invests $3,600 in the Security National Bank at 5%. How much additional money must she invest at 10% so that the total annual interest income will be equal to 8% of her entire investment?
    A. $2,400
    B. $3,600
    C. $1,200
    D. $3,000
    E. $5,400

28. A plane traveling 800 miles per hour is 40 miles from Kennedy Airport at 5:58 p.m. At what time will it arrive at the airport?
    A. 6:00 p.m.
    B. 6.01 p.m.
    C. 6:02 p.m.
    D. 6:03 p.m.
    E. 6:04 p.m.

29. Mr. Bridges can wash his car in 30 minutes, while his son Dave takes twice as long to do the same job. If they work together, how many minutes will the job take them?
    A. 5 min.
    B. 10 min.
    C. 20 min.
    D. 28 min.
    E. 36 min.

30. The sum of a number and eight equals four less than the product of four and the number. Find the number.
    A. x = 3
    B. x = 2
    C. x = 6
    D. x = 4
    E. x = 5

31. Sales decreases cause a department store to reduce its output by 25%. By what percent must the reduced sales be increased for production to be brought to normal?
    A. 33.3%
    B. 50%
    C. 66.7%
    D. 75%
    E. 100%

32. Edward leaves home for work, driving at 24 miles per hour. Fifteen minutes later his wife notices he left his brief case. She decides to catch him on the road. If his wife drives 40 miles per hour, how far must she drive before she catches up with him?
    A. 15 miles
    B. 30 miles
    C. 45 miles
    D. 60 miles
    E. 25 miles

33. There are three consecutive even integers such that the third of the three even integers is eight more than the sum of the first and second. Find the third even integer.
    A. –10
    B. –8
    C. –6
    D. –4
    E. –2

34. Elizabeth has \$5.50 in nickels and dimes. She has five more nickels than dimes. How many dimes does she have?
A. 35
B. 30
C. 25
D. 20
E. 40

35. If the ratio of P to Q is 3/4 and the ratio of Q to R is 12/19, what is the ratio of P to R?
A. 9/19
B. 1/4
C. 17/19
D. 3/19
E. 1/3

36. Find the equation of the line that contains the point (– 1, 0) and has slope 2.
A. $y = 2x - 1$
B. $y = 2x + 2$
C. $y = 2x$
D. $y = 2x - 3$
E. $y = 2x + 1$

37. The following right triangles ABC and DEF are similar. How long is DF?

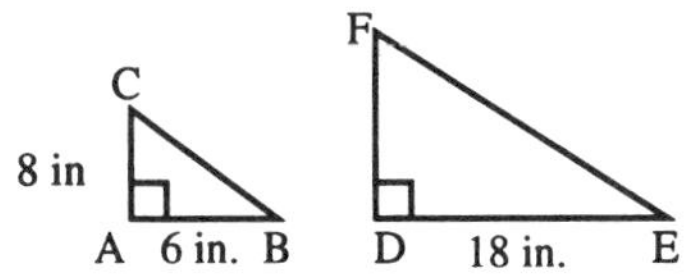

A. 24 in
B. 20 in
C. 16 in
D. 12 in
E. 8 in

38. Which of the following is equal to $-2 < \frac{x}{3} \leq 2$?
A. $-3 < x \leq 3$
B. $-4 < x \leq 4$
C. $-9 < x \leq 9$
D. $-6 < x \leq 6$
E. $-8 < x \leq 8$

39. Which of the following is identically equal to sin 2A?
A. $1 - \cos^2 2A$
B. $2 \sin A \cos A$
C. $\frac{1}{\sec 2A}$
D. $2 \sin A$
E. $1 - \cos 2A$

40. If $\sin \theta = 1/3$, then $\cos \theta = ?$
A. $\frac{1}{3}$
B. $-\frac{1}{3}$
C. $-\sqrt{\frac{2}{3}}$
D. $\sqrt{\frac{2}{3}}$
E. $\frac{\pm 2\sqrt{2}}{3}$

7.3 SURVEY OF THE NATURAL SCIENCES

DIRECTIONS: For each question, read all the choices carefully. Then select the answer that you consider correct or most nearly correct. Blacken the answer space corresponding to your best choice just as you would do on the actual examination. **This examination is comprised of 100 items: Biology (1–40), General Chemistry (41–70), and Organic Chemistry (71–100).**

Time limit: 90 minutes

1. Which of the following organelles is incorrectly matched with its function?
- **A.** Mitochondria – fermentation
- **B.** Chloroplast – fixation of CO_2
- **C.** Lysosome – storage of hydrolytic enzymes
- **D.** Golgi Apparatus – packaging and secretion of glycoprotein
- **E.** Nucleus – location of genetic material

2. The corpus luteum secretes:
- **A.** LH.
- **B.** progesterone.
- **C.** FSH.
- **D.** hCG.
- **E.** oxytocin.

3. When members of two species both benefit from living together in close association, the relationship is called
- **A.** mutualism.
- **B.** commensalism.
- **C.** parasitism.
- **D.** predation.
- **E.** a society.

4. Which substance has the highest energy content per gram?
- **A.** Proteins
- **B.** Fats
- **C.** Carbohydrates
- **D.** Phospholipids
- **E.** Monosaccharides

5. Cyanide blocks cellular production of energy at which stage?
- **A.** Glycolysis
- **B.** Citric acid cycle
- **C.** Electron transport system
- **D.** Oxidative phosphorylation
- **E.** Krebs cycle

6. Lysosomes
- **A.** are the site of protein synthesis.
- **B.** form the rough endoplasmic reticulum.
- **C.** contain digestive enzymes.
- **D.** contain the enzymes for oxidative phosphorylation.
- **E.** function to destroy the cells no longer useful to the organism.

7. Which of the following conditions will cause a gene frequency to depart from the equilibrium expected from the Hardy-Weinberg law?
- **A.** Random assortment
- **B.** Nonrandom mating
- **C.** Large population
- **D.** No mutation
- **E.** No migration

8. Which of the following substances is NOT secreted into the human digestive tract?
- **A.** Bile
- **B.** Insulin
- **C.** Ptyalin
- **D.** Pepsinogen
- **E.** Trypsinogen

9. Which of the following is a characteristic of both eukaryotic animal cells and animal viruses?
- **A.** The ability to undergo mutation.
- **B.** The ability to reproduce through mitosis.
- **C.** The ability to produce proteins.
- **D.** The ability to enter other cells and cause lysis.
- **E.** The ability to replicate nucleic acids independently.

10. One of the major differences between fungi and bacteria is that only fungi
- **A.** are photosynthetic.
- **B.** can produce spores.
- **C.** are always diploid.
- **D.** can undergo meiosis and mitosis.
- **E.** have a cell wall.

11. Blood that is pumped from the left ventricle of the heart
- **A.** is highly oxygenated.
- **B.** flows into the aorta.
- **C.** is under high pressure.
- **D.** all of the above.
- **E.** both **A** and **C.**

12. Muscles are bound to joints by
- **A.** cartilage.
- **B.** tendons.
- **C.** ligaments.
- **D.** myosin fibers.
- **E.** bone spurs.

13. The development of the ovarian follicle is initiated by
- **A.** FSH.
- **B.** LH.
- **C.** estrogen.
- **D.** progesterone.
- **E.** oxytocin.

14. In the immune system, B cells
A. are lymphocytes that release antibodies.
B. are special phagocytic neutrophils.
C. are transformed into macrophages at the site of inflammation.
D. are lymphocytes that destroy foreign cells.
E. release histamines at the site of tissue damage.

15. One species benefitting and the other being harmed in a relationship is called
A. mutualism.
B. socialism.
C. commensalism.
D. parasitism.
E. none of the above.

16. Translation of the genetic code does not directly require
A. activated tRNA - AA.
B. mesosomes.
C. mRNA.
D. DNA.
E. all of the above.

17. What is the correct hierarchy (from the highest to lowest) of given levels of taxonomy?
A. Class, order, family, genus
B. Order, family, genus, class
C. Family, genus, class, order
D. Family, class, order, genus
E. Genus, class, order, family

18. "Under certain conditions gene frequencies and genotypic frequencies remain constant from generation to generation in sexually reproducing populations" was put forth by
A. Dalton.
B. Hardy-Weinberg.
C. Mendel.
D. Mendeleev.
E. Darwin.

19. Given the following representative pedigree, what is the most likely pattern of inheritance (blackened symbol means trait is present)?

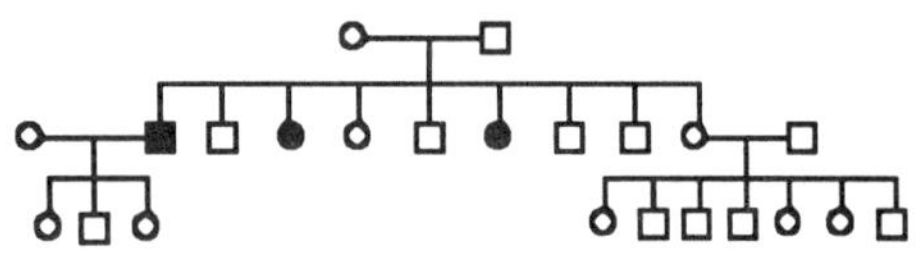

A. Autosomal dominant
B. Autosomal recessive
C. Sex-influenced
D. Triglycerides
E. Sodium and chloride ions

20. Which of the following substances is NOT generally absorbed into the blood capillaries of the intestinal villi?
A. Water
B. Glucose
C. Amino acids
D. Triglycerides
E. Sodium and chloride ions

21. Which of the following is required for the conversion of fructose-6-phosphate to fructose 1, 6- diphosphate during glycolysis?
A. Oxygen
B. An excess of fructose-6-phosphate
C. A kinase enzyme, specific for fructose-6-phosphate
D. Any of the enzymes that catalyze the reactions of glycolysis
E. A small amount of the single enzyme that catalyzes all the reactions of glycolysis

22. A membrane may be found on all of the following structures except
A. Golgi complex.
B. lysosomes.
C. endoplasmic reticulum.
D. mitochondria.
E. centrioles.

23. During facilitated diffusion
A. carrier substances carry molecules across the membrane.
B. molecules can go against the concentration gradient.
C. molecules require energy.
D. saturation kinetics is not observed.
E. phagocytosis takes place.

24. If red blood cells are put in a hypertonic solution, they will
A. remain the same.
B. hemolyze.
C. crenate.
D. swell up.
E. move to a more suitable environment.

25. What anatomical structure(s) is (are) used to prevent the bronchi from collapsing?
A. Cartilage rings
B. Alveolus
C. Bony rings
D. Epiglottis
E. None of the above

26. The greatest resistance to blood flow is in the
A. capillaries.
B. veins.
C. arteries.
D. arterioles.
E. aorta.

27. Bacteriophages
   A. cause disease in humans.
   B. contain both DNA and RNA.
   C. are viruses.
   D. are bacteria.
   E. can reproduce by binary fission.

28. Which structure may protect a bacterium from phagocytosis by white blood cells?
   A. Mesosome
   B. Cilia
   C. Capsule
   D. Nucleoid
   E. Cell wall

29. The chromosomes become coiled and visible and the nuclear membrane disintegrates. This is what phase of mitosis?
   A. Anaphase
   B. Telophase
   C. Prophase
   D. Metaphase
   E. Interphase

30. The genetic code is composed of sequences of
   A. three nucleotides.
   B. three nucleosides.
   C. three amino acids.
   D. two amino acids.
   E. two DNA molecules.

31. The following is one strand of a double helix of DNA (showing only nitrogen bases). What is the structure of its complementary strand? (A = adenine, G = guanine, T = thymine, C = cytosine, U = uracil)

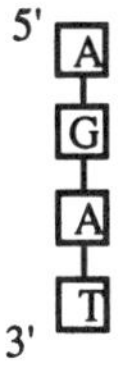

A. 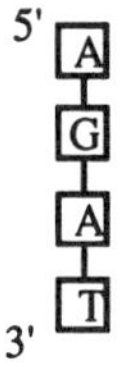

B. 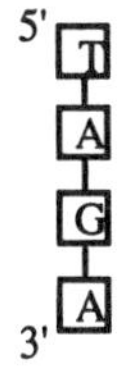

C. 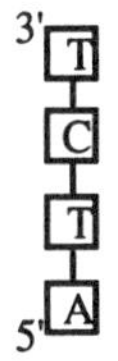

D. 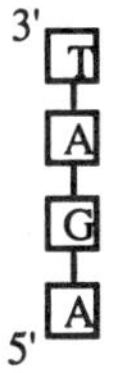

E. 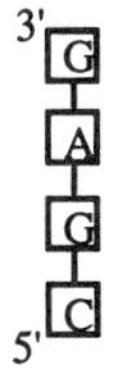

32. Which of the following is involved in the immune system?
   A. Neutrophils
   B. Platelets
   C. Lymphocytes
   D. Basophils
   E. DNA

33. All are part of the kidney except
   A. glomerulus.
   B. loop of Henle.
   C. Bowman's capsule.
   D. Malpighian tubules.
   E. collecting ducts.

34. Reabsorption of most of the water, glucose, amino acids, sodium, and other nutrients occurs at the
A. loop of Henle.
B. small intestines.
C. collecting duct.
D. distal convoluted tubules.
E. proximal convoluted tubules.

35. Control of body temperature is localized in the
A. skin.
B. heart.
C. cerebrum.
D. hypothalamus.
E. medulla.

36. Which of the following is not a feature of the unit membrane model of the cell membrane?
A. Continuous lipid bilayer present
B. Globular proteins floating in lipids
C. Hydrophobic ends of lipids in contact with water
D. Continuous protein bilayers outside lipid layer
E. Poorly defined pores for movement of large and/or non-lipid molecules.

37. If a cell is placed in a solution that causes it to shrink because of water loss, that solution is said to be
A. hypotonic.
B. isotonic.
C. hypertonic.
D. homeostatic.
E. equilibrated.

38. The term glycolysis, which is the first series of reactions in the oxidative breakdown of glucose, is sometimes used as a synonym for the
A. Kreb's cycle.
B. Calvin cycle.
C. Embden-Meyerhof Pathway.
D. electron transport system.
E. photosynthetic pathway.

39. Fertilization of an ovum by sperm normally occurs in the
A. uterus.
B. vagina.
C. oviduct.
D. fallopian tube.
E. ovary.

40. Which of the following is not a function of the liver?
A. Synthesis of insulin
B. Synthesis of carbohydrates, proteins, and fats
C. Detoxification of drugs
D. Synthesis of bile
E. Regulation of blood glucose

41. A neutral atom that has 53 electrons and an atomic mass of 111 has
A. no other isotopes.
B. an atomic number of 58.
C. a nucleus containing 58 neutrons.
D. a nucleus containing 53 neutrons.
E. a nucleus containing 58 protons.

42. Which of the following measurements or techniques can be used to find the atomic weight, or molecular weight of a substance?
A. Heat of combustion
B. Boiling point elevation
C. Boiling point of the pure substance
D. Electrical conductivity
E. Density of the liquid state

43. How many grams of HCl are required to react completely with 32.5 grams of Zn (producing zinc chloride and hydrogen)?
A. 9 g
B. 18 g
C. 36 g
D. 72 g
E. 90 g

44. What is the sum of the coefficients of all species in the balanced equation

$$Pb(NO_3)_2 \rightarrow NO_2 + PbO + O_2$$

A. 18
B. 15
C. 12
D. 9
E. 6

45. Estimate the boiling point of a solution of a nonelectrolyte in acetic acid. The boiling point of acetic acid is 118°C.
A. 115°
B. 118°
C. 120°
D. 100°
E. 130°

46. Given that the standard heats of formation of SO_2 and SO_3 are –70 and –95 kcal/mole respectively, find the heat of reaction for

$$SO_2 + 1/2\ O_2 \rightarrow SO_3$$

A. –25 kcal
B. –165 kcal
C. 25 kcal
D. 165 kcal
E. 190 kcal

47. If 50 mL of 2.0 M NaOH is mixed with 50 mL of 4.0 M nitric acid, what is the pH of the final solution?
A. 1.00
B. 7.00
C. 14.00
D. 10.00
E. not enough information to solve.

48. What is the volume occupied by 0.50 moles of an ideal gas at 760 torr and 0°C?
A. 2.24 L
B. 11.2 L
C. 22.4 L
D. 44.8 L
E. 75.6 L

49. What volume of HI can be made if 14.2 L of hydrogen and 23.5 L of iodine react at STP?

$$H_2 + I_2 \rightarrow 2\,HI$$

A. 14.2 L
B. 23.5 L
C. 28.4 L
D. 47.0 L
E. 53.8 L

50. A gas mixture contains equal numbers of CO molecules and CO_2 molecules, and no others. Assuming ideal gas behavior, which of the following statements is true?
A. The total mass of CO_2 and CO is the same.
B. The partial pressure of CO_2 and CO is the same.
C. Since carbon dioxide molecules have more mass, they have more inertia and contribute more to the total pressure.
D. The density of CO_2 and CO is the same.
E. The molecular weights of CO_2 and CO are the same.

51. Which of the following compounds is incorrectly named?
A. $TiSe_2$; titanium selenide
B. $V(ClO_3)_3$; vanadium (III) chlorate
C. $Na_2C_2O_4$; sodium oxalate
D. $AlPO_4$; aluminum phosphate
E. $KHSO_4$; Krypton bisulfate

52. Fe metal adopts a body-center cube structure. How many Fe atoms are present in the unit cell?
A. 1
B. 2
C. 4
D. 6
E. 8

53. Which of the following combinations of quantum numbers DO NOT represent permissible solutions of the Schroedinger wave equation for the hydrogen atom?

	n	l	m	s
(i)	9	0	0	–5/2
(ii)	2	1	0	–1/2
(iii)	1	3	3	1/2

A. (i)
B. (iii)
C. (i) and (ii)
D. (i) and (iii)
E. (ii) and (iii)

54. Atom A has 3 valence electrons and atom B has 7 valence electrons. The formula expected for an ionic compound of A and B is
A. AB.
B. AB_3.
C. AB_2.
D. A_2B.
E. A_3B.

55. Which of the following trends in first ionization potential is NOT correct?
A. Rb<Sb<Cl<Ne
B. Na<Mg<P<Cl
C. Be<Sb<P<N
D. F<N<B<Li
E. Te<Se<S<O

56. In which of the following molecules is the octet rule violated?
A. $SnCl_2$
B. $PbCl_4$
C. F_2
D. All of the above.
E. None of the above.

57. Which of the following oxidation states would not be expected?
A. Ar(0)
B. Pb(IV)
C. Nb(V)
D. N(VI)
E. All of the above are not expected.

58. Which of the following molecules would be expected to be polar?

1. NO 2. $GaCl_3$ 3. HF 4. $COCl_2$

A. 1
B. 2 and 4
C. 1, 3, and 4
D. 1, 2, and 3
E. All of the above.

59. What is the pH of a 0.0100 molar HNO_3 aqueous solution?
A. 7.00
B. 12.00
C. 2.00
D. 2.76
E. 4.60

60. Given the following hypothetical half-reactions,

$$M^{2+} + e^- \rightarrow M^+ \quad E° = -0.579\ V$$
$$M^{3+} + e^- \rightarrow M^{2+} \quad E° = 0.735\ V$$

Which of the following is true?
A. M^{2+} is reduced.
B. M^{3+} is reduced.
C. This reaction is never spontaneous.
D. More information is needed.
E. M^{3+} is oxidized.

61. If 75% of a radioactive isotope decays in 300 days, what is its half-life?
A. 100 days
B. 150 days
C. 200 days
D. 300 days
E. 350 days

62. Which of the following arrangements of atoms is most likely?

A. O—C—O—O

B. 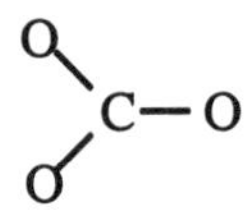

C. 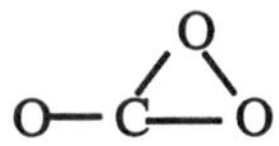

D. 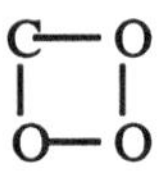

E. C - C - O - O

63. A compound was found to have an empirical formula of NO and a molecular mass of 90g/mole. What is the molecular formula?
A. NO
B. N_2O_2
C. N_3O_3
D. N_4O_4
E. N_4O_5

64. An element with this electron configuration, $1s^2 2s^2 2p^4$, will form which of the following ions?
A. +2
B. +4
C. −2
D. −4
E. −3

65. Element A exists in three isotopic forms with masses of 21.0, 25.0, and 26.0 amu, respectively. Element B also exists in three isotopic forms with masses of 22.0, 24.0, and 26.0 amu respectively. It is true that
A. element A has a higher atomic mass than B.
B. element B has a higher atomic mass than A.
C. A and B have identical atomic masses since the sum of their isotopic masses are equal.
D. you cannot predict which atomic mass is greater from the data given.
E. elements A and B have identical chemical structures.

66. Which of the following oxidation states would not be expected?
A. Ar(0)
B. Ag(I)
C. S (VII)
D. Na(III)
E. All of the above

67. Which one of the following gives the correct hybridization for the central atom in the molecule?

	$AlCl_3$	N_3^-	CS_2
A.	sp^3	sp^2	sp^2
B.	sp^3	sp	sp^2
C.	sp	sp^3	sp^2
D.	sp^2	sp	sp^2
E.	All of the above.		

68. The biological effect of radiation is measured in units of
A. geigers.
B. electron volts.
C. curies.
D. rems.
E. newtons.

69. When sulfuric acid is added to sodium chloride, the gas given off has the formula
A. Cl_2.
B. HCl.
C. H_2S.
D. SO_3.
E. SO_2.

70. Which species cannot behave as a reducing agent?
A. ClO^-
B. ClO_2^-
C. ClO_3^-
D. ClO_4^-
E. All of the above

71. Which of the following carbon backbones forms the structure of 2,3,6-trimethyloctane?

A. 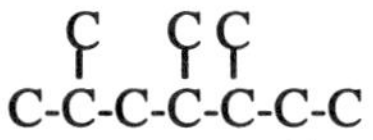

B. 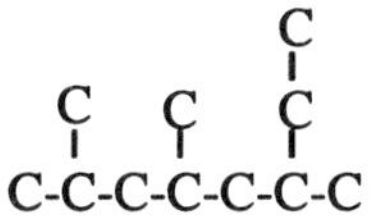

C. 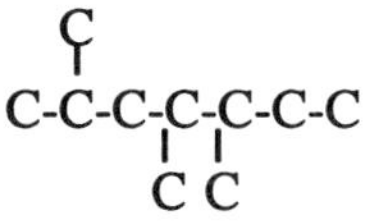

D. 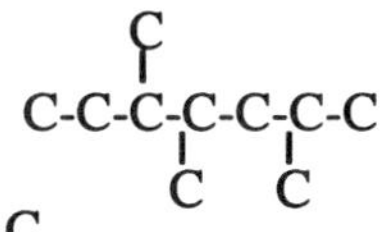

E. 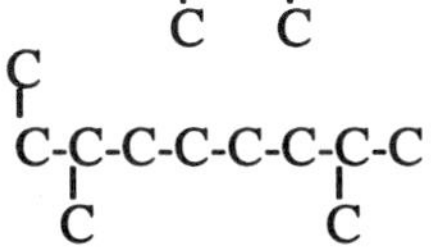

72. Which of the following compounds has the highest dipole moment?

A. 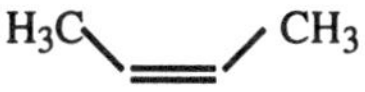

B. 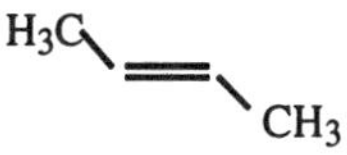

C. $H_3C-\equiv-CH_3$

D. 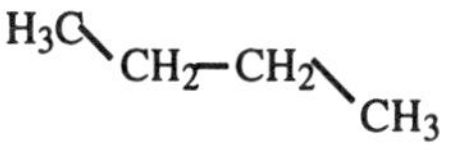

E. $H_3C{-}CH{\equiv}HC-CH_3$

73. What is the product of the reaction between 1,1,1-tribromo-2-butene and HBr?

A. 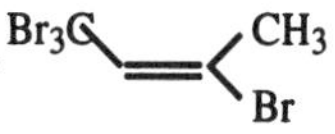

B. 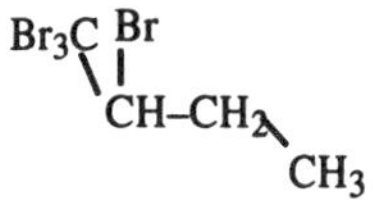

C. $Br_3C-\equiv-CH_3$

D. 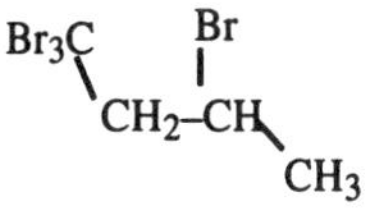

E. $CBr_3-CH{\equiv}CH-CBr_3$

74. What is the product of the reaction between Br^+ and anisole?

A. 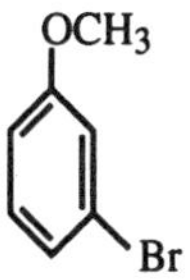

B. 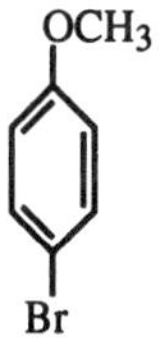

C. 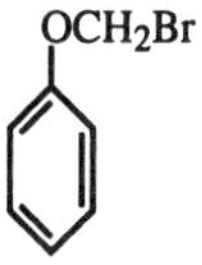

D. 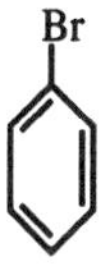

E. 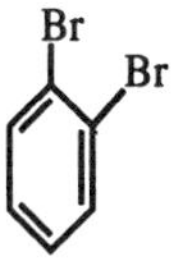

75. Which of the following is the strongest acid?
A. Isopropanol
B. Sec-butanol
C. Tert-butanol
D. Propanol
E. Methanol

76. Which of the following is the least soluble in water?

A. Methanol
B. Ethanol
C. Propanol
D. Butanol
E. Pentanol

77. Which of the following alcohols is most likely to undergo S_N2 substitutions?

A. CH_3OH
B. CH_3CH_3OH
C. $(CH_3)_2CHOH$
D. $(CH_3)_3COH$
E. C_6H_5OH

78. What is the relationship between these straight-chain aldoses?

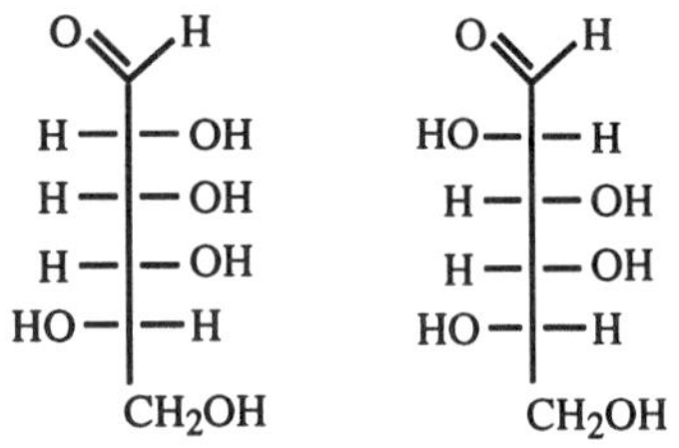

A. Anomers
B. Enantiomers
C. Epimers
D. Racemers
E. Isomers

79. Which of the following is not a product of this reaction?

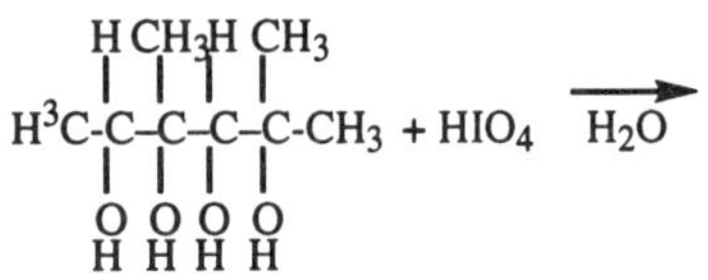

A. H_3CCH (with C=O)

B. $H_2C{=}O$

C. $(CH_3)_2C{=}O$

D. $(CH_3)_3COH$

E. H–C(H)=O

80. Name the following compound.

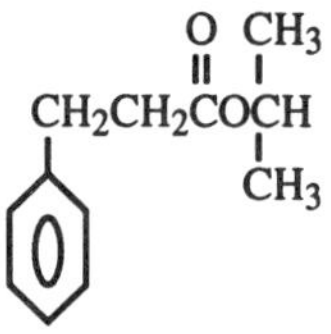

A. Isopropyl benzoate
B. Benzyl isopropyl ester
C. Isopropyl-3-phenylproponate
D. Isoalkyl chloride
E. None of the above

81. What is the product of the following reaction?

$(CH_3)_3CCH_2CH_2OH + KMnO_4 \rightarrow$

A. $(CH_3)_3CCH_2CH$ (with C=O)

B. $(CH_3)_3CCH{=}CH_2$

C. $(CH_3)_3CCCH_3$ (with C=O)

D. CH_3COOH

E. No reaction occurs

82. Which of the following is not a property of phenols?

A. More acidic than alcohols, but less acidic than carboxylic acids.
B. Most reactions involve breaking the O–H bond.
C. Cannot be dehydrated.
D. Easily oxidized to ketones.
E. All of the above.

83. Which of the following reagents is used in a Fridel-Crafts acylation?

A. CuX
B. RX and $AlCl_3$
C. $KMnO_4$
D. RC(=O)X and $AlCl_3$
E. $CuSO_4$

84. Which of the following sugars is a furanose?

A. 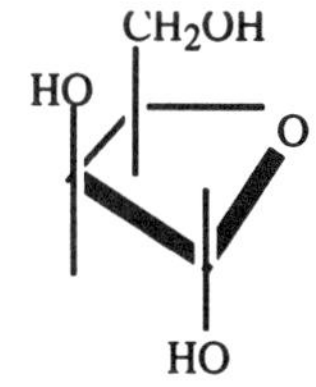

B. 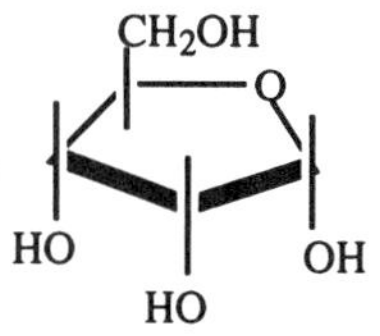

C. 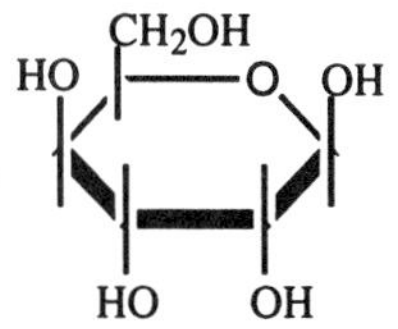

D. 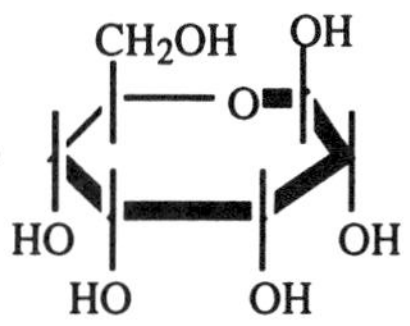

E. 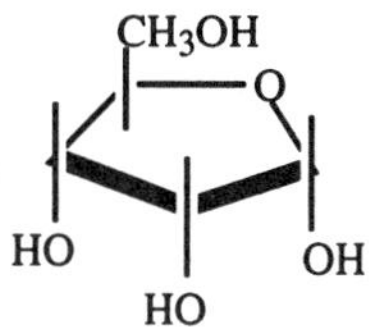

85. Which of the following structures is consistent with this IR and ^{1}H NMR data?

IR: 3620 cm^{-1} broad peak; 2980 cm^{-1} strong peak; no other strong peaks

NMR: 1.1 doublet, area 6; 2.6 broad, area 1; 3.9 septet, area 1

Mass Spec: C_3H_8O

A. 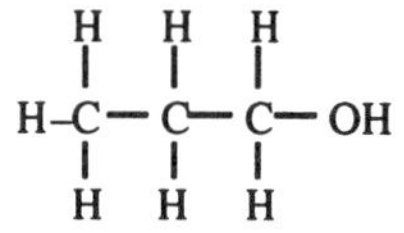

B. 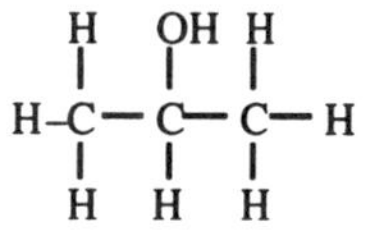

C. 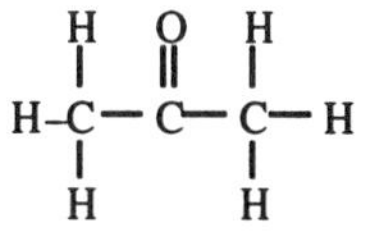

D. 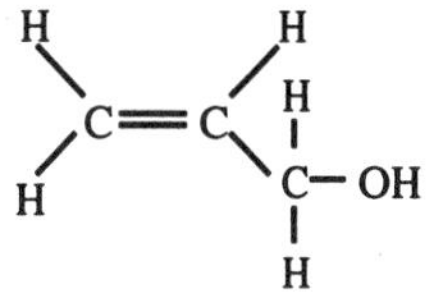

E. 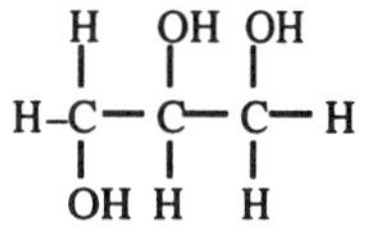

86. Aldehydes and ketones react with secondary amines to form compounds called

A. amides.
B. enamines.
C. lipids.
D. barbiturates.
E. amino acids.

87. Which of the following best describes a *transesterification* reaction?

A. High boiling ester + high-boiling alcohol → higher-boiling ester + low-boiling alcohol.
B. High boiling ester + low-boiling alcohol → higher-boiling ester + high-boiling alcohol.
C. Low boiling ester + high-boiling alcohol → high-boiling ester + low-boiling alcohol.
D. Low-boiling ester + low-boiling alcohol → high-boiling ester + high-boiling alcohol.
E. High boiling ester + low-boiling alcohol → low-boiling ester + high-boiling alcohol.

88. What is the product of the following reaction?

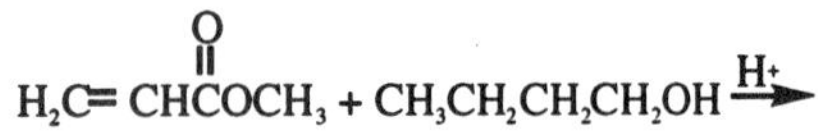

A. 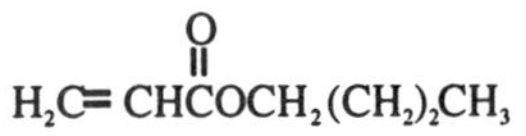

B. 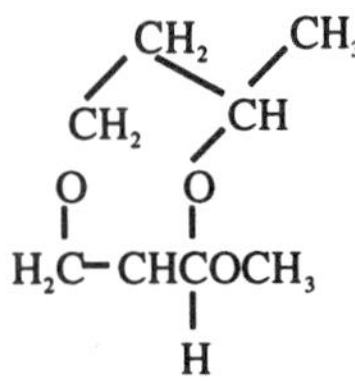

C. 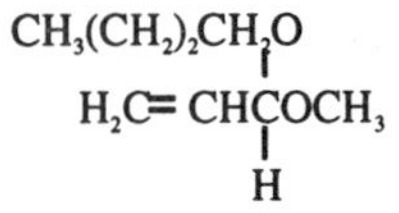

D. 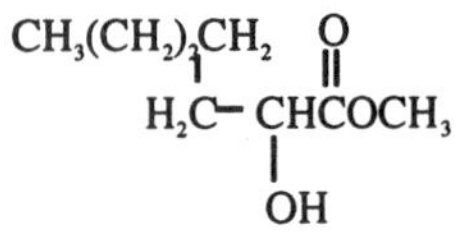

E. 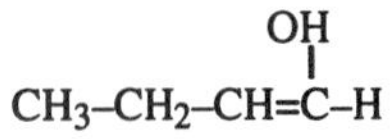

89. Which of the following steps is not a chain-propagating step for a radical reaction?

A. $(C_6H_5)_3C\bullet + O_2$ Æ $(C_6H_5)_3C\text{-}O\text{-}O\bullet$

B. $(C_6H_5)_3C\text{-}O\text{-}O\bullet + (C_6H_5)_3CH$ Æ $(C_6H_5)_3C\bullet + (C_6H_5)_3C\text{-}O\text{-}OH$

C. $(C_6H_5)_3C\bullet + (C_6H_5)_3C\text{-}O\text{-}OH$ Æ $(C_6H_5)_3C\text{-}O\text{-}O\bullet + (C_6H_5)_3CH$

D. $(C_6H_5)_3C\bullet + (C_6H_5)_3C\bullet$ Æ $(C_6H_5)_3C\text{-}C(C_6H_5)_3$

E. $(C_6H_5)_3C\text{-}O\text{-}O\bullet + (C_6H_5)_3C\bullet + O_2$

90. Reduction of an organic compound usually entails

A. a decrease in its oxygen content.

B. an increase in its oxygen content.

C. a decrease in the length of the longest carbon chain.

D. an increase in the length of the longest carbon chain.

E. none of the above.

91. A compound with an empirical formula of $C_5H_{10}O$ showed the following spectral characteristics: IR: strong peak near 1710 cm^{-1}, NMR: doublet at 1.10 ppm (6H), singlet at 2.10 ppm (3H), and a septet and 2.50 ppm (1H). Which of the following compounds agrees best with this data?

A. 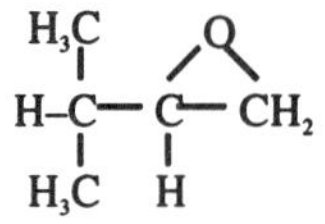

B. 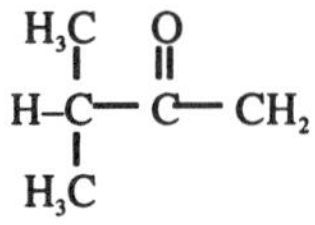

C. 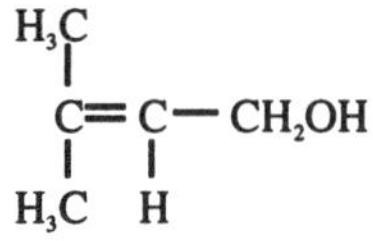

D. 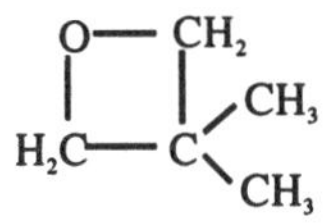

E. 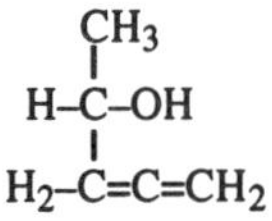

92. Which of the following is the major product for the reaction

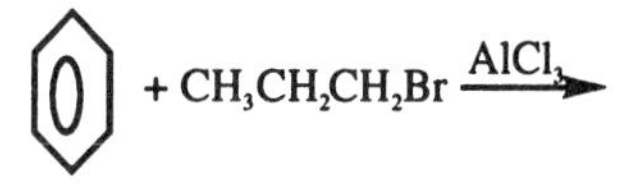

A. 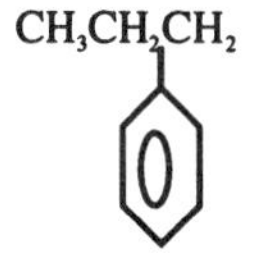

B. 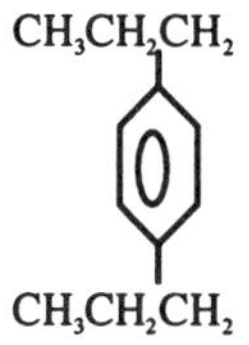

C. 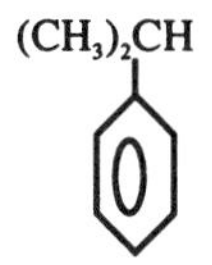

D. 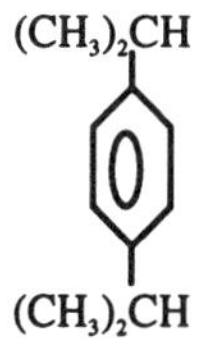

E. 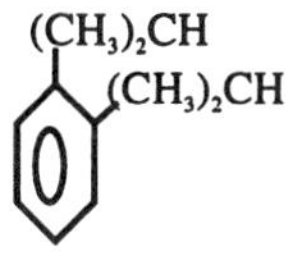

93. Which of the following substituent groups functions as a meta-director on electrophilic aromatic substitution reactions?
A. $-NH_2$
B. $-CH_3$
C. $-CF_3$
D. –F
E. –Cl

94. Cyclooctatetrene reacts with 2 equivalents of potassium to yield the very stable compound, $K_2C_8H_8$. The NMR spectrum of this compound indicates all of the hydrogens are equivalent. Which of the following statements best accounts for these observations?
A. The compound is ionic.
B. The compound is cyclic.
C. The compound is planar.
D. The compound is aromatic.
E. The compound is aliphatic.

95. Which of the following sets of reactants would produce

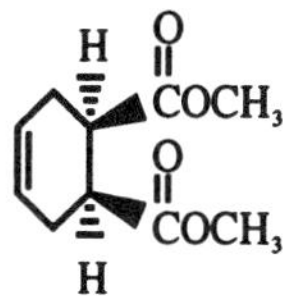

A. 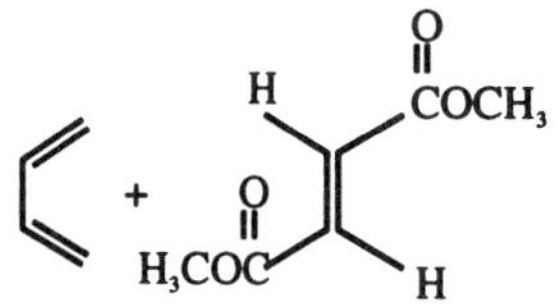

B. 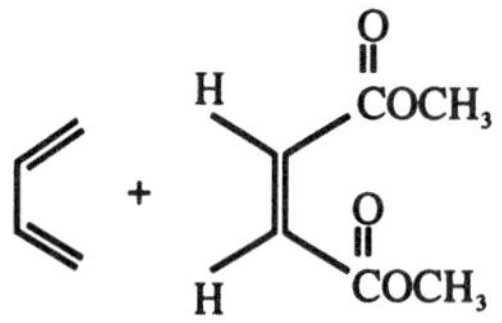

C. 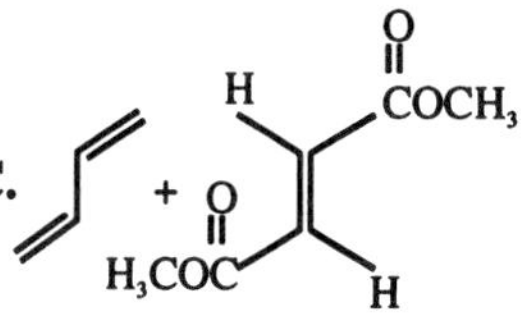

D. 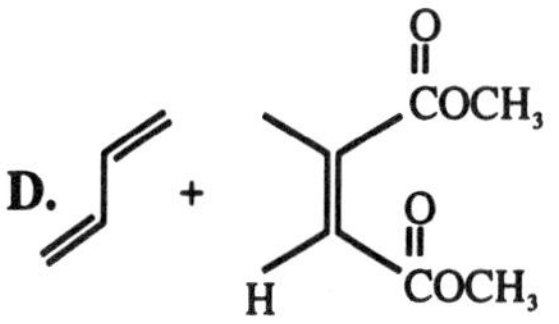

E. 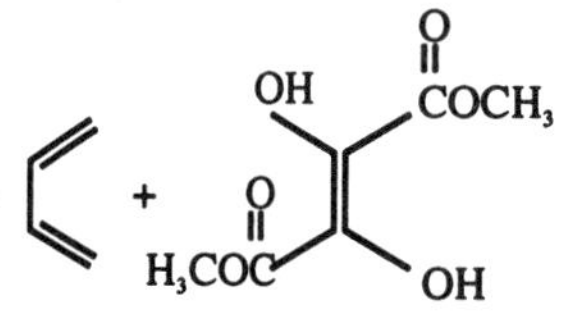

96. Which of the following is the strongest carbon acid?
A. Acetylene
B. Ethene
C. Ethane
D. Methane
E. Ethylene

97. Which of the following compounds is drawn as a “Trans” isomer?

A. 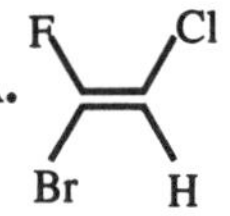

B. 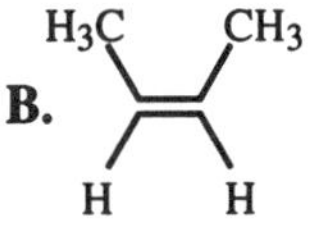

C. 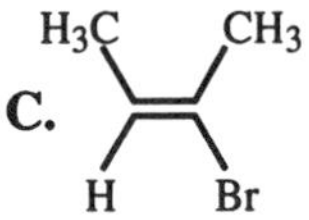

D. 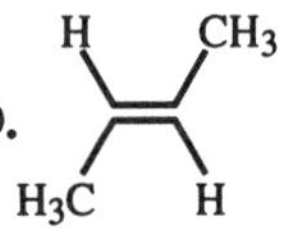

E. 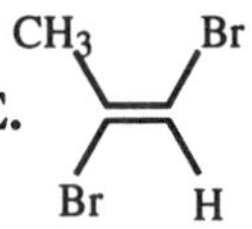

98. In the following reaction

$$(-)CH_3\underset{\substack{|\\OH}}{C}HCHO + Br_2 \xrightarrow{H_2O} CH_3\underset{\substack{|\\OH}}{C}HCOOH$$

What occurs to the configuration of the chiral carbon?

A. Retention
B. Inversion
C. Racemization
D. Chirality is lost
E. Chirality is inverted

99. Which of the following are cis-isomers?

1. 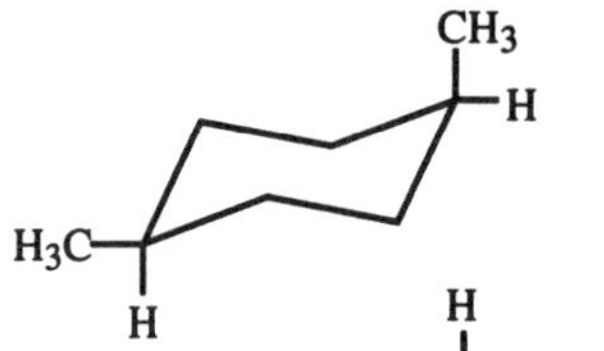

2. 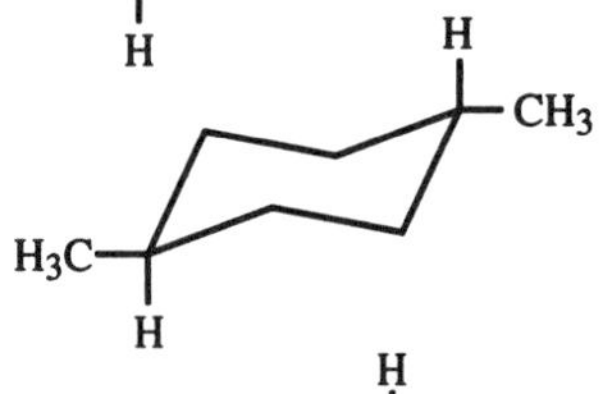

3. 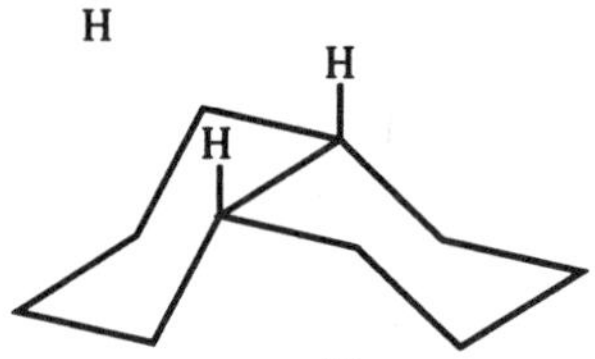

4. 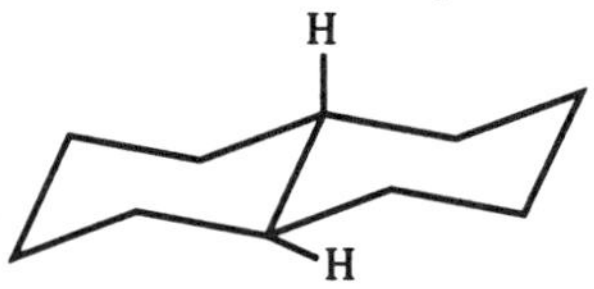

A. 1 and 2
B. 1 and 3
C. 1 and 4
D. 2 and 3
E. 3 and 4

100. A Grignard reagent reacts with esters to form
A. primary alcohols.
B. secondary alcohols.
C. tertiary alcohols.
D. ketones.
E. aldehydes.

7.4 PHYSICS

The following test is a model of the Physics Test on the OAT. The problems here are of similar format to those on the actual OAT. The test items in Physics are followed by either four or five multiple-choice responses. All other parts of the OAT are followed by five multiple-choice responses. Read specific directions or data provided on graphs or sketches. There are actually 40 items on the Physics test to be completed within 50 minutes.

1. What are the x- and y-components of A + B?

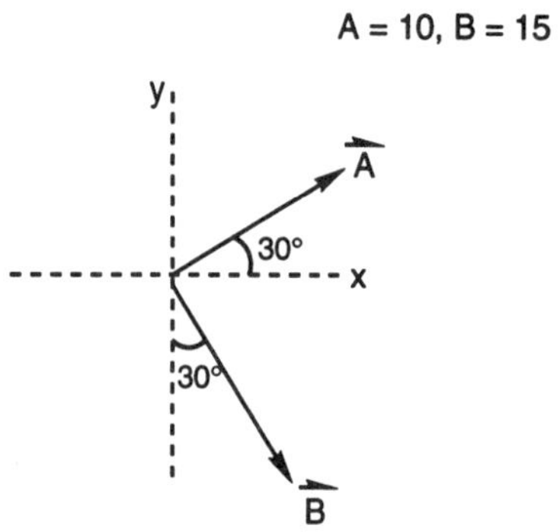

A. $A_x = 7.5, B_y = 5.0$
B. $A_x = 5.0, B_y = 5\sqrt{3}$
C. $A_y = 6.0, B_x = -7.5\sqrt{3}$
D. $A_x = 5\sqrt{3}, B_y = -7.5\sqrt{3}$
E. $A_y = -7.5\sqrt{3}, B_x = 6.0$

Use the following velocity-time graph for Questions #2 and #3. The motion is in a straight line.

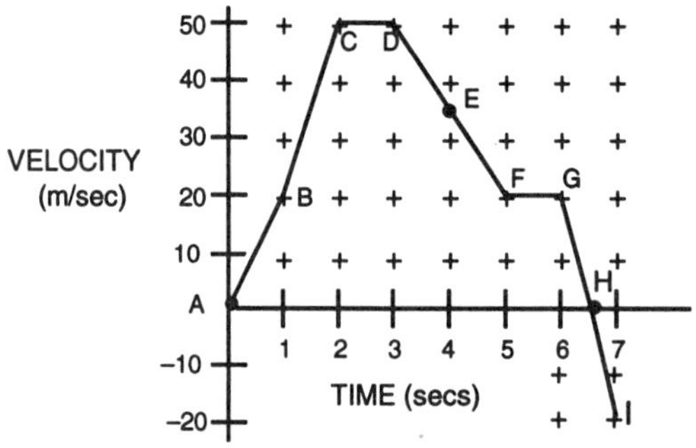

2. The instantaneous acceleration at point E is
A. 15 m/sec^2
B. –15 m/sec^2
C. 30 m/sec^2
D. –30 m/sec^2
E. –25 m/sec^2

3. The total distance traveled by the particle from t = 0 to t = 7 seconds is approximately
A. –145 m
B. 125 m
C. 185 m
D. 350 m

Use the following information for Questions #4 and #5.

An object is thrown with an initial speed of 19.6 m/sec at an angle of 30° with the horizontal.

4. The maximum height the object reaches is
A. 2.45 m
B. 4.9 m
C. 9.8 m
D. 98 m
E. 19.6 m

5. The range (horizontal distance) of the object is
   A. 19.6 m
   B. $19.6\sqrt{3}$ m
   C. 9.8 m
   D. $9.8\sqrt{3}$ m
   E. 52m

6. An object first begins to slip down an inclined plane when the angle with the horizontal is 45°. The coefficient of static friction (μ_s) of the object-surface is
   A. 0.5
   B. $1/\sqrt{2}$
   C. $\sqrt{2}/2$
   D. need more information
   E. 1.0

7. A force of 15 newtons acting upon a 5 kg object will produce an acceleration equal to
   A. $\frac{1}{3}$ m/sec^2
   B. $\frac{1}{75}$ m/sec^2
   C. 3 m/sec^2
   D. 75 m/sec^2

8. If a force is acting on an object, but off an axis, what type of motion results?
   A. rotational
   B. translational
   C. frictional
   D. projectile
   E. vibrational

9. The net force (in newtons) on the following object (answers in nts) is:

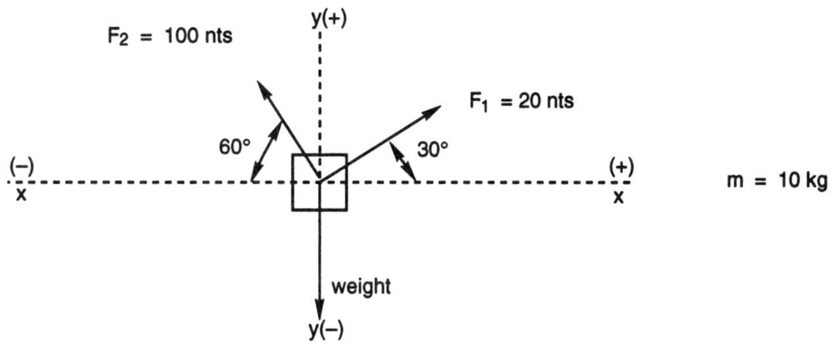

   A. zero
   B. 32.7 nts
   C. 99.5 nts
   D. 127.9 nts

10. The object below is in static and rotational equilibrium. What are the components of the force, F_1?

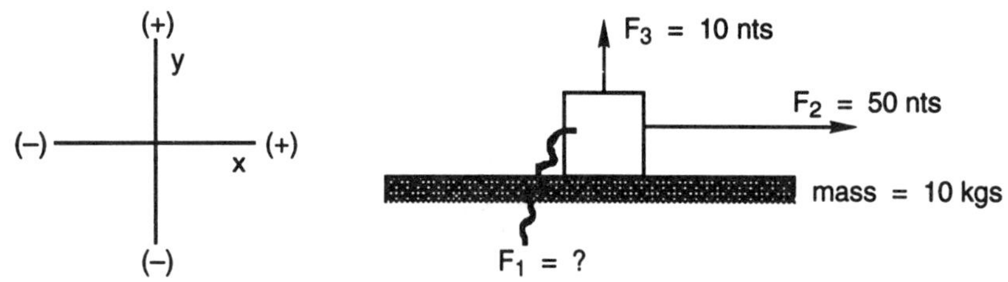

A. F_x = –50 nts; F_y = –10 nts
B. F_x = –50 nts; F_y = +88 nts
C. F_x = +50 nts; F_y = –108 nts
D. F_x = +50 nts; F_y = –88 nts
E. None of the above

11. The product of force times the perpendicular moment arm is the
A. energy.
B. work.
C. torque.
D. force.

12. The object below is in rotational equilibrium. What force, F_1, is required for this equilibrium (neglect the weight)?

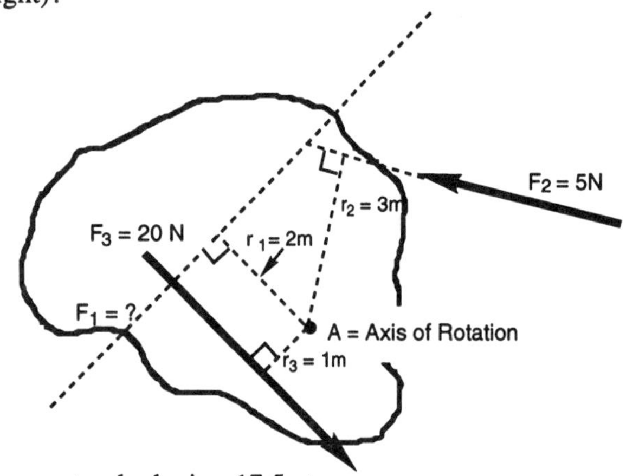

A. counterclockwise, 17.5 nts
B. clockwise, 5 nts
C. clockwise, 35 nts
D. counterclockwise, 25.0 nts
E. none of the above

13. When a system does work or work is done on a system
A. the force of the systems changes.
B. the momentum of the system changes.
C. the torque of the system changes.
D. the energy of the system changes.

14. A 5 kg object is moving in a straight line at an average velocity of 4 meters/sec. The kinetic energy (K) is
A. 40 joules
B. 20 joules
C. 10 joules
D. 80 joules

15. A force of 20 newtons is used to move an object 20 meters in 10 seconds; the power (P) used is
A. 40,000 watts.
B. 4,000 watts.
C. 400 watts.
D. 40 watts.

16. How much work is performed to move the box in the diagram below?

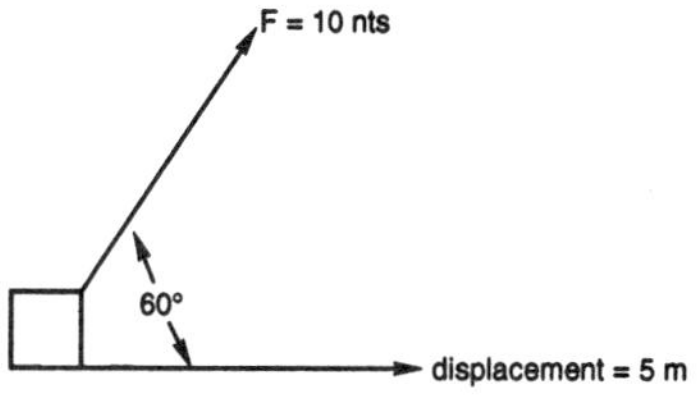

A. 50 joules
B. 50 cos 30° joules
C. 25 joules
D. 50 sin 60° joules

17. A 5 kg object moving at 4 m/sec strikes a second object. After the collision, the first object is moving at 2 m/sec. Assuming all the energy (E) was used to perform work (W) on the second object, the work performed is
A. 30 joules.
B. 60 joules.
C. 90 joules.
D. 120 joules.

18. Condensations and rarefactions would be found in
A. light waves.
B. water waves.
C. transverse waves.
D. longitudinal waves.
E. electromagnetic waves.

19. Select the *incorrect* relationship between the energy (E) of a wave and the parameters given: (f = frequency, λ = wavelength, A = amplitude)
A. $E \propto f$
B. $E \propto A^2$
C. $E \propto 1/\lambda$
D. All are correct.

20. The speed of light (c) is 3.0×10^{10} cm/sec. If the wavelength (λ) of red light is approximately 400 nm (nm = 10^{-9} m), then the frequency (f) of red light is
A. 7.5×10^{12}/sec.
B. 7.5×10^{14}/sec.
C. 7.5×10^{4}/sec.
D. 7.5×10^{6}/sec.

Use the following data for Question #21.
The particle of mass = 2 kg below is oscillating about the fixed point O as shown. Given are some values of the force on the particle at different values of displacement (x) from O. The maximal displacement from O in any one direction is ± A and A = 5 m.

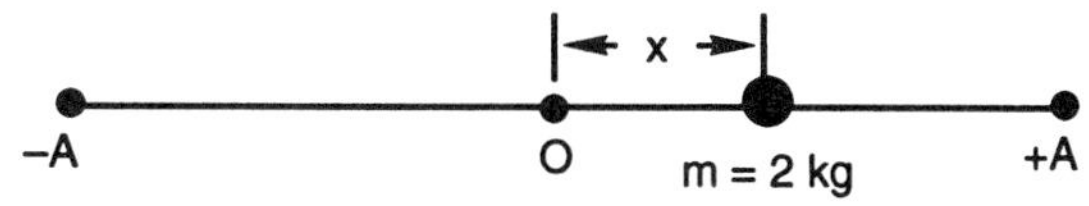

x (meters)	+3	+1	–2	–4
F (newtons)	–0.6	–0.2	+0.4	+0.8

21. The value of F at A = –5m is
A. 0.2 nts.
B. 0.5 nts.
C. 1.0 nts.
D. 5 nts.

22. If an object is moved from a depth of 4 meters to a depth of 8 meters beneath the surface of a large tank of water, the pressure on it will
A. remain the same.
B. quadruple.
C. halve.
D. double.

23. At a depth of 10 meters in a large container of water, 3 sheets of glass are placed parallel to the surface. Sheet A is 3m × 5m, sheet B is 4 × 4 and sheet C is 2 × 9. Which sheet has the greatest fluid pressure on its surface?
A. A
B. B
C. C
D. All are equal.

24. The buoyant force (F_B) of an object that has a mass of 10 gms (assume $g = 980$ cm/sec^2), a volume of 10 mls and displaces 2 mls of a liquid with a density of 5 gms/ml is
A. 10 dynes.
B. 9800 dynes.
C. 1000 dynes.
D. 40 dynes.

25. The conversion of 10 grams of a solid to 10 grams of its liquid at the freezing point (25°C) requires 100 cals of heat. The heat of fusion of this substance is
A. 0.40 cals/gm•°C.
B. 40 cals•gm/°C.
C. 10 cals/gm.
D. 250 cals•°C/gm.

26. A temperature of 50°C (Celsius) corresponds to what temperature Fahrenheit (F)?
A. 122°F
B. 90°F
C. 82°F
D. 27.8°F

27. Heat is being conducted through a square-faced metal block 4 meters long with sides 2 meters in length. If another block of the same metal is constructed but with a square face of 4 meters on a side and 8 meters long, what is the rate of heat conduction through it, compared with the first block, for a given temperature difference? *Note:* the heat is passing through the square faces along the complete length.
A. The second rate is four times the first rate.
B. The second rate is twice the first rate.
C. The second rate is one-half the first rate.
D. The second rate is one-fourth the first rate.

28. The net force on charge C (q_c) is:

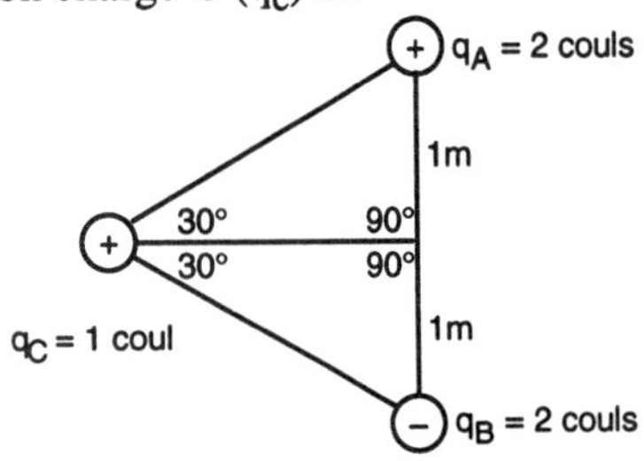

assume k = dielectric constant

A. zero.
B. horizontal and to the right, 0.5k nts.
C. horizontal and to the left, 0.5k nts.
D. vertical and up, 0.5k nts.
E. vertical and down, 0.5k nts.

29. What is the work done in moving a charge q_1 from A to B?

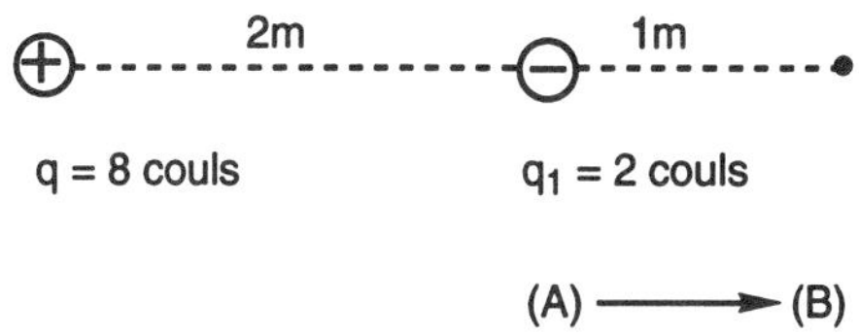

A. -10π joules
B. $+10\pi$ joules
C. (+8k/3) joules
D. (–8k/3) joules

30. Some of the shortest electromagnetic waves are
A. microwaves.
B. x-rays.
C. AM-radio waves.
D. FM-radio waves.

31. In a circuit with a voltage of 10 volts and a resistance of 10 ohms and a current passing for 10 secs, the maximum possible number of joules of heat produced is
A. 100 joules.
B. 1000 joules.
C. 1 joule.
D. 10 joules.
E. 50 joules

32. The voltage (V) of the following battery is (neglect internal resistance of battery)

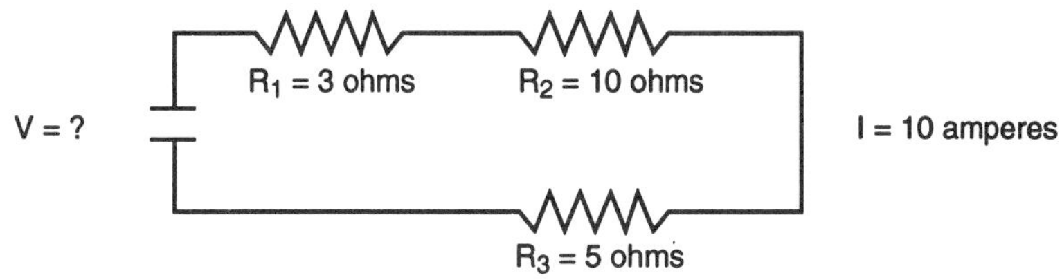

A. 180 volts.
B. 18 volts.
C. 1.8 volts.
D. 0.55 volts.
E. 36 volts

33. Determine the current (I) in the following circuit:

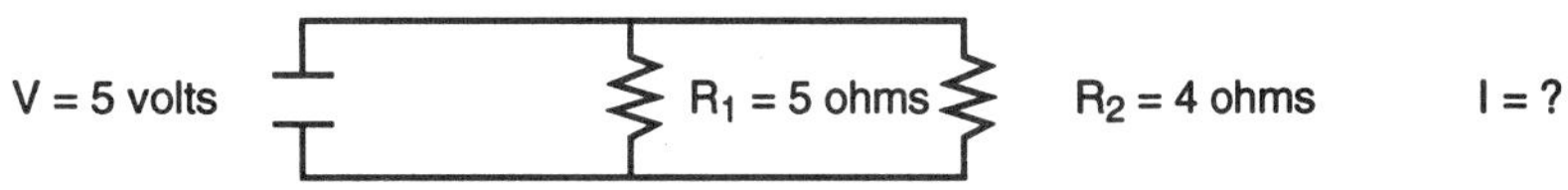

A. 5/9 amperes
B. 1.8 amperes
C. 2.25 amperes
D. 45 amperes

34. If f = focal length, R = radius of curvature of a spherical mirror, then
A. $f = 2R$.
B. $f = R/2$.
C. $f = R^2$.
D. $f = \sqrt{R}$.
E. $f = I/R$.

35. Given the diagram below for refraction of light, the correct relationship between the angles (θ) shown and the indices of refraction (n) in the media is

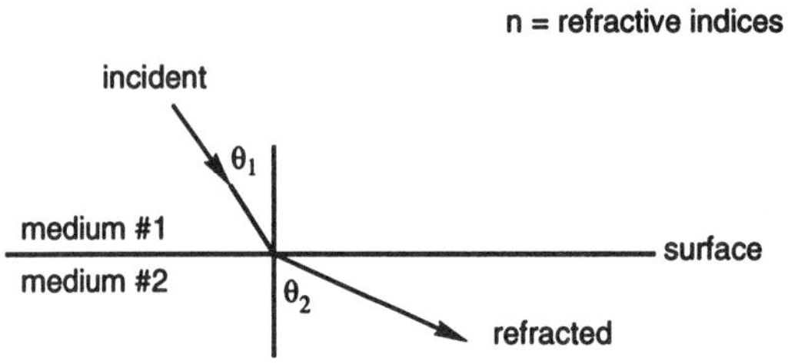

A. $n_2 \sin\theta_1 = n_1 \sin\theta_2$.
B. $n_1\,\theta_1 = n_2\theta_2$.
C. $\sin\theta_1/\sin\theta_2 = n_2/n_1$.
D. $\theta_1/\theta_2 = n_1/n_2$.

36. An object 10 cms tall is placed 20 cms from a concave lens with a focal length of 5 cms. The image is
A. virtual, inverted, 40 cms from lens and 20 cms tall
B. virtual, erect, 10 cms from lens and 40 cms tall
C. real, inverted, 10 cms from lens and 40 cms tall
D. real, erect, 4 cms from lens and 4 cms tall

37. Select the correct path of light through the eye (anterior to posterior):
A. cornea, aqueous humor, lens, vitreous humor, retina
B. lens, aqueous humor, cornea, vitreous humor, retina
C. cornea, vitreous humor, lens, aqueous humor, retina
D. retina, cornea, aqueous humor, lens, vitreous humor

38. The half-life of a substance called JUNKIUM is 11.5 hours. How much time will it take to lose 25% of its original starting mass?
A. 2.88 hours
B. 46 hours
C. 5.75 hours
D. 4.77 hours

39. The equation for the force F of gravity is:

$$F = k\frac{m_1 m_2}{r^2},$$

where m_1 and m_2 are masses and r is the distance between them.

What are the units in terms of mass (m), length (l), and time (t) of the constant k?
A. $l^3\,m^{-1}\,t^{-2}$
B. $l^3\,m^{-2}\,t^{-3}$
C. $l^2\,m^{-1}\,t^{-2}$
D. $l^2\,m^{-2}\,t^{-3}$

40. Lewis and Matt work on a job together and finish it in 4 hours. If Lewis and Matt work together for 2 hours and then Matt leaves, it takes Lewis 3 more hours to finish the job alone. Find the time taken by each man to finish the job alone.
A. L = 5 hours; M = 7 hours
B. L = 12 hours; M = 6 hours
C. L = 8 hours; M = 4 hours
D. L = 6 hours; M = 12 hours
E. L = 4 hours; M = 8 hours

7.5 OAT SAMPLE TEST ANSWER KEYS

7.5.1 Reading Comprehension

1. D
2. D
3. B
4. D
5. A
6. E
7. B
8. A
9. C
10. C
11. B
12. B
13. D
14. B
15. D
16. B
17. B
18. C
19. D
20. C
21. D
22. E
23. A
24. C
25. B
26. D
27. D
28. B
29. C
30. D
31. C
32. C
33. D
34. B
35. A
36. C
37. C
38. D
39. A
40. D
41. B
42. B
43. D
44. C
45. C
46. D
47. C
48. C
49. A
50. B

7.5.2 Quantitative Reasoning

1. D
2. A
3. B
4. A
5. D
6. E
7. B
8. C
9. D
10. D
11. B
12. A
13. C
14. A
15. B
16. A
17. D
18. A
19. D
20. B
21. A
22. D
23. C
24. B
25. B
26. D
27. E
28. B
29. C
30. D
31. A
32. A
33. E
34. A
35. A
36. B
37. A
38. D
39. B
40. E

7.5.3 Natural Sciences

Biology		General Chemistry		Organic Chemistry	
1. A	**21.** C	**41.** C	**56.** A	**71.** B	**86.** B
2. B	**22.** E	**42.** B	**57.** D	**72.** A	**87.** A
3. A	**23.** A	**43.** C	**58.** C	**73.** D	**88.** A
4. B	**24.** C	**44.** D	**59.** C	**74.** B	**89.** D
5. C	**25.** A	**45.** C	**60.** B	**75.** D	**90.** A
6. C	**26.** D	**46.** A	**61.** B	**76.** E	**91.** B
7. B	**27.** C	**47.** A	**62.** B	**77.** A	**92.** C
8. B	**28.** C	**48.** B	**63.** C	**78.** C	**93.** C
9. A	**29.** C	**49.** A	**64.** C	**79.** D	**94.** D
10. D	**30.** A	**50.** B	**65.** D	**80.** C	**95.** B
11. D	**31.** C	**51.** E	**66.** D	**81.** A	**96.** A
12. B	**32.** C	**52.** B	**67.** B	**82.** D	**97.** D
13. A	**33.** D	**53.** D	**68.** D	**83.** D	**98.** A
14. A	**34.** E	**54.** B	**69.** B	**84.** B	**99.** B
15. D	**35.** D	**55.** D	**70.** D	**85.** B	**100.** C
16. B	**36.** B				
17. A	**37.** C				
18. B	**38.** C				
19. B	**39.** D				
20. D	**40.** A				

7.5.4 Physics

1. D	**9.** B	**17.** A	**25.** C	**33.** C
2. B	**10.** B	**18.** D	**26.** A	**34.** B
3. C	**11.** C	**19.** D	**27.** B	**35.** C
4. B	**12.** E	**20.** B	**28.** E	**36.** B
5. B	**13.** D	**21.** C	**29.** C	**37.** A
6. E	**14.** A	**22.** D	**30.** B	**38.** D
7. C	**15.** D	**23.** D	**31.** A	**39.** A
8. A	**16.** C	**24.** B	**32.** A	**40.** D

7.6 REFERENCES

1. Optometry Admission Test Preparation Materials, Department of Testing Services, Optometry Admission Testing Program, 1990.

Appendix A

Scope of Examinations

This "Scope of Examinations" was produced in its entirety from the AOA-Optometry Admission Test application brochure, 1991. There are four examinations included in the Optometry Admission Testing Program. The actual OAT requires approximately 5 hours for administration. The scope of examinations is described on the following pages.

A.1 QUANTITATIVE REASONING

Quantitative Reasoning	
1. algebraic equations	Mathematics Problems
2. fractions	Mathematics Problems
3. conversions	Mathematics Problems
(a) ounces	Mathematics Problems
(b) pounds	Mathematics Problems
(c) inches	Mathematics Problems
(d) feet	Mathematics Problems
4. percentages	Mathematics Problems
5. exponential notation	Mathematics Problems
6. probability and statistics	Mathematics Problems
7. geometry	Mathematics Problems
8. trigonometry	Mathematics Problems
9. word problems (type not specified but the test preparation materials reflect the type of items typically used).	Applied Mathematics Problems

The quantitative reasoning content appears on the examination with the following distribution of items:

1. Mathematics Problems (20 items)
2. Applied Mathematics Problems (20 items)

A.2 PHYSICS

Physics	
1. units of measurement	Units and Vectors
(a) length	Units and Vectors
(b) mass	Units and Vectors
(c) time	Units and Vectors
(d) derived units	Units and Vectors
(e) conversions	Units and Vectors
2. vectors and scalars	Units and Vectors
3. graphical addition of vectors	Units and Vectors
4. resolution of vectors	Units and Vectors
5. equations of translational motion	Kinematics
6. angular velocity	Kinematics
7. angular acceleration	Kinematics
8. equilibrium	Statics and Dynamics
9. moment of a force	Statics and Dynamics
10. center of mass	Statics and Dynamics
11. types of levers	Statics and Dynamics
12. force, weight	Statics and Dynamics
13. momentum	Statics and Dynamics
(a) linear	Statics and Dynamics
(b) angular	Statics and Dynamics
14. gravitation, gravity	Statics and Dynamics
15. Newton's Laws of motion	Statics and Dynamics
16. dynamic equilibrium	Statics and Dynamics
17. work and power	Energy and Momentum
18. energy	Energy and Momentum
(a) potential	Energy and Momentum
(b) kinetic	Energy and Momentum
19. impulse-momentum equation	Energy and Momentum
20. colliding objects	Energy and Momentum
(a) elastic	Energy and Momentum
(b) inelastic	Energy and Momentum
21. oscillations, vibrations	Waves
22. characteristics of waves	Waves
(a) wave length	Waves
(b) wave period	Waves
(c) wave amplitude	Waves
(d) wave period, frequency	Waves
(e) wave velocity	Waves
23. pendulum	Simple Harmonic Motion

24. resonance	Simple Harmonic Motion
25. properties of solids	Fluid Statics
26. fluid statics	Fluid Statics
27. fluid dynamics (optional)	Fluid Statics
28. the human ear	Sound (optional)
29. speed of sound	Sound (optional)
30. sound intensity	Sound (optional)
31. Doppler effect	Sound (optional)
32. ultrasonics	Sound (optional)
33. heat and temperature	Thermal Energy and Heat Transfer
34. temperature scales and conversions	Thermal Energy and Heat Transfer
35. heat transfer	Thermal Energy and Heat Transfer
(a) conduction	Thermal Energy and Heat Transfer
(b) convection	Thermal Energy and Heat Transfer
(c) radiation	Thermal Energy and Heat Transfer
36. calorie, BTU	Thermal Energy and Heat Transfer
37. laws of thermodynamics	Thermal Energy and Heat Transfer
(a) first law	Thermal Energy and Heat Transfer
(b) second law	Thermal Energy and Heat Transfer
38. entropy	Thermal Energy and Heat Transfer
39. enthalpy	Thermal Energy and Heat Transfer
40. electrical charge	Electrostatics
41. coulomb definition	Electrostatics
42. conductors/insulators	Electrostatics
43. Coulomb's law	Electrostatics
44. electric resistance	D.C. Circuits
45. electric current	D.C. Circuits
46. electric potential	D.C. Circuits
47. Ohm's law	D.C. Circuits
48. capacitance	D.C. Circuits
49. single-loop circuits	D.C. Circuits
50. magnetic field	Magnetism
51. units of measurement	Magnetism
52. electromagnetism	Magnetism
53. magnetic properties of materials	Magnetism
(a) paramagnetic	Magnetism
(b) diamagnetic	Magnetism
(c) ferromagnetic	Magnetism
54. the human eye	Optics
55. reflection and mirrors	Optics
56. refraction and lenses	Optics

57. the lens equation	Optics
58. optical instruments	Optics
(a) microscope	Optics
(b) telescope	Optics
(c) colonfiberscope	Optics
(d) periscope	Optics
(e) modern optical instruments	Optics
59. fission	Atomic and Nuclear
60. fusion	Atomic and Nuclear
61. half life	Atomic and Nuclear
62. radioactivity	Atomic and Nuclear

The physics content appears on the examination with the following distribution of items:

1. Units and Vectors (3 items)
2. Kinematics (4 items)
3. Statics and Dynamics (5 items)
4. Rotational Motion (2 items)
5. Energy and Momentum (4 items)
6. Simple Harmonic Motion (2 items)
7. Waves (2 items)
8. Fluid Statics (2 items)
9. Thermal Energy and Heat Transfer (2 items)
10. Thermodynamics (3 items)
11. Electrostatics (1 item)
12. D.C. Circuits (3 items)
13. Magnetism (1 item)
14. Optics (4 items)
15. Modern Physics (Atomic and Nuclear) (2 items)

Biology	
1. origin of life	Cell and Molecular Biology
2. cell metabolism (including photosynthesis)	Cell and Molecular Biology
3. enzymology	Cell and Molecular Biology
4. thermodynamics	Cell and Molecular Biology
5. organelle structure and function	Cell and Molecular Biology
6. biological organization and relationship of major taxa using the five-kingdom system	Diversity of Life
(a) Monera	Diversity of Life
(b) angiosperms	Diversity of Life
(c) arthropods	Diversity of Life
(d) chordates	Diversity of Life
7. structure and function of vertebrate systems	Vertebrate Anatomy and Physiology
(a) integumentary	Vertebrate Anatomy and Physiology
(b) skeletal	Vertebrate Anatomy and Physiology
(c) muscular	Vertebrate Anatomy and Physiology
(d) circulatory	Vertebrate Anatomy and Physiology
(e) immunological	Vertebrate Anatomy and Physiology
(f) digestive	Vertebrate Anatomy and Physiology
(g) respiratory	Vertebrate Anatomy and Physiology
(h) urinary	Vertebrate Anatomy and Physiology
(i) nervous	Vertebrate Anatomy and Physiology
(j) endocrine	Vertebrate Anatomy and Physiology
(k) reproductive	Vertebrate Anatomy and Physiology
8. Embryology	Development Biology
(a) fertilization	Development Biology
(b) descriptive embryology	Development Biology
(c) development mechanisms	Development Biology
9. Genetics	Genetics
(a) Mendelian inheritance	Genetics
(b) chromosomal genetics	Genetics
(c) meiosis	Genetics
(d) molecular genetics	Genetics
(e) human genetics	Genetics
10. Evolution, Population	Evolution, Ecology, and Behavior
(a) natural selection	Evolution, Ecology, and Behavior
(b) population genetics	Evolution, Ecology, and Behavior
(c) speciation	Evolution, Ecology, and Behavior
(d) population and community ecology	Evolution, Ecology, and Behavior
(e) animal behavior (including social behavior)	Evolution, Ecology, and Behavior

The biology content appears on the examination with the following distribution of items:

1. Cell and Molecular Biology (13 items)
2. Diversity of Life (4 items)
3. Vertebrate Anatomy and Physiology (8 items)
4. Development Biology (4 items)
5. Genetics (7 items)
6. Evolution, Ecology, and Behavior (4 items)

General Chemistry	
1. percent of composition	Stoichiometry
2. empirical formulas from percent of composition	Stoichiometry
3. balancing equations	Stoichiometry
4. weight/weight, weight/volume, and density problems	Stoichiometry
5. kinetic molecular theory of gases	Gases
6. Graham's law	Gases
7. Dalton's law	Gases
8. Boyle's law	Gases
9. Charles's law	Gases
10. ideal gas law	Gases
11. intermolecular forces	Liquids and Solids
12. phase diagrams	Liquids and Solids
13. vapor pressure	Liquids and Solids
14. molecular structures	Liquids and Solids
15. polarity of chemical bonds	Liquids and Solids
16. colligative properties	Solutions
17. concentration calculations	Solutions
18. molecular equilibrium	Chemical Equilibrium
19. acid/base equilibrium	Chemical Equilibrium
20. base/acid equilibrium	Chemical Equilibrium
21. precipitation calculations	Chemical Equilibrium
22. equilibria calculations	Chemical Equilibrium
23. laws of thermodynamics	Thermodynamics and Thermochemistry
24. Hess's law	Thermodynamics and Thermochemistry
25. spontaneity prediction	Thermodynamics and Thermochemistry
26. rate laws	Chemical Kinetics
27. activation energy	Chemical Kinetics
28. half-life	Chemical Kinetics
29. balancing equations	Oxidation-Reduction Reactions
30. determinations of oxidation numbers	Oxidation-Reduction Reactions
31. electro-chemical calculations	Oxidation-Reduction Reactions
32. electro-chemical concepts	Oxidation-Reduction Reactions
33. electron configuration	Atomic and Molecular Structure
34. orbital types	Atomic and Molecular Structure
35. Lewis-Dot diagrams	Atomic and Molecular Structure
36. atomic theories	Atomic and Molecular Structure
37. molecular geometry	Atomic and Molecular Structure
38. bond types	Atomic and Molecular Structure

39. quantum mechanics	Atomic and Molecular Structure
40. nonmetals	Periodic Properties
41. transition metals	Periodic Properties
42. nontransition metals	Periodic Properties
43. nuclear reactions	Nuclear Reactions

The general chemistry content appears on the examination with the following distribution of items:

1. Stoichiometry (4 items)
2. Gases (2 items)
3. Liquids and Solids (1 item)
4. Solutions (3 items)
5. Acids and Bases (3 items)
6. Chemical Equilibrium (3 items)
7. Thermodynamics and Thermochemistry (2 items)
8. Chemical Kinetics (2 items)
9. Oxidation-Reduction Reactions (3 items)
10. Atomic and Molecular Structure (4 items)
11. Nuclear Reactions (1 item)
12. Periodic Properties (2 items)

Organic Chemistry	
1. energetics	Mechanisms
2. structure and stability of intermediates	Mechanisms
(a) S_N1, S_N2	Mechanisms
(b) elimination	Mechanisms
(c) addition	Mechanisms
(d) free radical mechanisms	Mechanisms
(e) substitution mechanisms	Mechanisms
3. stability	Chemical and Physical Properties of Molecules
4. solubility	Chemical and Physical Properties of Molecules
5. polarity	Chemical and Physical Properties of Molecules
6. intermolecular forces	Chemical and Physical Properties of Molecules
7. intramolecular forces	Chemical and Physical Properties of Molecules
8. separation techniques	Chemical and Physical Properties of Molecules
9. introductory infrared	Organic Analysis
10. ^{1}H NMR spectroscopy	Organic Analysis
11. simple chemical tests	Organic Analysis
12. conformational analysis	Stereochemistry
13. optical activity	Stereochemistry
14. chirality	Stereochemistry
15. chiral centers	Stereochemistry
16. planes of symmetry	Stereochemistry
17. enantiomers	Stereochemistry
18. diastereomers	Stereochemistry
19. meso compounds	Stereochemistry
20. IUPAC rules	Nomenclature
21. identification of functional groups on molecules	Nomenclature
22. prediction of reaction products	Reactions of the Major Functional Groups
23. important mechanistic generalities	Reactions of the Major Functional Groups
24. resonance effects	Acid-Base Chemistry
25. inductive effects	Acid-Base Chemistry
26. prediction of products	Acid-Base Chemistry
27. prediction of equilibria	Acid-Base Chemistry
26. atomic orbitals	Bonding
27. molecular orbitals	Bonding
28. hybridization	Bonding

29. Lewis structures	Bonding
30. bond angles	Bonding
31. bond lengths	Bonding
32. concept of aromaticity	Aromatics
33. electrophilic aromatic substitution	Aromatics
34. identification of the product of, or the reagents used in, a simple sequence of reactions	Synthesis

The organic chemistry content appears on the examination with the following distribution of items:

1. Mechanisms (6 items)
2. Chemical and Physical Properties of Molecules and Organic Analysis (3 items)
3. Stereochemistry (3 items)
4. Nomenclature (2 items)
5. Reactions of the Major Functional Groups (8 items)
6. Acid-Base Chemistry (3 items)
7. Aromatics and bonding (3 items)
8. Synthesis (2 items)